computers
in the
medical office

SUSAN M. SANDERSON, CPEHR

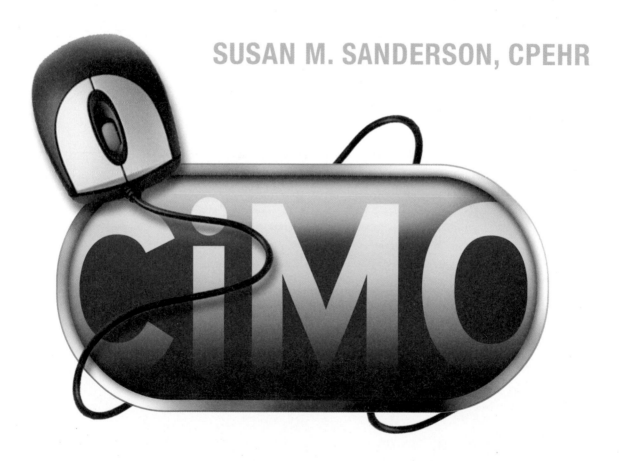

Seventh Edition

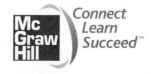

Connect
Learn
Succeed™

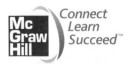

COMPUTERS IN THE MEDICAL OFFICE, SEVENTH EDITION

Published by McGraw-Hill, a business unit of The McGraw-Hill Companies, Inc., 1221 Avenue of the Americas, New York, NY, 10020. Copyright © 2011 by The McGraw-Hill Companies, Inc. All rights reserved. Previous editions © 1995, 1999, 2002, 2005, 2007, and 2009. No part of this publication may be reproduced or distributed in any form or by any means, or stored in a database or retrieval system, without the prior written consent of The McGraw-Hill Companies, Inc., including, but not limited to, in any network or other electronic storage or transmission, or broadcast for distance learning.

Some ancillaries, including electronic and print components, may not be available to customers outside the United States.

This book is printed on acid-free paper.

1 2 3 4 5 6 7 8 9 0 DOW/DOW 1 0 9 8 7 6 5 4 3 2 1 0

ISBN   978-0-07-337460-4
MHID   0-07-337460-1

Vice president/Editor in chief: *Elizabeth Haefele*
Vice president/Director of marketing: *John E. Biernat*
Publisher: *Kenneth S. Kasee Jr.*
Senior sponsoring editor: *Natalie J. Ruffatto*
Managing developmental editor: *Michelle L. Flomenhoft*
Executive marketing manager: *Roxan Kinsey*
Lead digital product manager: *Damian Moshak*
Director, Editing/Design/Production: *Jess Ann Kosic*
Project manager: *Marlena Pechan*

Buyer II: *Debra R. Sylvester*
Senior designer: *Marianna Kinigakis*
Senior photo research coordinator: *Lori Hancock*
Digital development editor: *Kevin White*
Media project manager: *Cathy L. Tepper*
Typeface: *11/13.5 Palatino*
Compositor: *Aptara, Inc.*
Printer: *R. R. Donnelley*
Cover and interior design: *Gino Cieslik*

Cover credit: Gino Cieslik; Mouse: ©Yuri Arcurs/Getty Images
Credits: The credits section for this book begins on page 492 and is considered an extension of the copyright page.
Codeveloped by McGraw-Hill Higher Education and Chestnut Hill Enterprises, Inc. chestnuthl@aol.com

Medisoft® is a registered trademark of McKesson Corporation and/or one of its subsidiaries. Screenshots and material pertaining to Medisoft® Software used with permission of McKesson Corporation. © 2010 McKesson Corporation and/or one of its subsidiaries. All Rights Reserved.

The Medidata (student data file), illustrations, instructions, and exercises in *Computers in the Medical Office* are compatible with the Medisoft Advanced Version 16 Patient Accounting software available at the time of publication. Note that Medisoft Advanced Version 16 Patient Accounting software must be available to access the Medidata. It can be obtained by contacting your McGraw-Hill sales representative.

All brand or product names are trademarks or registered trademarks of their respective companies.

CPT five-digit codes, nomenclature, and other data are copyright 2009 American Medical Association. All Rights Reserved. No fee schedules, basic units relative values, or related listings are included in CPT. The AMA assumes no liability for the data contained herein.

CPT codes are based on CPT 2010.
ICD-9-CM codes are based on ICD-9-CM 2010.

All names, situations, and anecdotes are fictitious. They do not represent any person, event, or medical record.

Library of Congress Cataloging-in-Publication Data

Sanderson, Susan M.
    Computers in the medical office/Susan M. Sanderson.—7th ed.
        p. ; cm.
    Includes index.
    ISBN-13: 978-0-07-337460-4 (pbk. : alk. paper)
    ISBN-10: 0-07-337460-1 (pbk. : alk. paper)
    1. Medical offices—Automation. 2. MediSoft. I. Title.
    [DNLM: 1. MediSoft. 2. Office Automation—Problems and Exercises. 3. Practice
Management, Medical—Problems and Exercises. 4. Software—Problems and Exercises.
W 18.2 S216c 2011]
    R864.S26 2011
    651′.9610285—dc22
                                                                2010018339

The Internet addresses listed in the text were accurate at the time of publication. The inclusion of a Web site does not indicate an endorsement by the authors or McGraw-Hill, and McGraw-Hill does not guarantee the accuracy of the information presented at these sites.

www.mhhe.com

brief contents

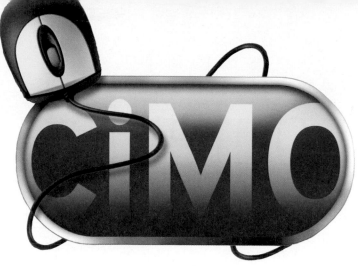

contents

part 2

cimo

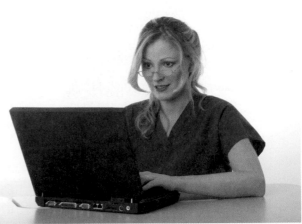

CiMO

chapter 10

chapter 11

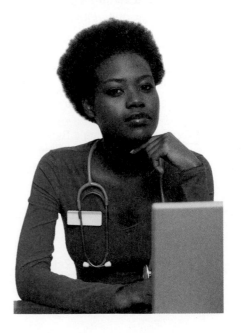

part 3

CiMO

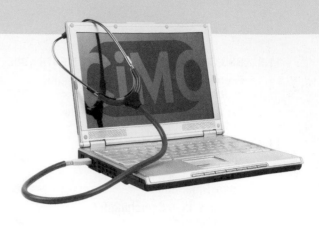

part 4

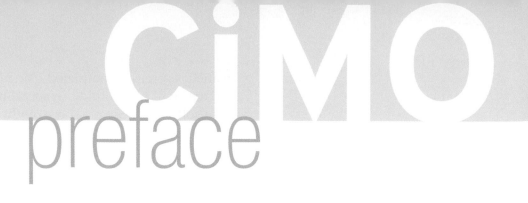

CiMO™: THE STEP-BY-STEP, HANDS-ON APPROACH

Welcome to the seventh edition of *Computers in the Medical Office* (*CiMO*)! This product introduces your students to the concepts and skills they will need for a successful career in medical office billing. Medical billers are in high demand, and theirs remains one of the ten fastest-growing allied health/health profession occupations. *CiMO* provides instruction on key tasks that students throughout the health professions curriculum, such as those studying medical assisting, health information management, and health information technology, will need to be competent and to move forward. Teaching this material to your students may be challenging because of the diverse student population that takes this course—some students may be very technology-savvy and move through the book quickly, while others may be computer novices and need more help. No matter what your students' skill levels are, *CiMO* gives not only the step-by-step instructions they need to learn, but also the "why" behind those steps.

Here's what you and your students can expect from *CiMO*:

- Coverage of Medisoft® Advanced Version 16 patient billing software, a full-featured software program, including screen captures showing how the concepts described in the book actually look in the medical billing software

- Both a tutorial and a simulation of Medisoft®, using a medical office setting, Family Care Center, and related patient data

- Detailed, easy-to-understand explanations of concepts balanced by step-by-step, hands-on exercises

- The necessary building blocks for students to establish a strong skill set and gain confidence to attain the jobs they want

- Realistic exercises, completed using Medisoft®, that cover what students will see working in actual medical practices, no matter what software those practices might use
- An understanding of the medical billing cycle and how completing the related tasks will positively affect the financial well-being of a medical practice

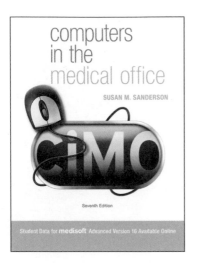

ABOUT THE COVER

Throughout the past fifteen years, *Computers in the Medical Office* (as well as author Susan Sanderson) has become a brand unto itself—*CiMO*. The text has become iconic; in fact, because it has been so well-received, the course was named after it! With the cover of the seventh edition, we wanted to present our logo as a symbol of the product's essential goal: to provide a step-by-step, hands-on experience for students. We tried to give the logo a three-dimensional feel—like a button or a key on the computer keyboard that you can reach out and press to get the information you need.

HERE'S HOW YOUR COLLEAGUES HAVE DESCRIBED *CiMO*

"I think the author did a great job in organizing the chapters and the flow of them as they relate very closely to the normal flow in an office setting. . . . I'm a firm believer in applying realistic scenarios to boost the student's understanding and this book does an EXCELLENT job at attaining that goal."
Wanda D. Strayhan M.S., CBCS, CMA, Florida Career College

"A book worth looking at. It [covers] all learning styles by the approach that is given in the chapters. It also allows the instructor with experience to use this text to its fullest potential."
Tom Wesley, Minnesota School of Business

"The practical hands-on [approach] shows students what happens in a medical office on a day to day basis. In addition, when students make errors, the process of correcting the error(s) also helps them learn how what they do in the medical office affects different people they work with."
Amy L. Blochowiak, MBA, ACS, AIAA, AIRC, ARA, FLHC, FLMI, HCSA, HIA, HIPAA, MHP, PCS, SILA-F, Northeast Wisconsin Technical College

ORGANIZATION OF CiMO, 7E

CiMO is divided into four parts:

Part	Coverage
1: Introduction to Computers in the Medical Office	Covers the medical billing cycle and the role that computers play in that cycle. Also covers the use of health information technology, electronic health records, HIPAA, and the HITECH Act.
2: Medisoft Advanced Training	Teaches the student how to start Medisoft®; enter patient information; work with cases; enter charges, payments, and adjustments; create claims; post insurance payments; create patient statements; create reports; create collection letters; and schedule appointments. The sequence takes the student through Medisoft® in a clear, concise manner. Each chapter includes a number of exercises that are to be done at the computer.
3: Applying Your Skills	Completes the learning process by requiring the student to perform a series of tasks using Medisoft®. Each task is an application of knowledge required in the medical office.
4: Source Documents	Gives the student the data needed to complete the exercises. The patient information form, encounter form, and other forms are similar to those used in medical offices.

NEW TO THE SEVENTH EDITION!

One of the first things you may notice, if you are familiar with earlier editions, is that the design of *CiMO* has been updated and refreshed. The changes made to the design are a direct result of customer feedback. They include yellow highlighting of key terms to make them easier to find; a clear indication of where exercises start and stop, along with titles for all exercises; the renaming of the "On Your Own" exercises to "Applying Your Skills" to eliminate the perception that these exercises are optional; and the addition of an end-of-chapter summary for easier review.

Key content changes include:

- Software (*Items with the * symbol relate to Medisoft® changes from Version 14 to Version 16.*)

  - *Medisoft® Version 16 is used for all databases and illustrations (screen captures). There are major changes in the appearance of the program, but not in the functionality. See the icons on the toolbar and Activities menu to the right and on page xiv.

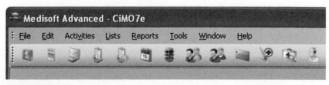

New icons on toolbar

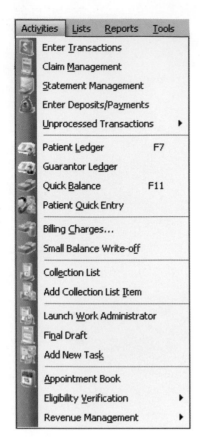

New look for menus

- HIPAA-Related
  - 2010 ICD-9-CM and CPT/HCPCS codes are used.
  - HITECH rules are incorporated.
- Pedagogy
  - In-chapter exercises are titled and, when new tasks are applied, contain completed screen keys so that students can check that they are working correctly.
  - Learning Outcomes are revised to reflect the revised version of Bloom's Taxonomy.
  - Major chapter heads are structured to reflect the Learning Outcomes and are numbered accordingly.
  - End-of-chapter elements are keyed to Learning Outcomes.
  - New chapter summaries created in tabular, step-by-step format with page references.
  - New "Thinking About It" exercises at the end of each chapter provide more critical thinking opportunities.
- Chapter by Chapter
  - Chapter 1: New key terms—documentation, electronic health record, and medical record; future change to ICD-10-CM introduced; and Step 4: Check Out Patients, incorporates topics on EHR
  - Chapter 2: New key terms—computer-assisted coding, HITECH (Health Information Technology for Economic and Clinical Health) Act, personal health records, workflow; new content on electronic health records (definitions of EHR, EMR, PHR; functions of EHRs, advantages of EHRs); new content on the impact of HIT on documentation and coding; and updated HIPAA information to include HITECH content
  - Chapter 3: New key terms—access rights, Auto Log Off, Medisoft Program Date; new steps under "The Medisoft Menus" on how to determine which version of Medisoft® is in use; addition of Windows 7 content to section on changing the program date; to address former confusion on this topic, "Changing the Medisoft Program Date" is covered at the major head level; and new major head "Using Medisoft Security Features to Ensure HIPAA Compliance"
  - Chapter 4: New additional search exercise: one now uses the Field option, whereas the other uses Locate buttons; and separate editing exercise (previously part of search exercise)
  - Chapter 5: Expanded section on understanding cases, with examples of when to create a new case; and tabs are taught in a different order—now grouped by Patient and Account

Information, Insurance Information, Health Information, and Other Information

- Chapter 6: New key term—NSF checks; new concept— explanation of need for refunds to patients; new section on the procedure for processing a refund; and new section on the procedure for processing NSF checks, reinforced by a new exercise

- Chapter 7: New exercise on using the List Only feature to select specific claims; and information on submitting electronic claims using the new Revenue Management feature

- Chapter 8: Simplification of difficult topic of capitation— single exercise divided into three separate exercises

- Chapter 9: *New Reports data selection entry dialog box; and *new content and exercises using Medisoft Reports (formerly an external product called Focus Reports), a collection of additional reports added to Version 16 of Medisoft®

- Chapter 10: New concept—payments from a collection agency; and new section on the procedure for posting collection agency payments, reinforced by a new exercise

- Chapter 11: New content and exercise on creating a report that shows which patients with upcoming appointments have outstanding balances

- Chapters 12–15: New introduction on the purpose of these chapters; and inclusion of chapter and page references with "What You Need to Know" for each of these chapters to make it easier for students to find where they first learned each task

For a detailed transition guide between the sixth and seventh editions of *CiMO*, visit www.mhhe.com/cimo7e.

TO THE INSTRUCTOR

McGraw-Hill knows how much effort it takes to prepare for a new course. Through focus groups, symposia, reviews, and conversations with instructors like you, we have gathered information about what materials you need in order to facilitate successful courses. We are committed to providing you with high-quality, accurate instructor support.

USING MEDISOFT® ADVANCED VERSION 16 WITH CiMO

CiMO features Medisoft® Advanced Version 16 patient accounting software. Students who complete *CiMO* find that the concepts and activities in the textbook are general enough to cover most administrative software used by health care providers. McGraw-Hill has partnered with Medisoft® from the very beginning, going back fifteen years to when the software was DOS-based! The support you receive

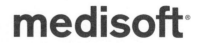

when you are using a McGraw-Hill text with Medisoft® is second to none.

Your students will need the following:

- Minimum System Requirements
  - Pentium III
  - 500 MHz (minimum) or higher processor
  - 500 MB available hard disk space
  - 512 MB RAM
  - 32-bit color display (minimum screen display of 1024 × 768)
  - Windows XP Professional SP3 or higher 32-bit
  - Windows Vista Business SP1 or higher 32-bit
  - Windows 7 Ultimate
- External storage device, such as a USB flash drive, for storing backup copies of the working database
- Medisoft® Advanced Version 16 patient billing software
- Student patient data, available for download from the book's Online Learning Center, www.mhhe.com/cimo7e. (More details on how to download the software can be found on the STOP pages between Chapters 2 and 3.)

Instructor's Software: Medisoft® Advanced Version 16 CD-ROM

Instructors who use McGraw-Hill Medisoft-compatible titles in their courses receive a fully working version of Medisoft® Advanced Version 16 software, which allows a school to place the live software on laboratory or classroom computers. Only one copy is needed per campus location. Your McGraw-Hill sales representative will help you obtain Medisoft® for your campus.

Medisoft-Compatible Titles Available from McGraw-Hill:

- Sanderson, *Computers in the Medical Office (CiMO), 7e*
  0073374601, 9780073374604

- Sanderson, *Case Studies for Use with Computers in the Medical Office, 6e*
  007337489X, 9780073374895

- Valerius/Bayes/Newby/Seggern, *Medical Insurance: An Integrated Claims Process Approach, 5e*
  0073374911, 9780073374918

- Valerius, *Workbook for Use with Medical Insurance: An Integrated Claims Process Approach, 5e*
  0077364333, 9780077364335

- Bayes/Becklin/Crist, *Medical Office Procedures, 7e*
  0073401986, 9780073401980

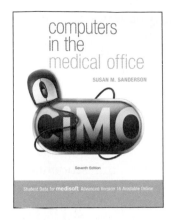
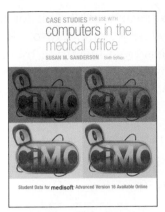
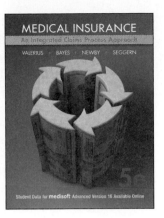
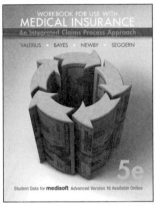
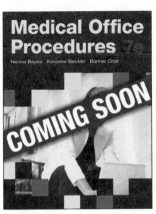

THE McGRAW-HILL GUIDE TO SUCCESS FOR MEDISOFT® ADVANCED VERSION 16

We want your transition to Medisoft® Advanced Version 16 to be a snap! In *The McGraw-Hill Guide to Success for Medisoft® Advanced Version 16,* the following topics are addressed:

- Software installation procedures for both the Instructor Version and the Student At-Home Version of Medisoft®

- Student data files installation procedures

- Use of flash drives

- Backup and restore processes

- Frequently asked questions (FAQs)

- Instructor resources

- Technical support

Ask your McGraw-Hill sales representative to send you a copy, or visit www.mhhe.com/cimo7e to review the materials online.

> "I feel this is their [instructors'] manual to give them the confidence to be successful. It is a tool that can help them prepare, and show them how to set the students up for a successful class. It is the mini 'bible' for Medisoft."
> *Cheryl Miller, MBA/HCM, Westmoreland County Community College*

"This guide is an invaluable tool for helping students and instructors get started with Medisoft. It covers all steps in the Medisoft process from installing the software to obtaining the student files from the Online Learning Center."
Nikita Carr, CPC, CMBS, Centura College

INSTRUCTORS' RESOURCES

After you install the software and are ready for your students to begin using Medisoft® Advanced Version 16, you can rely on the following materials to help you and your students work through the exercises in the book:

- Instructor Edition of the Online Learning Center at www.mhhe.com/cimo7e. Your McGraw-Hill sales representative can provide you with access and show you how to "go green" with our online instructor support.

  - Instructor's Manual with course overview; information on ordering Medisoft® Advanced Version 16; lesson plans; sample syllabi; transition guides; answer keys for worksheets, end-of-chapter questions, and software exercises; and correlations to competencies from several organizations such as ABHES, CAAHEP, and CAHIIM. More details can be found in the IM and at the book's website, www.mhhe.com/cimo7e.

  - A PowerPoint slide presentation for each chapter, containing teaching notes keyed to Learning Outcomes. Each presentation seeks to reinforce key concepts and provide a visual for students. The slides are excellent for in-class lectures.

  - Test bank and answer key for use in classroom assessment. The comprehensive test bank includes a variety of question types, with each question linked directly to its Learning Outcome, Bloom's Taxonomy, and difficulty level. Both a Word version and a computerized version (EZ Test) of the test bank are provided.

  - Conversion Guide with a chapter-by-chapter breakdown of how the content has been revised between editions. The guide is helpful if you are currently using *CiMO* and moving to the new edition, or if you are a first-time adopter.

  - Instructor Asset Map to help you find the teaching material you need with a click of the mouse. These online chapter tables are organized by Learning Outcomes, and allow you to find instructor notes, PowerPoint slides, and even test bank suggestions with ease! The Asset Map is a completely integrated tool designed to help you plan and instruct your courses efficiently and comprehensively. It labels and organizes course material for use in a multitude of learning applications.

- **Important!** End-of-chapter Medisoft® backup files for Chapters 4 through 15. There is a tool for data restoration should a student enter incorrect answers (data) and if, as the semester continues, incorrect answers prohibit the student from moving forward effectively with the software. The chapter-by-chapter backup files will allow you to restore the Medisoft® data on your students' computers to the beginning of any chapter. Medisoft® backup files always have the .mbk file extension, and each file represents a completed chapter. For example, CIMO7eCh9.mbk is the completed Chapter 9 file that will allow your student to start with Chapter 10.

- Print Instructor's Manual (0077390601, 9780077390600). Also available through your McGraw-Hill sales representative.

- Additional options

  - *Student At-Home Medisoft® Advanced Version 16 (0077390598, 9780077390594).* A great option for online courses or students who wish to practice at home. Available individually or packaged with the textbook—it's up to you!

  - *Case Studies for Use with Computers in the Medical Office, 6e.* This book provides a capstone simulation using Medisoft® Advanced Version 16. It offers students enhanced training that is meant to improve their qualifications for a variety of medical office jobs. Extensive hands-on practice with realistic source documents teach students to input information, schedule appointments, and handle billing, reports, and other essential tasks. The book provides additional activities, including more complex activities for advanced students.

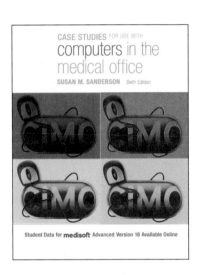

"I like how *CiMO* teaches the software step-by-step with exercises at the computer for every chapter. I like how *Case Studies* puts it all together making it a real-life situation with the exercises at the end of the chapters that can be graded and assess the progress of the student."
Stacey Wilson, CMA (AAMA), MT/PBT (ASCP), MHA, Cabarrus College of Health Sciences

- Connect *Plus*⁺ McGraw-Hill Connect *Plus*⁺ is a revolutionary online assignment and assessment solution, providing instructors and students with tools and resources to maximize their success. Through Connect *Plus*⁺, instructors enjoy simplified course setup and assignment creation. Robust, media-rich tools and activities, all tied to the textbook Learning Outcomes ensure you'll create classes geared toward achievement. You'll have more time with your students and spend less time agonizing over course planning.

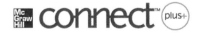

- McGraw-Hill LearnSmart for Medical Insurance, Billing, and Coding: LearnSmart diagnoses students' skill levels to determine what they're good at and where they need help.

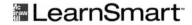

Then, it delivers customized learning content based on their strengths and weakness. The result: Students get the help they need, right when they need it—instead of getting stuck on lessons, or being continually frustrated with stalled progress.

NEED HELP? CONTACT THE DIGITAL CARE SUPPORT TEAM

Visit our Digital CARE Support website at www.mhhe.com/support. Browse the FAQs (frequently asked questions) and product documentation, and/or contact a CARE support representative.

The Digital CARE Support Team is available Sunday through Friday.

Susan M. Sanderson, Senior Technical Writer for Chestnut Hill Enterprises, Inc., has authored all Windows-based editions of *Computers in the Medical Office*. She has also written *Case Studies for Use with Computers in the Medical Office* and *Electronic Health Records for Allied Health Careers*. To accompany the latter title, she developed interactive digital learning content for Practice Partner, a McKesson electronic health record program.

In her more than ten years' experience with Medisoft®, Susan has participated in alpha and beta testing, worked with instructors to site-test materials, and provided technical support to McGraw-Hill customers.

In 2009, Susan earned her CPEHR (Certified Professional in Electronic Health Records) certification. In addition, she is a member of the Healthcare Information and Management Systems Society (HIMSS). Susan is a graduate of Drew University with further study at Columbia University.

CiMO
to the student

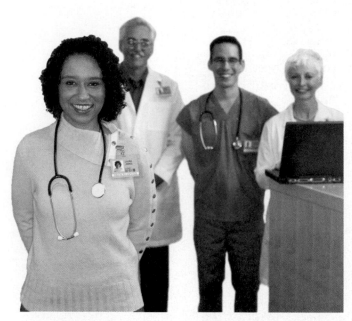

CAREERS IN MEDICAL BILLING

Medical billers play important roles in the financial well-being of every health care business. Billing for services in health care is more complicated than in other industries. Government and private payers pay different amounts for the same services, and health care providers deliver services to beneficiaries of several insurance companies at any one time. Medical billers must be familiar with the rules and guidelines of each health care plan in order to submit the proper documentation so the office receives the maximum appropriate reimbursement for services provided. Without an effective billing staff, a medical office would have no cash flow!

Medical billers come in contact with clients, insurance companies, and patients. They also work with other staff members such as medical assistants, nurses, and doctors. In addition to having specialized knowledge about medical billing and computer skills, medical billers must possess excellent customer service skills to succeed in this field. Even though they are not involved in providing medical care, they play a key role in a client's experience at a medical office.

Medical billing is a challenging, interesting career. Billers are compensated according to their skill level and how effectively they put their skills to use. Those with the right combination of skills and abilities may have the opportunity to advance to management positions, such as patient account manager, physician office supervisor, and medical office manager. The more education the individual has, the more employment options and advancement opportunities are available. Individuals who have practical experience in using computers and patient billing software will find themselves well prepared to enter this ever-changing field.

Computers in the Medical Office includes a tutorial and a simulation. Once you learn how to operate the Medisoft® Advanced

Version 16 program by completing the tutorial, you can practice those skills by working through the simulation. Both the tutorial and the simulation use a medical office setting, Family Care Center, to provide a realistic environment in which you can learn how to use the software.

Medisoft® is a popular patient billing and accounting software program. It enables health care practices to maintain their billing data as well as to generate report information. The software handles all the basic tasks that a medical biller needs in order to effectively perform the job. As a result, Medisoft® is an excellent training tool for anyone interested in working as a medical biller.

Even if you do not use Medisoft® on the job, the skills you learn here will be similar to the skills needed to use almost any medical accounting program. You will learn how to

- Enter patient information
- Work with cases
- Enter charges, payments, and adjustments
- Create claims
- Post insurance payments
- Create patient statements
- Produce reports
- Create collection letters
- Schedule

walkthrough

Many pedagogical tools have been incorporated throughout the book to help students learn.

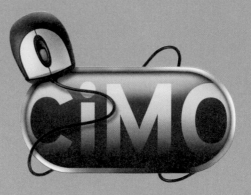

CiMO

key terms

access rights
Auto Log Off
backup data
database
knowledge base
Medisoft Program Date
MMDDCCYY format
packing data
purging data
rebuilding indexes
recalculating balances
restoring data

learning outcomes

When you finish this chapter, you will be able to:

3.1 List the six databases Medisoft uses to store information.

3.2 List the menus in Medisoft.

3.3 Explain the function of the Medisoft toolbar.

3.4 Explain how to enter, edit, save, and delete data in Medisoft.

3.5 Describe how to change the Medisoft Program Date.

3.6 Discuss three types of help available in Medisoft.

3.7 Explain how to create and restore backup files in Medisoft.

3.8 Describe the functions of the file maintenance utilities in Medisoft.

3.9 Describe the Medisoft security features used to ensure compliance with HIPAA and HITECH regulations.

what you need to know

To use this chapter, you need to know how to:
- Start your computer and Microsoft Windows.
- Use the keyboard and mouse.

CHAPTER OPENER

The **chapter opener** sets the stage for what will be learned in the chapter.

Key Terms

Key terms are first introduced in the chapter opener so the student can see them all in one place.

Learning Outcomes

Learning Outcomes are written to reflect the revised version of Bloom's Taxonomy, and to establish the key points the student should focus on in the chapter. In addition, major chapter heads are structured to reflect the Learning Outcomes and are numbered accordingly.

What You Need to Know

What You Need to Know lets students check whether they understand and recall the information they learned in previous chapters. Mastery of the information listed here is necessary to complete the current chapter.

responsibility for the procedure. For example, if the fee for a procedure is $80 and the patient is responsible for 20 percent of charges, the patient may be asked to pay $16 at check-in. Since it is not always possible to accurately estimate a patient's financial obligation at check-in, offices usually base the patient's share on the average charge for the scheduled service. The prepayment amounts are usually accurate enough that few patients overpay.

documentation a record of health care encounters between the physician and the patient, created by the provider

medical record a chronological record of a patient's medical history and care that includes information that the patient provides, as well as the physician's assessment, diagnosis, and treatment plan

1.4 STEP 4: CHECK OUT PATIENTS

Every time a patient is treated by a health care provider, a record of the encounter, known as **documentation**, is made. This chronological **medical record**, or chart, includes information that the patient

CiMO glossary

a

access rights security option that determines the areas of the program a user can access, and whether the user has rights to enter or edit data

accounting cycle the flow of financial transactions in a business

accounts receivable (AR) monies that are flowing into a business

adjudication series of steps that determine whether a claim should be paid

adjustments changes to patients' accounts that alter the amounts charged or paid

capitation payments payments made to physicians on a regular basis for providing services to patients in a managed care plan

case a grouping of transactions that share a common element

charges amounts a provider bills for the services performed

chart a folder that contains all records pertaining to a patient

chart number a unique number that identifies a patient

clean claims claims with all the correct information necessary for payer processing

OPENING A PATIENT OR CASE
The quickest way to open a patient or case is to double click on the line associated with a patient or case.

about patients, and the right side of the window contains information about cases. Cases are covered in Chapter 5.

On the upper-right side of the Patient List dialog box, there are two radio buttons: Patient and Case. When the Patient radio button is clicked, the left side of the window becomes active. Correspondingly, when the Case radio button is clicked, the right side of the window becomes active. The command buttons at the bottom of the dialog box vary, depending on which side of the window is active. When the Patient window is active, the command buttons at the bottom of the screen include Edit Patient, New Patient, Delete Patient, Print Grid, Quick Entry, and Close.

LEARNING AIDS

Key Terms
Key terms are defined in the margin so that students will become familiar with the language necessary to perform medical billing tasks.

Glossary
The **Glossary** at the back of the book also makes it easy to find a term's definition.

Shortcuts
Marginal **Shortcuts** suggest ways to be a more efficient user of the software.

EXERCISES

Chapter Exercises
Exercises within the chapter provide students with hands-on practice using a medical billing software program. The exercises offer step-by-step instructions for completing each task. They must be completed in order!

Applying Your Skills
Applying Your Skills exercises let students see how well they have learned the medical billing tasks in the chapter.

EXERCISE 5-6   EDITING A CASE

John Fitzwilliams, an established patient, has just divorced. Edit the information in his Case dialog box to reflect this change.

Date: October 3, 2016

1. Click in the Search for field and press the backspace key to delete the *T* that was entered to search for Hiro Tanaka. The Patient List once again displays the complete list of patients.
2. Enter *F* in the Search for field. All patients who have last names beginning with the letter *F* are displayed. Click anywhere in the listing for John Fitzwilliams to select his entry.
3. Click the Case radio button. Verify that Acute Gastric Ulcer is listed in the Case area of the dialog box.
4. Click the Edit Case button.
5. In the Personal tab, change the entry in the Marital Status box from Married to Divorced.
6. Check your work for accuracy.
7. Save the changes.
8. Close the Patient List dialog box.   CiMO

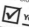 **You have completed Exercise 5-6.**

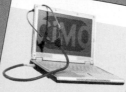

APPLYING YOUR SKILLS
2: CREATING A CASE FOR A NEW PATIENT

October 3, 2016
Lisa Wright is a new patient who has just arrived for her office visit with Dr. Jessica Rudner. Dr. Rudner accepts assignment from Blue Cross/Blue Shield. Using Source Document 2, complete the Personal, Account, and Policy 1 tabs in the Case dialog box. In the Policy 1 tab, enter 100 in all the Insurance Coverage by Service Classification boxes. (Note: Not all tabs and text boxes will have entries.)

Remember to create a backup of your work before exiting Medisoft! To help you keep track of your work, name the backup file after the chapter you are working on, for example, StudentID-c5.mbk.

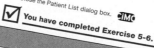

ELECTRONIC HEALTH RECORD EXCHANGE

Electronic Health Record Exchange boxes explore how billing programs and electronic health records share data and improve productivity.

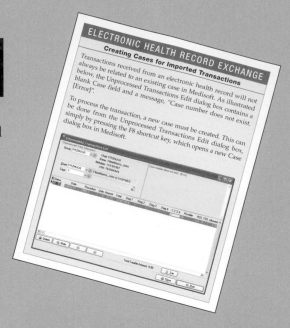

ELECTRONIC HEALTH RECORD EXCHANGE
Creating Cases for Imported Transactions

Transactions received from an electronic health record will not always be related to an existing case in Medisoft. As illustrated below, the Unprocessed Transactions Edit dialog box contains a blank Case field and a message, "Case number does not exist. [Error]".

To process the transaction, a new case must be created. This can be done from the Unprocessed Transactions Edit dialog box, simply by pressing the F8 shortcut key, which opens a new Case dialog box in Medisoft.

END-OF-CHAPTER RESOURCES

Chapter Summary

The **Chapter Summary** is in a tabular, step-by-step format with page references to help with review of the material.

Worksheet

The student **Worksheet** contains objective questions that require students to accurately complete the computer exercises in each chapter.

Chapter Review

The **Chapter Review** contains the following exercises, all tagged by Learning Outcome: Using Terminology, Checking Your Understanding, Applying Knowledge, Thinking About It, and At the Computer. All the exercises reinforce the content the student has just learned.

SOURCE DOCUMENTS

The **Source Documents** are examples of typical documents and forms that one would work with in a real medical practice. These documents provide students with the information they need to complete the software exercises in the book.

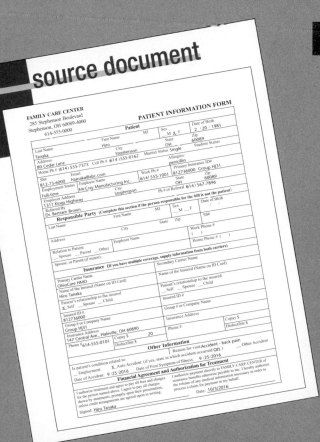

CiMO
acknowledgments

Suggestions have been received from faculty and students throughout the country. This is vital feedback that is relied upon with each edition. Each person who has offered comments and suggestions has our thanks.

The efforts of many people are needed to develop and improve a product. Among these people are the reviewers and consultants who point out areas of concern, cite areas of strength, and make recommendations for change. In this regard, the following instructors provided feedback that was enormously helpful in preparing the seventh edition of *CiMO*.

We would like to extend special thanks to the people at Corinthian Colleges, Inc. for all of their valuable feedback during the development of the new edition. We also greatly appreciate the feedback from the people at Career Education Corporation throughout the development process.

SYMPOSIA

An enthusiastic group of trusted faculty members active in this course area attended symposia to provide crucial feedback.

Amelia Island, Florida

- Stacey Ashford, CPC, Remington College
- Bonnie J. Crist, BS, CMA (AAMA), Harrison College
- Jill Ferrari, MA MT MLT (ASCP), Sullivan University
- Cindy Glewwe, M.Ed., RHIA, Rasmussen College
- Shelly Halper, A.A.S., NCMA, RMA, NCPT, NCICS, Fox College
- Jennifer L. Holmes, Concorde Career Colleges, Inc.
- Michelle Knighton, MBA, RHIA, Herzing University Online
- Angela Massengill, RMA (AMT), Institute of Business and Medical Careers
- Michelle R. McClatchey, BS, Westwood College

- Debra L. Soucy, CPC, The Salter School
- Stacey Wilson, CMA (AAMA), MT/PBT (ASCP), MHA, Cabarrus College of Health Sciences

Tucson, Arizona

- Amy L. Blochowiak, MBA, ACS, AIAA, AIRC, ARA, FLHC, FLMI, HCSA, HIA, HIPAA, MHP, PCS, SILA-F, Northeast Wisconsin Technical College
- Nikita Carr, CPC, CMBS, Centura College
- Robin Maddalena, CMT, Branford Hall Career Institute
- Cheryl Miller, MBA/HCM, Westmoreland County Community College
- Tammy L. Shick, Great Lakes Institute of Technology
- Lynn A. Skafte, CMA, Rasmussen College
- Heidi Weber, BS, CMA (AAMA), RMA, Globe University

WORKSHOPS

In 2009 and 2010, McGraw-Hill has conducted fifteen allied health workshops, providing an opportunity for more than six hundred faculty members to gain continuing education credits as well as to provide feedback on our products.

BOOK REVIEWS

More than a hundred instructors reviewed the sixth edition once it was published and provided valuable feedback that directly affected the development of the seventh edition.

- Phillip M. Abbatiello, A.A., B.S., Lincoln Technical Institute
- Ruth Anderson, BS, Westmoreland County Community College
- Stacey Ashford, CPC, Remington College
- Diane Roche Benson, CMA (AAMA), BSHCA, MSA, CFP, CMRS, CPC, CDE, NSC-SCFAT, ASE, AHA BCLS/First Aid-Instructor, PALS, CAAM-I, ACLS, Wake Technical Community College and University of Phoenix
- Amy L. Blochowiak, MBA, ACS, AIAA, AIRC, ARA, FLHC, FLMI, HCSA, HIA, HIPAA, MHP, PCS, SILA-F, Northeast Wisconsin Technical College
- Gerry A. Brasin, AS, CMA (AAMA), CPC, Premier Education Group
- Deborah S. Briones, MSN, Taller San Jose Medical Careers Academy and Argosy University

- Teresa M. Buglione, CHI, CMA, Cert. EKG Tech, CPC Bachelors HealthCare Admin, MBA, Martinsburg Institute, SME, Career Tech Schools
- Lisa Bynoe, ASA College
- Angela M. Chisley, AHI, RMA, College of Southern Maryland
- Ursula Cole, CMA (AAMA), CCS-P, Platt College
- Michelle H. Cranney, MBA, RHIT, CCS-P, CPC, Virginia College, Online division
- Bonnie J. Crist, BS, CMA (AAMA), Harrison College
- Laurie Dennis, CBCS, Florida Career College
- Jane W. Dumas, MSN, CCMA, CHI (NHA), Remington College
- Rhonda K. Epps, CMA (AAMA), RMA, AS, National College of Business and Technology
- Sheila Gawne, Blue Cliff College
- Elizabeth Hoffman, MA Ed., CMA (AAMA), CPT, (ASPT), Baker College of Clinton Township
- Geraldine Hotz, RHIA, CCS-P, St. Cloud Technical College
- Karen A. King, CNA, CMA, ADN, Everest College
- Jody A. Kirk, BS, CCS-P, Cambria Rowe Business College
- Mary F. Koloski, CBCS, CHI, HIBC Team Lead, Florida Career College
- Amy D. Lawrence, CCA, MBA/HR, Everest University
- Rhonda LeMora, MPA, Remington College
- Gregory A. Martinez, MS, CMBS, Wichita Technical Institute
- Danielle Mbadu, MA, M.Ed., Kaplan Higher Education Campuses
- Wilsetta McClain, RMA (AMT), NCPT, MBA, ABD, Baker College of Auburn Hills
- Michelle R. McClatchey, BS, Westwood College
- Lane Miller, MBA/HCM, Medical Careers Institute
- Lisa M. Myers, RMA, Everest University
- Angela Parmley-Williams, MBA, CBCS, CHI, Sanford Brown Institute
- Natelle A. Pollidore, RMA, Sanford Brown Institute
- Janette Rodriguez, RN, RMA, Wood Tobe Coburn School
- Shelley C. Safian, CCS-P, CPC-H, CPC-I, Herzing University Online
- Rosemarie Scaringella, Bachelors in Education, CBCS, CMAA, Hunter Business School
- Bridget Smalls, Sanford-Brown Institute

- Lisa Smith, B.S., RMA/AMT, BMO/FL, Keiser University
- Wanda D. Strayhan, M.S., CBCS, CMA, Florida Career College
- Tammy Lee Summerson, RMA
- Terrina Thomas, CHES, Sentara Healthcare
- Lynn M. Tuck, MAEd, Corinthian Colleges
- Joyce S. Waters, MA, RHIA, CCS, Atlanta Technical College
- Michael Weinand, Kaplan Higher Education
- Tom Wesley, Minnesota School of Business
- Stacey Wilson, CMA (AAMA), MT/PBT (ASCP), MHA, Cabarrus College of Health Sciences
- Jane F. Yakicic, CMA, CCP-S, Cambria Rowe Business College

TECHNICAL EDITING/ACCURACY PANEL

A panel of instructors completed a technical edit and review of all content in the book page proofs to verify its accuracy, especially in relation to Medisoft®.

- Stacey Ashford, CPC, Remington College
- Amy L. Blochowiak, MBA, ACS, AIAA, AIRC, ARA, FLHC, FLMI, HCSA, HIA, HIPAA, MHP, PCS, SILA-F, Northeast Wisconsin Technical College
- Nikita Carr, CPC, CMBS, Centura College
- Jill Ferrari, MA MT MLT (ASCP), Sullivan University
- Cindy Glewwe, M.Ed., RHIA, Rasmussen College
- Michelle Knighton, MBA, RHIA, Herzing University Online
- Robin Maddalena, CMT, Branford Hall Career Institute
- Cheryl Miller, MBA/HCM, Westmoreland County Community College
- Tammy L. Shick, Great Lakes Institute of Technology
- Debra L. Soucy, CPC, The Salter School
- Stacey Wilson, CMA (AAMA), MT/PBT (ASCP), MHA, Cabarrus College of Health Sciences

SURVEYS

Nearly one hundred people participated in a survey about the software they use in this course.

- Kathryn G. Aguirre, NCMA, International Education Corporation & UEI Colleges
- Velma Alexander, Southwestern Community College

- Risha Ali-Baldeo, Certified Coder Associate, Florida Career College
- Stacey Ashford, CPC, Remington College
- Cindi Brassington, MS CMA, Quinebaug Valley Community College
- Marion Bucci, Montgomery County Community College
- Angela M. Chisley, AHI, RMA, College of Southern Maryland
- Patricia D. Christian, MS, MCAS, Southwest Georgia Technical College
- Bonnie J. Crist, BS, CMA, (AAMA), Harrison College
- Ursula Cole, CMA (AAMA), CCS-P, Platt College
- Anita Denson, CMA (AAMA), National College
- John Dingle, Butler Business College
- Robin J. Douglas, B.S., M.S., Holmes Community College
- Vanessa D. Escalante, MPA, BSC, LA College International
- Cynthia Ferguson, Texas State Technical College
- William C. Fiala, MA, CCS-P, University of Akron
- Savanna Garrity, MPA, Madisonville Community College
- Bonita Gregg, MSEd, RN, Community College of Allegheny County
- Dan Guerra, Community Business College
- Carol Hinricher, University of Montana College of Technology
- Kathleen Holbrook, CMT, Andrews and Holbrook Training Corp.
- Jody Hurtt, MEd, East Central Community College
- JoAnn Kalessa, National College
- Mark Kapusta, BA, QM, CCA, Santa Clarita Medical Academy
- Katin Keirstead, Seacoast Career Schools
- Robin Kern, RN, BSN, Moultrie Technical College
- Cristine L. Kirtley, MSTE, BSTE, CMA (AAMA), Akron Institute of Herzing University
- Crystal Kitchens, CMT, MA, Richland Community College
- Dawn Klemish, MS, RHIA, Lakeshore Technical College
- Judy Kronenberger, Sinclair Community College
- Ann Kunze, BA CMA (AAMA), Medical Careers Institute
- Donna Kyle-Brown, RMA, CPC, Virginia College

- Rhonda LeMora, MPA, Remington College

- Marsha L. Logsdon, PhD, MA, BS, Owensboro Community and Technical College

- Vanessa May BS, MBA, Acadiana Technical College

- Linda C. McHenry, CPC, CPD-I, AAS, Fortis College Online

- Nancy Measell, Ivy Tech Community College

- Genny Melancon, M.Ed. Education, Acadiana Technical College

- Helen Mills, RN, RMA, BMO, Keiser University

- Tina Nolen, Ben Franklin Career Center

- Karen Patton, AAB, BA, CPC, CMC, CCP, Stautzenberger College

- Fred R. Pearson, PhD, Brigham Young University Idaho

- Marianne Pindar, Lackawanna College

- Andrea Potteiger, CCS, CCS-P, CPC, New Horizons, Harrisburg

- Diana Reeder, CMA (AAMA), Maysville Community and Technical College

- Rebecca J. Rodenbaugh, CMA (AAMA), MBA, Baker College of Cadillac

- Janette Rodriguez, RN, RMA, Wood Tobe-Coburn School

- Darcy Roy, Brevard Community College

- Cindy Saloky, OIC Training Academy

- Rosemarie Scaringella, Bachelors in Education, CBCS, CMAA, Hunter Business School

- Gene Simon, RHIA, RMD, Florida Career College

- Juanita Smith, BA, MA, Central Texas College

- Amanda Snyder, YMCA

- Helen Spain, BS, MSEd., Wake Technical Community College

- Christine Sproles, RN, CMT, BSN, MS, Pensacola Christian College

- Brenda Ream Stover, RHIT, CCS, RMT, South Hills School of Business and Technology

- Debra Tymcio, BA, RT(R), RMA, National College

- Mary B. Valencia, CPC, CMC, CMOM, University of Texas at Brownsville/Texas Southmost College

- Katrina Varner, Centura College

- Karen Weil, MEd, McLennan Community College

- Deborah Womack, AAS, LPN, RMA, Tennessee Technology Center at McMinnville
- Jane F. Yakicic, CMA, CCP-S, Cambria Rowe Business College
- Brandy G. Ziesemer, RHIA, CCS, Lake-Sumter Community College
- Susan Zolvinski, BS, MBA, Brown Mackie College

ACKNOWLEDGMENTS FROM THE AUTHOR

To the students and instructors who use this book, your feedback and suggestions have made *CiMO* a better learning tool for all.

I especially want to thank the editorial team at McGraw-Hill—Liz Haefele, Ken Kasee, Natalie Ruffatto, and Michelle Flomenhoft—for their enthusiastic support and their willingness to go the extra mile to take a successful book to the next level.

Hats off to Tamiko Cooper and the Digital CARE Team at McGraw-Hill for providing outstanding technical assistance to students and instructors. Thank you also to Kevin White for stepping in when we needed him. The EDP staff was also outstanding; senior designer Anna Kinigakis created a terrific new design which was implemented through the production process by Marlena Pechan, project manager, Debra Sylvester, production supervisor, Lori Hancock, senior photo research coordinator, and Cathy Tepper, media project manager.

This book would not be in its seventh edition were it not for the tireless efforts of Roxan Kinsey, Executive Marketing Manager, who believed in *Computers in the Medical Office* and Medisoft® from day one.

Finally, a great big thank you to my coworkers at Chestnut Hill Enterprises, Inc.—Cynthia Newby, Susan Magovern, Myrna Breskin, and Derek Noland—for their wisdom, dedication, and patience. This book is truly the result of a group effort.

A COMMITMENT TO ACCURACY

You have a right to expect an accurate textbook, and McGraw-Hill invests considerable time and effort to make sure that we deliver one. Listed below are the many steps we take to make sure this happens.

OUR ACCURACY VERIFICATION PROCESS

First Round—Development Reviews

STEP 1: Numerous **health professions instructors** review the current edition and the draft manuscript and report on any errors that they may find. The authors make these corrections in their final manuscript.

Second Round—Page Proofs

STEP 2: Once the manuscript has been typeset, the **authors** check their manuscript against the page proofs to ensure that all illustrations, graphs, examples, and exercises have been correctly laid out on the pages, and that all codes have been updated correctly.

STEP 3: An outside panel of **peer instructors** completes a technical edit/review of all content in the page proofs to verify its accuracy, especially in relation to Medisoft® Version 16. The authors add these corrections to their review of the page proofs.

STEP 4: A **proofreader** adds a triple layer of accuracy assurance in pages by looking for errors; then a confirming, corrected round of page proofs is produced.

Third Round—Confirming Page Proofs

STEP 5: The **author team** reviews the confirming round of page proofs to make certain that any previous corrections were properly made and to look for any errors they might have missed on the first round.

STEP 6: The **project manager,** who has overseen the book from the beginning, performs **another proofread** to make sure that no new errors have been introduced during the production process.

Final Round—Printer's Proofs

STEP 7: The **project manager** performs a **final proofread** of the book during the printing process, providing a final accuracy review.

In concert with the main text, all supplements undergo a proofreading and technical editing stage to ensure their accuracy.

RESULTS

What results is a textbook that is as accurate and error-free as is humanly possible. Our authors and publishing staff are confident that the many layers of quality assurance have produced books that are leaders in the industry for their integrity and correctness. *Please view the Acknowledgments section for more details on the many people involved in this process.*

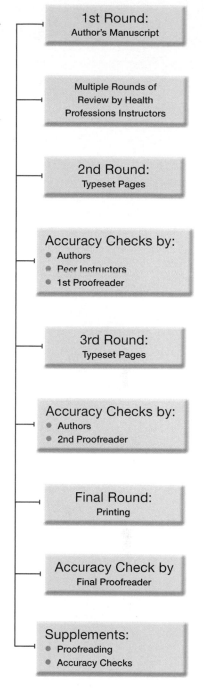

1st Round:
Author's Manuscript

Multiple Rounds of Review by Health Professions Instructors

2nd Round:
Typeset Pages

Accuracy Checks by:
- Authors
- Peer Instructors
- 1st Proofreader

3rd Round:
Typeset Pages

Accuracy Checks by:
- Authors
- 2nd Proofreader

Final Round:
Printing

Accuracy Check by
Final Proofreader

Supplements:
- Proofreading
- Accuracy Checks

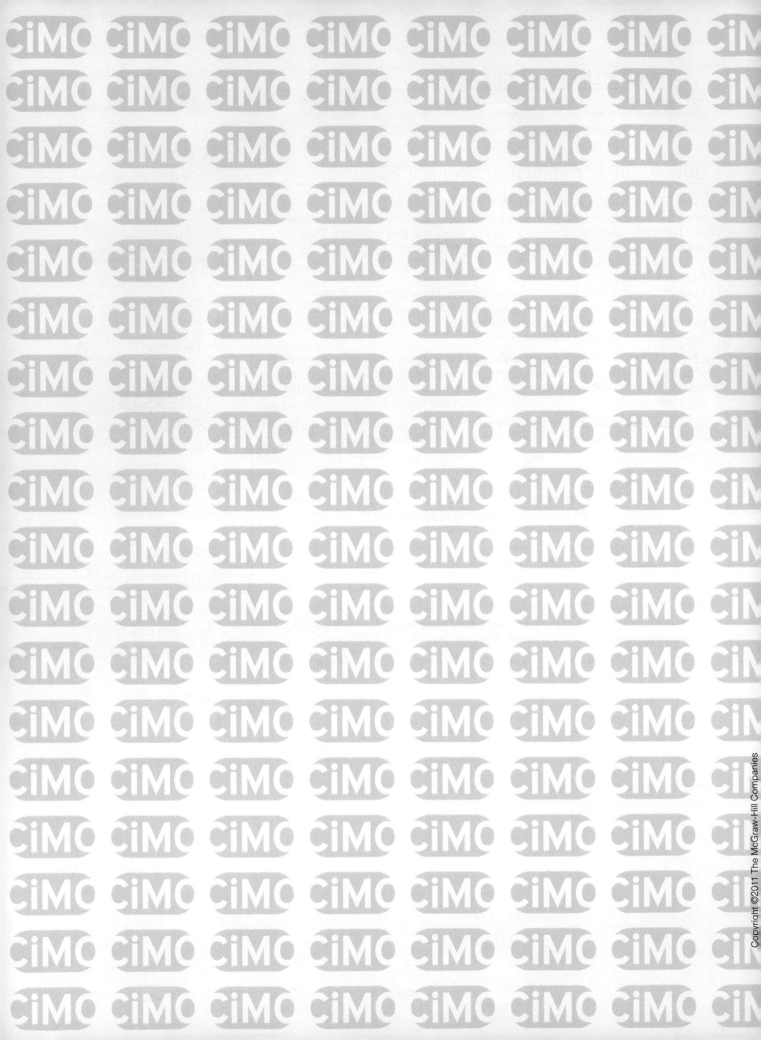

part 1

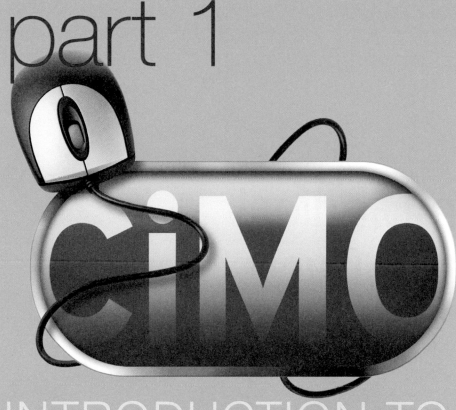

INTRODUCTION TO COMPUTERS IN THE MEDICAL OFFICE

Chapter 1:
The Medical Billing Cycle

Chapter 2:
The Use of Health Information
Technology in Physician Practices

The Medical Billing Cycle

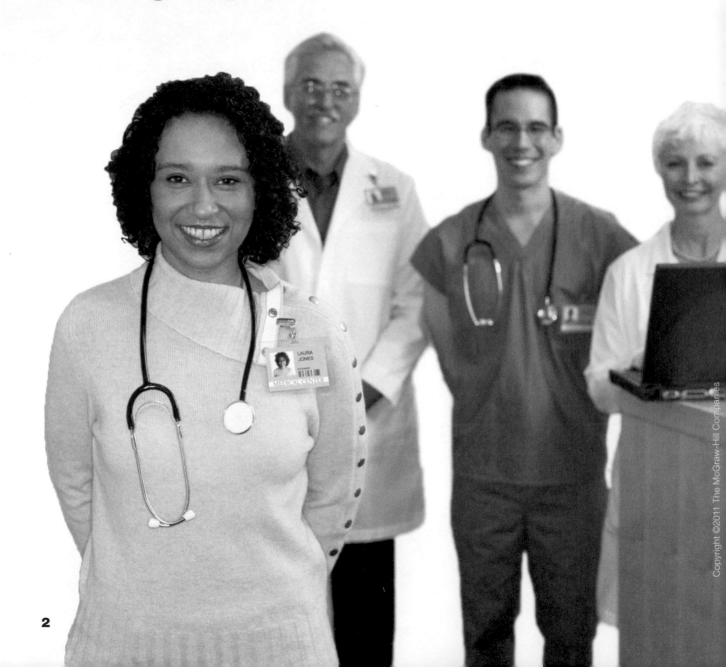

key terms

accounting cycle

accounts receivable (AR)

adjudication

capitation

coding

coinsurance

consumer-driven health
  plan (CDHP)

copayment

deductible

diagnosis

diagnosis code

documentation

electronic health record (EHR)

encounter form

explanation of benefits (EOB)

fee-for-service

health maintenance
  organization (HMO)

health plan

managed care

medical coder

medical necessity

medical record

modifier

patient information form

payer

policyholder

practice management
  program (PMP)

preferred provider
  organization (PPO)

premium

procedure

procedure code

remittance advice (RA)

statement

learning outcomes

When you finish this chapter, you will be able to:

1.1 Identify four types of information collected during preregistration.

1.2 Compare fee-for-service and managed care health plans, and describe three types of managed care approaches.

1.3 Discuss the activities completed during patient check-in.

1.4 Discuss the information contained on an encounter form at checkout.

1.5 Explain the importance of medical necessity.

1.6 Explain why billing compliance is important.

1.7 Describe the information required on an insurance claim.

1.8 List the information contained on a remittance advice.

1.9 Explain the role of patient statements in reimbursement.

1.10 List the reports created to monitor a practice's accounts receivable.

Medical Billing Cycle

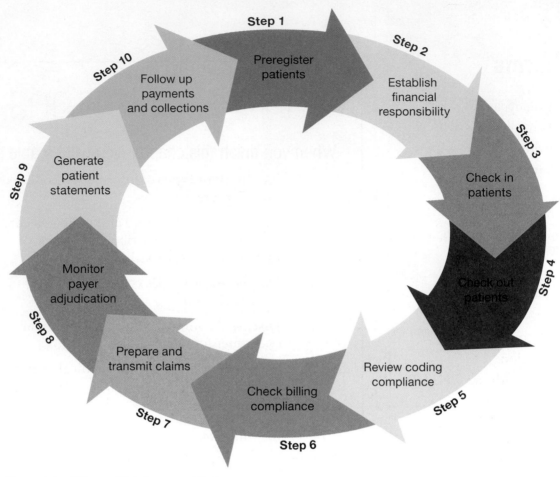

Figure 1-1   Billing and Reimbursement Cycle

From a business standpoint, the key to the financial health of a medical practice is billing and collecting fees for services. Without a steady flow of money coming in, payrolls cannot be met, supplies cannot be ordered, and utility bills cannot be paid. To maintain a regular cash flow, specific billing tasks must be completed on a regular schedule. The billing cycle consists of ten steps that result in timely payment for patients' medical services (see Figure 1-1).

1.1 STEP 1: PREREGISTER PATIENTS

The first step in the billing and reimbursement cycle is to gather information to preregister patients before their office visits. This information includes

- The patient's name.
- The patient's contact information; at the minimum, address and phone number.

- The patient's reason for the visit, such as a medical complaint or a need for an immunization.

- Whether the patient is new to the practice. According to the American Medical Association (AMA), a new patient has not received any services from the physician (or another physician of the same specialty in the practice) within the last three years, and an established patient has had an appointment within that time frame.

The information is obtained over the telephone or via the Internet, if the practice has a website.

1.2 STEP 2: ESTABLISH FINANCIAL RESPONSIBILITY FOR VISIT

Many patients are covered by some type of insurance. It is important to ask whether the patient has insurance and, if so, which specific plan. Usually this is done before the patient arrives for the appointment. The reason is that physicians often participate in some insurance plans and not in others. The information about whether the physician participates in the patient's plan must be provided to the patient before the office visit, since it will affect the amount the patient will pay. For example, if the physician does not participate in an insurance plan, the patient may be liable for all charges.

In most practices, the patient's insurance coverage is verified before the visit, so that it is clear what the patient will be responsible for paying under the terms of the medical insurance. Once the insurance information is obtained, the patient's current eligibility and benefits are verified with the payer. Verification may be done by telephone; it can also be done via the Internet.

MEDICAL INSURANCE BASICS

Medical insurance represents an agreement between a person or entity known as the **policyholder,** and a **health plan.** A health plan is any plan, program, or organization that provides health benefits; it may be an insurance company, also called a carrier, a government program, or a managed care organization (MCO). Payments made to the health plan by the policyholder for insurance coverage are called **premiums.** In exchange for the payments, the health plan agrees to pay for the insured's medical services according to the terms of the insurance policy or agreement.

There are many sources of medical insurance in the United States. Most insured people are covered by group policies, often through their employers. Some people have individual plans. Insurance coverage may be supplied by a private company, such as CIGNA, or by a government plan. CMS—Centers for Medicare and Medicaid

policyholder a person or entity who buys an insurance plan; the insured

health plan a plan, program, or organization that provides health benefits

premium the periodic amount of money the insured pays to a health plan for insurance coverage

Services—runs the Medicare and Medicaid programs. These are the most common government plans:

- **Medicare** Medicare is a federal health plan that covers persons aged sixty-five and over, people with disabilities and with end-stage renal disease (ESRD), and dependent widows.

- **Medicaid** People with low incomes who cannot afford medical care are covered by Medicaid, which is cosponsored by the federal and state governments. Qualifications and benefits vary by state.

- **TRICARE** TRICARE is a government program that covers medical expenses for dependents of active-duty members of the uniformed services and for retired military personnel. Formerly known as CHAMPUS, it also covers dependents of military personnel who were killed while on active duty.

- **CHAMPVA** The Civilian Health and Medical Program of the Veterans Administration is for veterans with permanent service-related disabilities and their dependents. It also covers surviving spouses and dependent children of veterans who died from service-related disabilities.

- **Workers' compensation** People with job-related illnesses or injuries are covered under workers' compensation insurance. Workers' compensation benefits vary according to state law.

Whether it is a private company or a government program, the health plan is called a **payer.** The term *third-party payer* is also used, because the primary relationship is between the provider and the patient, and the health plan is the third party.

payer private or government organization that insures or pays for health care on behalf of beneficiaries

FEE-FOR-SERVICE AND MANAGED CARE

Different types of medical insurance can be purchased. In a **fee-for-service** plan, policyholders are repaid for the costs of health care. The policy lists the medical services that are covered and the amounts that are paid. Usually, a **deductible**—an amount due before benefits begin—must be paid. Then the benefit may be for all or part of the charges. For example, the policy may indicate that 80 percent of charges for surgery are covered and that the policyholder is responsible for paying the other 20 percent. In this example, the portion of charges that an insured person must pay is known as **coinsurance.**

fee-for-service health plan that repays the policyholder for covered medical expenses

deductible amount due before benefits start

coinsurance percentage of charges that an insured person must pay for health care services after payment of the deductible amount

Another type of insurance is known as **managed care.** Most people who are insured through their employers are covered by some form of managed care. Managed care organizations control both the financing and the delivery of health care to policyholders. The managed care organization establishes contracts with physicians and other health care providers that control fees.

managed care a type of insurance in which the carrier is responsible for both the financing and the delivery of health care

Preferred Provider Organizations

The most common type of managed care health plan is a **preferred provider organization (PPO).** A PPO is a network of providers

preferred provider organization (PPO) managed care network of health care providers who agree to perform services for plan members at discounted fees

Copyright ©2011 The McGraw-Hill Companies

under contract with a managed care organization to perform services for plan members at discounted fees. Usually, members may choose to receive care from other doctors or providers outside the network, but they pay a higher cost.

Health Maintenance Organizations

Another common type of managed care system is a **health maintenance organization (HMO).** In one typical arrangement, providers are paid fixed rates at regular intervals, such as monthly, to provide necessary contracted services to patients who are plan members. This fixed payment is referred to as **capitation.**

The rate the provider is paid is based on several factors, including the number of plan members in the insured pool and their ages. The capitated rate per enrollee is paid to the provider even if the provider does not provide any medical services to the patient during the time period covered by the payment. Similarly, the provider receives the same capitated rate if a patient is treated more than once during the time period. In other plans, negotiated per-service fees are paid. These fees are less than the regular rate for a service that the provider normally charges.

In most HMOs, a patient also pays a **copayment**—a fixed fee, such as $20—at the time of an office visit. Usually, patients in an HMO must choose from a specific group of health care providers. If they seek services from a provider who is not in the health plan, the payer does not pay for the care.

Consumer-Driven Health Plans

A **consumer-driven health plan (CDHP)** is a type of managed care insurance in which a high-deductible low-premium insurance plan is combined with a pretax savings account to cover out-of-pocket medical expenses. These plans typically include three elements. The first is an insurance plan, usually a PPO, with a high deductible (such as $1,000), for which the policyholder pays a lower premium than for a plan with a lower deductible.

The second element is a designated health savings account (HSA) that is used to pay medical bills before the deductible has been met. The savings account, similar to an individual retirement account (IRA), lets people set aside untaxed wages to cover their out-of-pocket medical expenses. Some employers contribute to employees' accounts as a benefit. If money is left in the account at the end of a plan year, it rolls over to help cover the next year's health expenses.

The third element of a CDHP is access to informational tools that help consumers make informed decisions about their health care, such as plan-sponsored websites. The patient is purchasing health care services directly, and both insurance companies and employers believe that paying for medical services causes patients to be educated, efficient consumers.

health maintenance organization (HMO) a managed health care system in which providers agree to offer health care to the organization's members for fixed payments

capitation payment to a provider that covers each plan member's health care services for a certain period of time

copayment a fixed fee paid by the patient at the time of an office visit

consumer-driven health plan (CDHP) a type of managed care in which a high-deductible, low premium insurance plan is combined with a pretax savings account to cover out-of-pocket medical expenses

1.3 STEP 3: CHECK IN PATIENTS

When patients arrive in the office, additional information is collected if they are new patients and updated as needed if they are established patients.

COMPLETE OR UPDATE PATIENT INFORMATION

If they have not already done so, patients are asked to complete a patient information form. The **patient information form** contains the personal, employment, and medical insurance information needed to collect payment for the provider's services. This form, illustrated in Figure 1-2, becomes part of the patient's medical record and is updated when the patient reports a change, such as a new address or different medical insurance. Most offices ask all patients to update these forms periodically to ensure that the information is current and accurate.

The patient information form requires the patient's signature or the signature of a parent or guardian if the patient is a minor, mentally incapacitated, or incompetent. The signature also indicates that the patient accepts responsibility for payment of all charges not paid by the health plan, and authorizes the release of information required to process an insurance claim. The signature also authorizes the health plan or government program to send payments directly to the provider rather than to the patient.

VERIFY IDENTITY

During check-in, it is also common to photocopy or scan the patient's insurance identification card, front and back (see Figure 1-3), and a photo ID, such as a driver's license, to verify that the patient and the insured are in fact the same person. At this time, it is also important to make sure that the health plan's conditions for payment, such as pre-authorization requirements, are met before treatment is provided.

COLLECT TIME-OF-SERVICE PAYMENTS DUE BEFORE TREATMENT

A payment may be collected from the patient during check-in. Payments may be made by cash, check, or credit or debit card (if the practice accepts them). When a payment is made, a receipt is given to the patient. Copayments are routinely collected during check-in. In addition, if a patient owes a balance to the practice, this amount is also collected, or arrangements for payment are made. New patients receive information about the practice's financial policy so they understand that they are responsible for payment of charges that are not paid by their health plans.

While physician practices have always expected patients to pay copayments when they come in for care, some medical offices are now asking patients for partial payment of the office visit charges during check-in. The amount of the partial payment is the estimated patient

FAMILY CARE CENTER
285 Stephenson Boulevard
Stephenson, OH 60089-4000
614-555-0000

PATIENT INFORMATION FORM

Patient				

Last Name	First Name	MI	Sex __ M __ F	Date of Birth / /

Address	City		State	Zip

Home Ph # ( )	Cell Ph # ( )	Marital Status	Student Status

SS#	Email	Allergies

Employment Status	Employer Name	Work Ph # ( )	Primary Insurance ID#

Employer Address	City	State	Zip

Referred By	Ph # of Referral ( )

Responsible Party (Complete this section if the person responsible for the bill is not the patient)

Last Name	First Name	MI	Sex __ M __ F	Date of Birth / /

Address	City	State	Zip	SS#

Relation to Patient __ Spouse __ Parent __ Other	Employer Name	Work Phone # ( )

Spouse, or Parent (if minor):	Home Phone # ( )

Insurance (If you have multiple coverage, supply information from both carriers)

Primary Carrier Name	Secondary Carrier Name
Name of the Insured (Name on ID Card)	Name of the Insured (Name on ID Card)
Patient's relationship to the insured __ Self __ Spouse __ Child	Patient's relationship to the insured __ Self __ Spouse __ Child
Insured ID #	Insured ID #
Group # or Company Name	Group # or Company Name
Insurance Address	Insurance Address

Phone #	Copay $	Phone #	Copay $
	Deductible $		Deductible $

Other Information

Is patient's condition related to:	Reason for visit:

__ Employment   __ Auto Accident (if yes, state in which accident occurred: ___)   __ Other Accident

Date of Accident: / /   Date of First Symptom of Illness: / /

Financial Agreement and Authorization for Treatment

I authorize treatment and agree to pay all fees and charges for the person named above. I agree to pay all charges shown by statements, promptly upon their presentation, unless credit arrangements are agreed upon in writing.

I authorize payment directly to FAMILY CARE CENTER of insurance benefits otherwise payable to me. I hereby authorize the release of any medical information necessary in order to process a claim for payment in my behalf.

Signed: _____   Date: _____

Figure 1-2   Patient Information Form

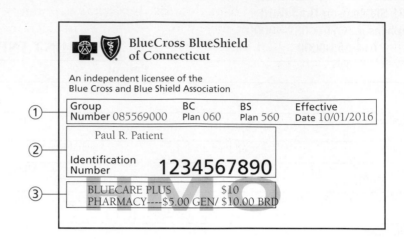

1. **Group identification number**
   The 9-digit number used to identify the member's employer.

   Blue Cross Blue Shield plan codes
   The numbers used to identify the codes assigned to each plan by the Blue Cross Blue Shield Association: used for claims submissions when medical services are rendered out-of-state.

   Effective date
   The date on which the member's coverage became effective.

2. **Member name**
   The full name of the cardholder.

   Identification number
   The 10-digit number used to identify each Anthem Blue Cross and Blue Shield of Connecticut or BlueCare Health Plan member.

3. **Health plan**
   The name of the health plan and the type of coverage; usually lists any copayment amounts, frequency limits or annual maximums for home and office visits; may also list the member's annual deductible amount.

   Riders (optional additional coverage)
   The type(s) of riders that are included in the member's benefits (DME, Visions).

   Pharmacy
   The type of prescription drug coverage; lists copayment amounts.

Figure 1-3   Sample Insurance Identification Card

responsibility for the procedure. For example, if the fee for a procedure is $80 and the patient is responsible for 20 percent of charges, the patient may be asked to pay $16 at check-in. Since it is not always possible to accurately estimate a patient's financial obligation at check-in, offices usually base the patient's share on the average charge for the scheduled service. The prepayment amounts are usually accurate enough that few patients overpay.

1.4 STEP 4: CHECK OUT PATIENTS

Every time a patient is treated by a health care provider, a record of the encounter, known as **documentation,** is made. This chronological **medical record,** or chart, includes information that the patient

documentation a record of health care encounters between the physician and the patient, created by the provider

medical record a chronological record of a patient's medical history and care that includes information that the patient provides, as well as the physician's assessment, diagnosis, and treatment plan

provides, such as medical history, as well as the physician's assessment, diagnosis, and treatment plan. Records also contain laboratory test results, X-rays and other diagnostic images, a list of medications prescribed, and reports that indicate the results of operations and other medical procedures.

DIAGNOSES AND PROCEDURES

Office visit documentation contains two very important pieces of information—the **diagnosis,** which is the physician's opinion of the nature of the patient's illness or injury, and the **procedures,** which are the services performed. When diagnoses and procedures are reported to health plans, code numbers are used in place of descriptions. **Coding** is the process of translating a description of a diagnosis or procedure into a standardized code. Standardization allows information to be shared among physicians, office personnel, health plans, and so on, without losing the precise meaning.

A patient's diagnosis is communicated to a health plan as a **diagnosis code,** a code found in the *International Classification of Diseases*, Ninth Revision, *Clinical Modification* (ICD-9-CM) (see Figure 1-4). Diagnosis codes

diagnosis physician's opinion of the nature of the patient's illness or injury

procedure medical treatment provided by a physician or other health care provider

coding the process of translating a description of a diagnosis or procedure into a standardized code

diagnosis code a standardized value that represents a patient's illness, signs, and symptoms

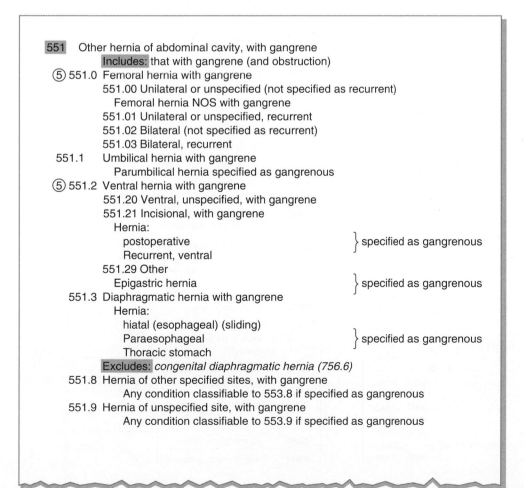

Figure 1-4   Sample of ICD Codes

provide health plans with very specific information about the patient's illness, signs, and symptoms. For example, the code for Alzheimer's disease is 331.0, and the code for influenza with other respiratory manifestations is 487.1. An updated diagnostic coding system, known as ICD-10-CM, must be implemented by physician practices on October 1, 2013.

procedure code a code that identifies a medical service

Similarly, each procedure the physician performs is assigned a **procedure code** that stands for the particular service, treatment, or test. This code is selected from the *Current Procedural Terminology* (CPT) (see Figure 1-5). A large group of codes cover the physician's

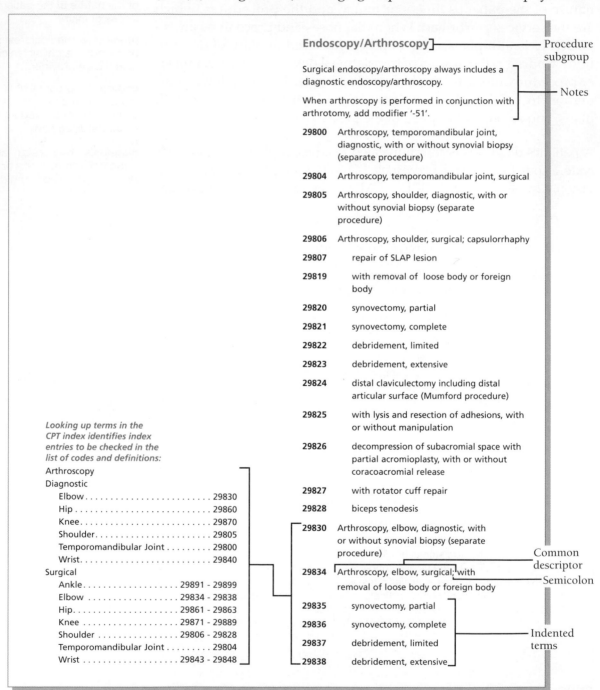

Figure 1-5   Sample of CPT Codes

evaluation and management of a patient's condition during an office visit or a visit at another location, such as a nursing home. Other codes cover groups of specific procedures, such as surgery, pathology, and radiology. For example, 99431 is the CPT code for the physician's examination of a newborn infant, and the code for a total hip replacement is 27130. These five-digit codes can also be followed by one or more modifiers. A CPT **modifier** is a two-digit character that is appended to a CPT code to report special circumstances involved with a procedure or service.

modifier a two-digit character that is appended to a CPT code to report special circumstances involved with a procedure or service

ENCOUNTER FORM

The diagnosis and procedure codes are recorded on an **encounter form,** also known as a superbill (see Figure 1-6). The encounter form may be electronic or paper-based. More and more physicians are turning to electronic health record programs to record information about patient encounters. An **electronic health record (EHR)** is a lifelong computerized health care record for an individual that incorporates data from providers who have treated the individual. An EHR includes information from a number of different physicians as well as from pharmacies, laboratories, hospitals, insurance carriers, and so on. Information is added to the record by health care professionals working in a variety of settings, and the record can be accessed by professionals in any location with computer access, twenty-four hours a day, seven days a week.

encounter form a list of the procedures and charges for a patient's visit

electronic health record (EHR) a computerized lifelong health care record for an individual that incorporates data from providers who treat the individual

In a provider's office that uses EHRs, procedure and diagnosis codes are transmitted electronically into the office's **practice management program (PMP).** A PMP is a software program that automates the administrative and financial tasks required to run a medical practice. For example, the PMP is used to process the financial transactions that result from patients' appointments. The program calculates charges for the office visit, estimates patient and insurance financial responsibilities, and creates insurance claims. The software is also used to record patients' payments and to print receipts. Later, when insurance payments are received, those payments are posted to patients' accounts. Once that step is complete, the program calculates the remaining balance that is the responsibility of the patient.

practice management program (PMP) a software program that automates many of the administrative and financial tasks in a medical practice

1.5 STEP 5: REVIEW CODING COMPLIANCE

Whether physicians are paid by health plans for treating patients depends in part on the diagnosis and procedure codes assigned to the office visit. The medical office staff member who does the coding must have specialized knowledge. In some medical practices, the physicians assign the codes; in others, a **medical coder** or a medical insurance specialist handles this task.

medical coder a person who analyzes and codes patient diagnoses, procedures, and symptoms

ENCOUNTER FORM

DATE _____   TIME _____

PATIENT NAME _____   CHART # _____

OFFICE VISITS - SYMPTOMATIC

NEW

99201	OF--New Patient Minimal	
99202	OF--New Patient Low	
99203	OF--New Patient Detailed	
99204	OF--New Patient Moderate	
99205	OF--New Patient High	

ESTABLISHED

99211	OF--Established Patient Minimal	
99212	OF--Established Patient Low	
99213	OF--Established Patient Detailed	
99214	OF--Established Patient Moderate	
99215	OF--Established Patient High	

PREVENTIVE VISITS

NEW

99381	Under 1 Year	
99382	1 - 4 Years	
99383	5 - 11 Years	
99384	12 - 17 Years	
99385	18 - 39 Years	
99386	40 - 64 Years	
99387	65 Years & Up	

ESTABLISHED

99391	Under 1 Year	
99392	1 - 4 Years	
99393	5 - 11 Years	
99394	12 - 17 Years	
99395	18 - 39 Years	
99396	40 - 64 Years	
99397	65 Years & Up	

PROCEDURES

12011	Simple suture--face--local anes.	
29125	App. of short arm splint; static	
29540	Strapping, ankle	
50390	Aspiration of renal cyst by needle	
71010	Chest x-ray, single view, frontal	

PROCEDURES

71020	Chest x-ray, two views, frontal & lateral	
71030	Chest x-ray, complete, four views	
73070	Elbow x-ray, AP & lateral views	
73090	Forearm x-ray, AP & lateral views	
73100	Wrist x-ray, AP & lateral views	
73510	Hip x-ray, complete, two views	
73600	Ankle x-ray, AP & lateral views	

LABORATORY

80019	19 clinical chemistry tests	
80048	Basic metabolic panel	
80061	Lipid panel	
82270	Blood screening, occult; feces	
82947	Glucose screening--quantitative	
82951	Glucose tolerance test, three specimens	
83718	HDL cholesterol	
84478	Triglycerides test	
85007	Manual differential WBC	
85018	Hemoglobin	
85651	Erythrocyte sedimentation rate--non-auto	
86580	TB Mantoux test	
87072	Culture by commercial kit, nonurine...	
87076	Culture, anaerobic isolate	
87077	Bacterial culture, aerobic isolate	
87086	Urine culture and colony count	
87430	Strep test	
87880	Direct streptococcus screen	

INJECTIONS

90471	Immunization administration	
90703	Tetanus injection	
96372	Injection	
92516	Facial nerve function studies	
93000	Electrocardiogram--ECG with interpretation	
93015	Treadmill stress test, with physician...	
96900	Ultraviolet light treatment	
99070	Supplies and materials provided	

FAMILY CARE CENTER
286 Stephenson Blvd.
Stephenson, OH 60089
614-555-0000

☐ DANA BANU, M.D.
☐ ROBERT BEACH, M.D.
☐ PATRICIA MCGRATH, M.D.

☐ JESSICA RUDNER, M.D.
☐ JOHN RUDNER, M.D.
☐ KATHERINE YAN, M.D.

NOTES

REFERRING PHYSICIAN	NPI	AUTHORIZATION #

DIAGNOSIS

PAYMENT AMOUNT

Figure 1-6   Encounter Form

In the area of coding, compliance involves following official guidelines of the American Hospital Association and the American Medical Association when codes are assigned. After they are selected, diagnosis and procedure codes must be checked for errors. Also, the diagnosis and the medical services that are documented in the patient's medical record should be logically connected, so that the **medical necessity** of the charges is clear to the insurance company.

Medical necessity is defined differently by different insurance plans. The American Medical Association (AMA) has defined medical necessity as "services or products that a prudent physician would provide to a patient for the purpose of preventing, diagnosing, or treating an illness, injury, or its symptoms in a manner that is: (1) in accordance with generally accepted standards of medical practice; (2) clinically appropriate in terms of type, frequency, extent, site, and duration; and (3) not primarily for the convenience of the patient, physician, or other health care provider." If medical necessity is not met, the physician will not receive payment from the health plan.

medical necessity treatment provided by a physician to a patient for the purpose of preventing, diagnosing, or treating an illness, injury, or its symptoms in a manner that is appropriate and is provided in accordance with generally accepted standards of medical practice

1.6 STEP 6: CHECK BILLING COMPLIANCE

Each charge, or fee, for a visit is represented by a specific procedure code. The provider's fees for services are listed on the medical practice's fee schedule. Most medical practices have standard fee schedules listing their usual fees. However, the fees listed on the master fee schedule are not necessarily the amount the provider will be paid. Many providers enter into contracts with insurance plans that require a discount from standard fees.

In addition, although there is a separate fee associated with each code, each code is not necessarily billable. Whether it can be billed depends on the payer's particular rules. Following these rules when preparing claims results in billing compliance. Some payers bundle groups of services under particular codes and do not permit billing those component codes separately. Medical billers apply their knowledge of payer guidelines to analyze what can be billed on health care claims.

1.7 STEP 7: PREPARE AND TRANSMIT CLAIMS

To receive payment, medical practices must produce documents for health plans and patients. One kind of document is an insurance claim. For a health plan to pay a claim, certain information about the patient must be shared. For example, a health plan needs to know the procedures the provider performed and the diagnosis that caused them to be needed, as well as the date and location of the visit.

Health plans also require basic information about the provider who is treating the patient, including the provider's name and identification number. Beyond the basic information requirements that are common to all payers, there are differences in what information is required on an insurance claim. A payer lists the required information in a provider's manual that is available to the medical office.

Using the information in the PMP, including the diagnosis and procedure coding information from the EHR, the PMP generates health care claims. These claims are then electronically transmitted to health plans for payment.

1.8 STEP 8: MONITOR PAYER ADJUDICATION

When the claim is received by the payer, it is reviewed following a process known as **adjudication**—a series of steps designed to judge whether it should be paid. A claim may be paid in full, partially paid, held for more information, or denied. The results of the adjudication process are explained in a document that is sent to the provider along with the payment. This document is called a **remittance advice (RA)** or **explanation of benefits (EOB)** (see Figure 1-7). The remittance advice provides details about each patient transaction, such as

- Date of service
- Services provided
- Patient name and control number
- Provider identifier number
- Amount allowed by contract
- Amount paid to provider
- Amount owed by patient

Usually, an RA is sent electronically to the provider; the patient receives a paper EOB. When the RA arrives at the provider's office, it is reviewed for accuracy. Each payment and explanation is compared with the claim to check that

- All procedures that were listed on the claim also appear on the payment transaction
- Any unpaid charges are explained
- The codes on the payment transactions match those on the claim
- The payment listed for each procedure is as expected

If any discrepancies are found when reviewing the RA, a request for a review of the claim is filed with the payer, following the payer's or the state's rules on seeking appropriate reimbursement for claims.

adjudication series of steps that determine whether a claim should be paid

remittance advice (RA) an explanation of benefits transmitted electronically by a payer to a provider

explanation of benefits (EOB) paper document from a payer that shows how the amount of a benefit was determined

EAST OHIO PPO
10 CENTRAL AVENUE
HALEVILLE, OH 60890

PROVIDER REMITTANCE

FAMILY CARE CENTER
285 STEPHENSON BLVD.
STEPHENSON, OH 60089

PAGE: 1 OF 1
DATE: 11/11/2016
ID NUMBER: 4679323

PROVIDER: PATRICIA MCGRATH, M.D.

PATIENT: BROOKS LAWANA   CLAIM: 234567890

FROM DATE	THRU DATE	PROC CODE	UNITS	AMOUNT BILLED	AMOUNT ALLOWED	DEDUCT	COPAY/ COINS	PROV PAID	REASON CODE
10/28/16	10/28/16	99212	1	54.00	48.60	.00	20.00	28.60	
10/28/16	10/28/16	73600	1	96.00	86.40	.00	.00	86.40	
	CLAIM TOTALS			150.00	135.00	.00	20.00	115.00	

PATIENT: HSU DIANE   CLAIM: 345678901

FROM DATE	THRU DATE	PROC CODE	UNITS	AMOUNT BILLED	AMOUNT ALLOWED	DEDUCT	COPAY/ COINS	PROV PAID	REASON CODE
10/28/16	10/28/16	99213	1	72.00	64.80	.00	20.00	44.80	
10/28/16	10/28/16	80048	1	50.00	45.00	.00	.00	45.00	
	CLAIM TOTALS			122.00	109.80	.00	20.00	89.80	

PROVIDER: DANA BANU, M.D.

PATIENT: PATEL RAJI   CLAIM: 567890123

FROM DATE	THRU DATE	PROC CODE	UNITS	AMOUNT BILLED	AMOUNT ALLOWED	DEDUCT	COPAY/ COINS	PROV PAID	REASON CODE
10/28/16	10/28/16	99212	1	54.00	48.60	.00	20.00	28.60	
	CLAIM TOTALS			54.00	48.60	.00	20.00	28.60	

PATIENT: SYZMANSKI MICHAEL   CLAIM: 678901234

FROM DATE	THRU DATE	PROC CODE	UNITS	AMOUNT BILLED	AMOUNT ALLOWED	DEDUCT	COPAY/ COINS	PROV PAID	REASON CODE
10/28/16	10/28/16	99212	1	54.00	48.60	.00	20.00	28.60	
	CLAIM TOTALS			54.00	48.60	.00	20.00	28.60	

PAYMENT SUMMARY		TOTAL ALL CLAIMS		EFT INFORMATION	
TOTAL AMOUNT PAID	262.00	AMOUNT CHARGED	380.00	NUMBER	4679323
PRIOR CREDIT BALANCE	.00	AMOUNT ALLOWED	342.00	DATE	11/11/16
CURRENT CREDIT DEFERRED	.00	DEDUCTIBLE	.00	AMOUNT	262.00
PRIOR CREDIT APPLIED	.00	COPAY	.00		
NEW CREDIT BALANCE	.00	COINSURANCE	80.00		
NET DISBURSED	262.00				

STATUS CODES:
A - APPROVED   AJ - ADJUSTMENT   IP - IN PROCESS   R - REJECTED   V - VOID

Figure 1-7   Remittance Advice

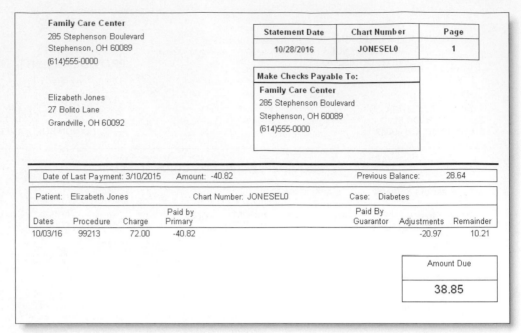

Figure 1-8 Patient Statement

Occasionally, an overpayment may be received, and a refund check is issued by the medical practice.

Once the RA is reviewed, the amount of the payment (whether a paper check or an electronic payment) is recorded in the PMP. Depending on the rules of the health plan, the patient may be billed for an outstanding balance. In other circumstances, a change is made in the software, and the patient is not billed.

1.9 STEP 9: GENERATE PATIENT STATEMENTS

statement a list of all services performed for a patient, along with the charges for each service

If charges are to be billed to the patient, a statement is created in the PMP and mailed to the patient. The **statement** lists all services performed, along with the charges for each service (see Figure 1-8). The statement lists the amount paid by the health plan and the remaining balance that is the responsibility of the patient.

Most medical practices have a regular schedule for sending statements to patients. For example, some practices bill half the patients on the fifteenth of the month and the other half on the thirtieth.

1.10 STEP 10: FOLLOW UP PATIENT PAYMENTS AND HANDLE COLLECTIONS

accounting cycle the flow of financial transactions in a business

The **accounting cycle** is the flow of financial transactions in a business—from making a sale to collecting payment for the goods or services delivered. In a medical practice, this is the cycle from

Family Care Center
Patient Day Sheet
Show all data where the Date From is between 9/5/2016, 9/5/2016

Entry	Date	Document	POS	Description		Provider	Code	Amount
ARLENSU0	**Arlen, Susan**							
359	09/05/2016	1009060000	11			5	99212	54.00
361	09/05/2016	1009060000	11			5	EAPCPAY	-20.00
			Patient Charges	Patient Receipts		Adjustments		Patient Balance
			$54.00	-$20.00		$0.00		$0.00
BELLHER0	**Bell, Herbert**							
362	09/05/2016	1009060000	11			2	99211	36.00
364	09/05/2016	1009060000	11			2	EAPCPAY	-20.00
			Patient Charges	Patient Receipts		Adjustments		Patient Balance
			$36.00	-$20.00		$0.00		$0.00
BELLJAN0	**Bell, Janine**							
365	09/05/2016	1009060000	11			3	99213	72.00
366	09/05/2016	1009060000	11			3	73510	124.00
368	09/05/2016	1009060000	11			3	EAPCPAY	-20.00
			Patient Charges	Patient Receipts		Adjustments		Patient Balance
			$196.00	-$20.00		$0.00		$0.00
BELLJON0	**Bell, Jonathan**							
369	09/05/2016	1009060000	11			3	99394	222.00
371	09/05/2016	1009060000	11			3	EAPCPAY	-20.00
			Patient Charges	Patient Receipts		Adjustments		Patient Balance
			$222.00	-$20.00		$0.00		$0.00
BELLSAM0	**Bell, Samuel**							
372	09/05/2016	1009060000	11			2	99212	54.00
374	09/05/2016	1009060000	11			2	EAPCPAY	-20.00
			Patient Charges	Patient Receipts		Adjustments		Patient Balance
			$54.00	-$20.00		$0.00		$0.00
BELLSAR0	**Bell, Sarina**							
375	09/05/2016	1009060000	11			3	99213	72.00
377	09/05/2016	1009060000	11			3	EAPCPAY	-20.00
			Patient Charges	Patient Receipts		Adjustments		Patient Balance
			$72.00	-$20.00		$0.00		$0.00

Figure 1-9   Sample Page from a Patient Day Sheet Report

treating the patient to receiving payments for services provided. Practice management programs (PMPs) are used to track **accounts receivable (AR)**—monies that are coming into the practice—and to produce financial reports.

accounts receivable (AR) monies that are flowing into a business

DAY SHEETS

At the end of each day, a day sheet report is generated that lists all charges, payments, and adjustments that occurred during that day (see Figure 1-9). To balance out a day, transactions listed on encounter forms (charges, payments, and adjustments) and totals from bank deposit entries are compared against the end-of-day report.

MONTHLY REPORT

A monthly report summarizes the financial activity of the entire month. This report lists charges, payments, adjustments, and the total accounts receivable for the month. It is possible to balance out the month by totaling the daily charges, payments, and adjustments and then comparing the totals to the amounts listed on the monthly report.

OUTSTANDING BALANCES

It is also good practice to print reports that list the outstanding balances owed to the practice by insurance companies and by patients. Regularly printing and reviewing the reports can alert the billing staff to accounts that require action to collect the amount due. A collection process is often started when patient payments are later than permitted under the practice's financial policy.

Overdue accounts require diligent follow-up to maintain the practice's cash flow. Insurance claims that are not paid in a timely manner also require follow-up to determine the reason for the nonpayment and to resubmit or appeal as appropriate.

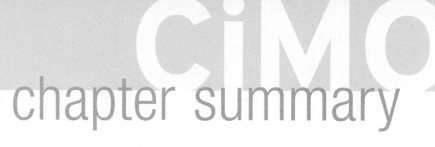
1.1 Identify four types of information collected during preregistration. Pages 4–5	- Patient's name - Contact information - Reason for visit - New or established patient

1.2 Compare fee-for-service and managed care health plans, and describe three types of managed care approaches. Pages 5–7	- Fee-for-service
	  Policyholders are reimbursed for a percentage of charges by the payer, and are responsible for the amount not paid by the insurer.
	- Managed care
	  A type of health plan in which the financing and delivery of health care is controlled by the payer.
	- Preferred provider organization (PPO)
	  A type of managed care plan in which providers contract with the organization to provide services to patients at a discounted fee.
	- Health maintenance organization (HMO)
	  A type of managed care plan in which providers are paid a predetermined amount at regular intervals to cover services they provide to patients.
	- Consumer-driven health plan (CDHP)
	  A type of managed care plan with a high deductible and a low premium, in which a policyholder uses a pretax savings account to cover medical expenses up to the deductible.

1.3 Discuss the activities completed during patient check-in. Pages 8–10	- Collect or update patient information form. - Photocopy/scan insurance card and driver's license to verify identity. - Collect any payments due.
1.4 Discuss the information contained on an encounter form at checkout. Pages 10–13	The encounter form contains diagnosis codes that provide health plans with very specific information about the patient's illness, signs, and symptoms. The encounter form also lists procedure codes that represent the services, treatments, or tests that the physician performed during the office visit.
1.5 Explain the importance of medical necessity. Pages 13–15	Insurance plans require that services provided be medically necessary. To be medically necessary, services must follow generally accepted standards of medical practice; be appropriate in terms of type, frequency, extent, site, and duration; and not be primarily for the convenience of the patient or the provider. If medical necessity is not met, the physician will not receive payment from the health plan.

1.6 Explain why billing compliance is important. Page 15	Even though each procedure code on an encounter form has a separate fee associated with it, the code is not necessarily billable. Whether it can be billed depends on each payer's rules. Some payers include particular codes in the payment for another code. Following these rules when preparing claims results in billing compliance.
1.7 Describe the information required on an insurance claim. Pages 15–16	- Health plans need to know the procedures the provider performed and the diagnosis, as well as the date and location of the visit. - Health plans also require basic information about the provider who is treating the patient, including the provider's name and identification number. - Beyond the basic information requirements that are common to all payers, there are differences in what information is required on an insurance claim. A payer lists the required information in a provider's manual that is available to the medical office.
1.8 List the information contained on a remittance advice. Pages 16–18	- Date of service - Services provided - Patient name and control number - Provider identifier number - Amount allowed by contract - Amount paid provider - Amount owed by patient
1.9 Explain the role of patient statements in reimbursement. Page 18	Patients' statements are used to collect payment from patients after insurance claims have been adjudicated. Statements list the amount paid by the health plan and the remaining balance that is the responsibility of the patient.
1.10 List the reports created to monitor a practice's accounts receivable. Pages 18–20	- Daily reports - Monthly reports - Outstanding balance reports

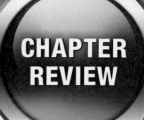
USING TERMINOLOGY

Match the terms on the left with the definitions on the right.

_____ **1.** *[LO 1.10]* accounting cycle

_____ **2.** *[LO 1.10]* accounts receivable (AR)

_____ **3.** *[LO 1.2]* capitation

_____ **4.** *[LO 1.2]* coinsurance

_____ **5.** *[LO 1.2]* copayment

_____ **6.** *[LO 1.4]* diagnosis code

_____ **7.** *[LO 1.4]* encounter form

_____ **8.** *[LO 1.8]* explanation of benefits (EOB)

_____ **9.** *[LO 1.2]* fee-for-service

_____ **10.** *[LO 1.2]* health maintenance organization (HMO)

_____ **11.** *[LO 1.2]* health plan

_____ **12.** *[LO 1.2]* managed care

_____ **13.** *[LO 1.3]* patient information form

_____ **14.** *[LO 1.2]* payer

_____ **15.** *[LO 1.2]* policyholder

_____ **16.** *[LO 1.2]* preferred provider organization (PPO)

a. A paper document from a health plan that lists the amount of a benefit and explains how it was determined.

b. A document that contains personal, employment, and medical insurance information about a patient.

c. A form listing procedures relevant to the specialty of a medical office, used to record the procedures.

d. Private or government organization that insures or pays for health care.

e. An electronic document from a health plan that lists the amount of a benefit and explains how it was determined.

f. A small fee paid by the patient at the time of an office visit.

g. An individual who has contracted with a health plan for coverage.

h. A payment made to a health plan by a policyholder for coverage.

i. A fixed amount that is paid to a provider in advance to provide medically necessary services to patients.

j. A type of insurance in which the carrier is responsible for the financing and delivery of health care.

k. A term used to describe money coming into a business.

l. A type of managed care system in which providers are paid fixed rates at regular intervals.

m. An insurance plan in which policyholders are reimbursed for health care costs.

n. Under an insurance plan, the portion or percentage of the charges that the patient is responsible for paying.

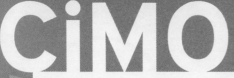
_____ **17.** *[LO 1.2]* premium

_____ **18.** *[LO 1.4]* procedure code

_____ **19.** *[LO 1.8]* remittance advice (RA)

o. A network of health care providers who agree to provide services to plan members at a discounted fee.

p. A value that stands for a patient's illness, signs, or symptoms.

q. A number that represents medical procedures performed by a provider.

r. The flow of financial transactions in a business.

s. A plan, program, or organization that provides health benefits.

CHECKING YOUR UNDERSTANDING

Write "T" or "F" in the blank to indicate whether you think the statement is true or false.

1. *[LO 1.3]* Many patient information forms contain a place for the patient to sign to authorize the patient's health plan to send payments directly to a provider. _____

2. *[LO 1.4]* CPT codes have eight digits. _____

3. *[LO 1.2]* "Coinsurance" refers to a fixed fee that must be paid by the patient at the time of an office visit. _____

Choose the best answer.

1. *[LO 1.3]* A patient information form contains information such as name, address, employer, and

   a. a procedure code

   b. insurance coverage information

   c. charges for procedures performed

2. *[LO 1.2]* A health maintenance organization (HMO) is one example of

   a. fee-for-service health plan

   b. government plan

   c. managed care health plan

3. *[LO 1.2]* In a managed care health plan, a _____ is usually collected from the patient at the office visit.

   a. deductible

   b. patient statement

   c. copayment

4. *[LO 1.4]* The most commonly used system of medical procedure codes is found in the

   a. CPT

   b. ICD

   c. CMS-1500

5. *[LO 1.4]* Information about a patient's medical procedures that is needed to create an insurance claim is found on the

   a. remittance advice

   b. encounter form

   c. patient information form

APPLYING YOUR KNOWLEDGE

Answer the question below in the space provided.

1.1. *[LO 1.1–1.10]* List the ten steps in the medical billing cycle.

_____

_____

THINKING ABOUT IT

Answer the questions below in the space provided.

1.1. *[LO 1.1]* Why is it important to verify a patient's insurance before the office visit?

_____

_____

1.2. *[LO 1.3]* Why is it necessary to collect estimated payments from patients during check-in?

_____

_____

The Use of Health Information Technology in Physician Practices

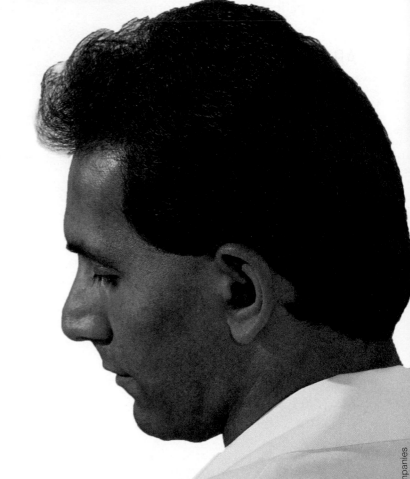

key terms

administrative safeguards

audit/edit report

audit trail

autoposting

breach

clearinghouse

CMS-1500 (08/05)

computer-assisted coding

electronic data interchange (EDI)

electronic funds transfer (EFT)

electronic medical records (EMRs)

electronic prescribing

evidence-based medicine

health information technology (HIT)

Health Information Technology for Economic and Clinical Health Act (HITECH)

Health Insurance Portability and Accountability Act of 1996 (HIPAA)

HIPAA Electronic Transaction and Code Sets standards

HIPAA Privacy Rule

HIPAA Security Rule

National Provider Identifier (NPI)

personal health records (PHRs)

physical safeguards

protected health information (PHI)

technical safeguards

walkout statement

workflow

X12-837 Health Care Claim (837P)

learning outcomes

When you finish this chapter, you will be able to:

2.1 Describe the functions of practice management programs.

2.2 Identify the core functions of an electronic health record program.

2.3 Discuss the advantages of electronic health records.

2.4 Describe the impact of health information technology on documentation and coding.

2.5 Discuss how the HIPAA Privacy Rule and Security Rule protect patient health information.

2.6 Explain how the measures put in place by the HITECH Act strengthen HIPAA privacy and security requirements.

In the 1980s few physicians' offices had a computer, and offices kept track of the paperwork associated with patients and insurance companies in a manual filing system. By the start of the twenty-first century, many offices used practice management programs (PMPs) for scheduling and billing. In recent years, more and more physicians have adopted electronic health records to replace the traditional paper-based patient chart as the health care industry migrates from paper-based to computer-based systems. **Health information technology (HIT)** is the term used to refer to the computer hardware, software, and networks that record, store, and manage patient health care information.

health information technology (HIT) technology that is used to record, store, and manage patient health care information

2.1 FUNCTIONS OF PRACTICE MANAGEMENT PROGRAMS

Most offices use a PMP to complete routine office tasks, including patient scheduling, recording patient information, creating and transmitting electronic claims, receiving electronic payments, billing patients, creating financial reports, and collecting on overdue accounts. Practice management programs are critical to a medical office's survival because accurate and timely records are required to determine whether the practice is profitable. These records are also important in meeting financial obligations and tax-reporting requirements.

Not all medical offices use the same PMP, but most programs operate in a similar manner. Initially, the program is prepared for use by entering basic facts about the practice. Often a computer consultant or an accountant helps set up these records. Information about many aspects of the business is recorded, including

- Information about each patient, such as name, address, contact telephone numbers, insurance coverage, and more

- Information about each provider, including referring providers and outside providers such as labs

- Data about the health plans used by the practice's patients

- Codes used by the practice to note a diagnosis and the treatment provided, as well as the facility where the treatment was provided

Once all these data are in the program, the software can be used to perform many of the daily tasks of a medical practice. Medisoft®, the practice management program used in *Computers in the Medical Office*, is one example of a PMP used in medical offices.

SCHEDULING

Practice management programs contain a computerized scheduling feature to keep track of patient appointments. (Chapter 11 covers this topic in depth.) When a patient telephones and requests an appointment, the program is used to search for an available time slot and enter the appointment. Figure 2-1 shows an example of a computerized physician schedule.

Family Care Center

Yan, Katherine			Monday, September 5, 2016	

Time	Name	Phone	Length	Notes
Monday, September 05, 2016				
8:00a	Staff Meeting		60	
9:00a	Ramos, Maritza	(614)315-2233	30	
10:00a	Fitzwilliams, Sarah	(614)002-1111	15	
10:30a	Gardiner, John	(614)726-9898	15	
10:45a	Jones, Elizabeth	(614)123-5555	30	
12:00p	Lunch		60	

Figure 2-1 Sample Computerized Physician Office Schedule

Each morning, the program prints a list of appointments for each provider in the practice. Appointments can easily be canceled or rescheduled, and the program also stores information about time reserved for hospital rounds, surgeries, seminars, lunches, vacations, and so on.

A major advantage of computerized scheduling is the ability to easily locate scheduled appointments. For example, if a patient calls to ask when her or his next appointment is scheduled, the medical office assistant enters the patient's name, and the program locates the appointment.

Computerized scheduling also simplifies the entry of repeated appointments. Rather than looking through an appointment book for acceptable dates and times, the computer program performs the search and displays the available times for the provider.

CLAIMS AND BILLING

The creation of accurate and timely insurance claims and patient statements is critical to a practice's cash flow. To generate claims and statements, a practice management program requires two basic types of information:

1. **Patient data** Personal information about the patient, as well as information about the patient's medical insurance coverage

2. **Transaction data** The date of the visit, the location of the treatment, the diagnosis and procedure codes, charges, and the payments made at the time of the office visit

When patient and transaction information has been entered in the PMP and checked for accuracy, the software creates insurance claims. To transmit electronic claims, a medical office may send claims directly to a health plan or may employ a clearinghouse. A **clearinghouse** is a company that collects electronic insurance claims from medical practices and forwards the claims to the appropriate health plans (see Figure 2-2). Clearinghouses also translate claim data to fit the standard format required for physician claims.

clearinghouse a company that receives claims from a provider, prepares them for processing, and transmits them to the payers in HIPAA-compliant format

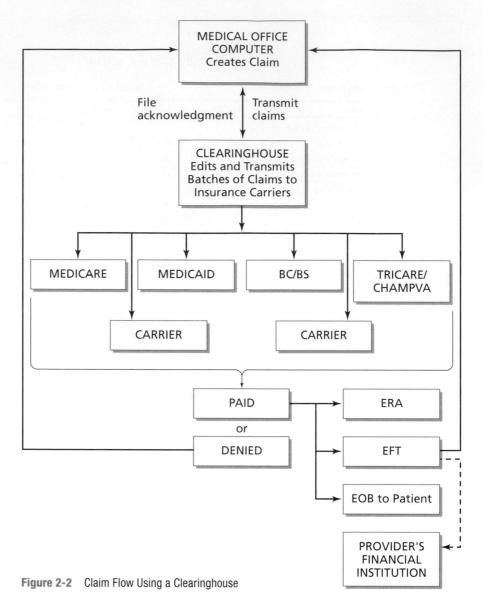

Figure 2-2   Claim Flow Using a Clearinghouse

When a clearinghouse receives a claim, it performs an edit—a check to see that all necessary information is included in the claim file. It checks for missing data and obvious errors, such as procedures performed on a date earlier than the patient's date of birth. After the basic edit is complete, an **audit/edit report** is sent from the clearinghouse to the practice. This report lists problems that need to be corrected before the claim can be sent to the health plan. Ensuring "clean" claims before transmission greatly reduces the number of claim rejections and speeds payment.

REIMBURSEMENT

Physicians receive reimbursement for services from health plans and from patients. If a patient makes a payment at the time of an office visit, the amount is entered into the practice management program, and a **walkout statement** is given to the patient. A walkout statement lists the procedures performed, the charges for the procedures, and the amount paid by the patient (see Figure 2-3).

audit/edit report a report from a clearinghouse that lists errors to be corrected before a claim can be submitted to the payer

walkout statement a document listing charges and payments that is given to a patient after an office visit

Family Care Center

285 Stephenson Boulevard
Stephenson, OH 60089
(614)555-0000

Page: 1

9/5/2016

Patient:	Susan Arlen	**Instructions:**
	310 Oneida Lane	Complete the patient information portion of your insurance claim form. Attach this bill, signed and dated, and all other bills pertaining to the claim. If you have a deductible policy, hold your claim forms until you have met your deductible. Mail directly to your insurance carrier.
	Stephenson, OH 60089	
Chart #:	ARLENSU0	
Case #:	24	

Date	Description	Procedure	Modify	Dx 1	Dx 2	Dx 3	Dx 4	Units	Charge
9/5/2016	OF--established patient, low	99212		466.0				1	54.00
9/5/2016	East Ohio PPO Copayment	EAPCPAY						1	-20.00

┌─ **Provider Information** ─┐

Provider Name:	Robert Beach MD
License:	84710
Insurance PIN:	
SSN or EIN:	199-99-9999

Total Charges:	$ 54.00
Total Payments:	-$ 20.00
Total Adjustments:	$ 0.00
Total Due This Visit:	**$ 34.00**
Total Account Balance:	$ 34.00

Assign and Release: I hereby authorize payment of medical benefits to this physician for the services described above. I also authorize the release of any information necessary to process this claim.

Patient Signature: _____   Date: _____

Figure 2-3   A Patient Walkout Statement

Payments from insurance companies are listed on a remittance advice (RA). If the RA is sent electronically rather than on paper, it is known as an *electronic remittance advice*, or *ERA*. The payments are entered in the practice management program (PMP) and applied to the relevant patients' accounts. This process may be done manually by the medical office assistant, who matches payments with individual patient transactions in the PMP and posts the payments in the program. Some practices use an automated process called **autoposting** to record the information in the program. In autoposting, the electronic data in the remittance advice are automatically posted to patient accounts in the PMP. While this approach saves the time that would be required to manually enter the information, the RA still must be reviewed by a person to identify any payments that are not as expected.

autoposting an automated process for entering information from a remittance advice (RA) into a practice management program

2.2 FUNCTIONS OF ELECTRONIC HEALTH RECORD PROGRAMS

Since the idea of computer-based medical records came about, they have been referred to by a number of different names. In the 1990s, they were known as electronic patient records (EPRs), computerized patient records (CPRs), and computerized medical records (CMRs). These terms gave way to the current names, which include electronic health records (EHRs), electronic medical records (EMRs), and personal health records (PHRs).

electronic medical records (EMRs) the computerized records of one physician's encounters with a patient over time

Electronic medical records (EMRs) are computerized records of one physician's encounters with a patient over time. They serve as the physician's legal record of patient care. While EMRs may contain information from external sources including pharmacies and laboratories, the information in an EMR reflects treatment of a patient by a single physician.

Electronic health records, on the other hand, can include information from the EMRs of a number of different physicians as well as from pharmacies, laboratories, hospitals, insurance carriers, and so on. Patients today use several providers to meet their health care needs, and each physician maintains a separate medical record for each patient. Unless the patient volunteers information, providers do not know whether the patient is being treated by another physician or what medications might have been prescribed. With an EHR, information is added to the record by health care professionals working in a variety of settings, and the record can be accessed by other professionals when needed.

personal health records (PHRs) private, secure electronic files that are created, maintained, and owned by the patient

Personal health records (PHRs) are private, secure electronic files that are created, maintained, and owned by the patient. The patient decides whether to share the contents with doctors or other health care professionals. PHRs typically include information on current medications and dosages, health insurance, immunizations, allergies, medical test results, past surgeries, family medical history, and more. Personal health records are created and stored on the Internet, but the files can easily be downloaded to a storage device such as a flash drive for portability.

While paper and electronic health records serve many of the same purposes, the electronic record is much more than a computerized version of a paper record. The Institute of Medicine has suggested that an EHR should include eight core functions (*Key Capabilities of an Electronic Health Record System*, 2003):

1. Health information and data elements

2. Results management

3. Order management

4. Decision support

5. Electronic communication and connectivity

6. Patient support

7. Administrative support

8. Population reporting and management

Table 2-1 highlights the differences among electronic medical records, electronic health records, and personal health records.

HEALTH INFORMATION AND DATA

An electronic health record must contain information about patients that enables health care providers to diagnose and treat injuries and illnesses. This includes demographic information about the patient, such as address and phone numbers, as well as clinical information about the patient's past and present health concerns (see Figure 2-4).

HEALTH INFORMATION AND DATA ELEMENTS

KEY DATA

- Problem list
- Procedures
- Diagnoses
- Medication list
- Allergies
- Demographics
- Diagnostic test results
- Radiology results
- Health maintenance
- Advance directives

CLINICAL AND PATIENT NARRATIVE

- Signs and symptoms
- Diagnoses
- Procedures
- Level of service
- Treatment plan

TABLE 2-1 | Defining the Terms

	Focus	Origin of Information	Access
EMR—Electronic Medical Record	• A computerized version of a paper chart with additional capabilities. • Documents episodes of illness or injury	• Created and maintained by a single provider	• Able to import data from external sources • Cannot be accessed by other providers
EHR—Electronic Health Record	• Broad focus on a patient's total health experience over the lifespan, rather than the documentation of episodes of illness or injury	• Created and maintained by multiple providers and facilities	• Can be viewed by multiple providers and facilities, including primary care physicians, specialists, hospitals, pharmacies, and laboratory and radiology facilities • Information can be added to the record by any of these providers or facilities
PHR—Personal Health Record	• A computerized record about an individual patient's health and health care, including medications, health insurance information, immunizations, allergies, medical test results, and family medical history	• Created and maintained by the individual patient	• Able to import data from providers and facilities • If permission is granted, providers can access limited data

RESULTS MANAGEMENT

Providers must have access to current and past laboratory, radiology, and other test results performed by anyone involved in the treatment of the patient. These computerized results can be accessed by multiple

RESULTS MANAGEMENT ELEMENTS

- Results reporting
- Results notification
- Multiple views of data/presentation
- Multimedia support (images, scanned documents)

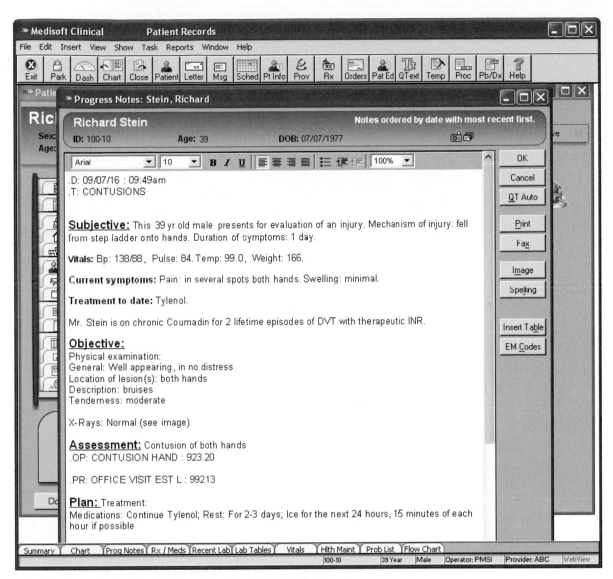

Figure 2-4 History and Physical Notes in an Electronic Health Record

providers when and where they are needed, which allows more prompt diagnosis and treatment decisions to be made (see Figure 2-5).

ORDER MANAGEMENT

EHR programs must be able to send, receive, and store orders for medications, tests, and other services by any provider involved in treating the patient. Staff members in different offices and facilities can access the orders, which eliminates unnecessary delays and duplicate testing. A major component of order management is **electronic prescribing**—the use of computers and handheld devices to transmit prescriptions to pharmacies in digital format (see Figure 2-6).

electronic prescribing the use of computers and handheld devices to transmit prescriptions in digital format

ORDER MANAGEMENT ELEMENT
- Computerized provider order entry (CPOE)—electronic prescribing, laboratory, pathology, X-ray, consultations

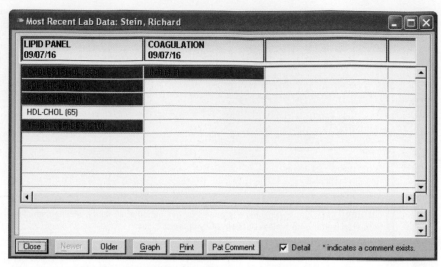

Figure 2-5   Laboratory Results in an Electronic Health Record

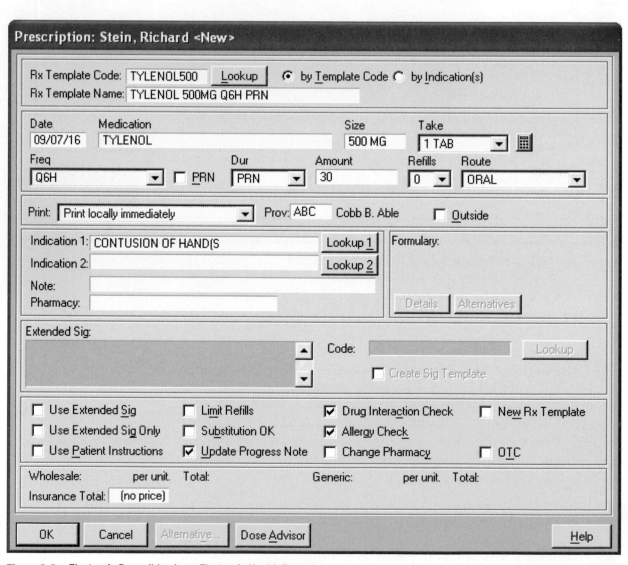

Figure 2-6   Electronic Prescribing in an Electronic Health Record

DECISION SUPPORT

As the practice of medicine becomes more complex, the amount of information available to physicians continues to grow. Hundreds of new studies are published on a daily basis. It is not possible for a physician to remember all this information or to be aware of all the latest, most effective treatments. The most up-to-date medical evidence is incorporated into care only 50 percent of the time.

Electronic health records give a physician who is examining a patient immediate access to the latest clinical research on diagnosis and treatment. The physician can also view the latest information on medications, including suggested doses, common side effects, and possible interactions.

In addition, electronic record systems provide a variety of alerts and reminders that physicians can use to improve a patient's health. Physicians can, for example, see a list of all women over fifty years of age who have not had mammograms in the past year. If the physician chooses, these women will all receive letters reminding them that they are due for this preventive screening.

DECISION SUPPORT ELEMENTS

- Access to knowledge sources
- Drug alerts
- Reminders
- Clinical guidelines and pathways
- Chronic disease management
- Clinician work list
- Diagnostic decision support
- Use of epidemiologic data
- Automated real-time surveillance

ELECTRONIC COMMUNICATION AND CONNECTIVITY

Today, a patient is typically treated by more than one provider in more than one facility. Physicians, nurses, medical assistants, referring doctors, testing facilities, and hospitals all need to communicate with one another to provide the safest and most effective care to patients. Insurance plans also need information from the health record to process claims for reimbursement. Electronic health record systems offer a number of mechanisms to facilitate these communications, including e-mail and the Internet.

ELECTRONIC COMMUNICATION AND CONNECTIVITY ELEMENTS

- Provider-provider
- Team coordination
- Patient-provider
- Medical devices
- External partners (pharmacy, insurer, laboratory, radiology)
- Integrated medical record (within setting, across settings, inpatient-outpatient)

PATIENT SUPPORT

Electronic health records offer patients access to appropriate educational materials on health topics, instructions for preparing for common medical tests, and the ability to report on home monitoring and testing to their physician.

PATIENT SUPPORT ELEMENTS

- Patient education (access to patient education materials)
- Family and informal caregiver education
- Data entered by patient, family, and/or informal caregiver (home monitoring, questionnaires)

ADMINISTRATIVE PROCESSES

The administrative area of health care also benefits from the use of EHRs. While most physician practices already use computers for billing and scheduling, an EHR streamlines the processes. In an office that uses a PMP and an EHR, some administrative tasks may be performed in either program.

ADMINISTRATIVE PROCESSES ELEMENTS

- Scheduling management (appointments, admissions, surgery and other procedures)
- Eligibility determination (insurance, clinical trials, drug recalls, chronic disease management)

REPORTING AND POPULATION MANAGEMENT

Electronic health record programs also enhance reporting capabilities both for internal use and for external reporting requirements. This makes it easier for physician offices and health care organizations to comply with federal, state, and private reporting requirements.

Electronic health records contain a wealth of information related to particular diseases and treatments. This information, as long as it does not include any patient's identity, can be used to advance medical knowledge through research. In addition, EHRs can assist in detecting threats to the health of the general population, such as bioterrorism or an outbreak of a new disease. For example, the immediate reporting of suspicious diseases to public health authorities may help identify a new influenza strain and prevent its spread.

REPORTING AND POPULATION MANAGEMENT ELEMENTS

- Patient safety and quality reporting
- Public health reporting
- Disease registries

2.3 ADVANTAGES OF ELECTRONIC HEALTH RECORDS

Electronic health records offer a number of advantages when compared to paper record-keeping systems. The most frequently cited advantages are increased patient safety, improved quality of care, and greater efficiency.

SAFETY

There is growing evidence that electronic record keeping can reduce medical errors and improve patient safety. The factors that contribute to greater safety include the following:

- Medication and physician order errors due to illegible handwriting are eliminated.

- Providers receive instant electronic alerts about patient allergies and possible drug interactions.

- Physicians receive alerts when medications deemed unsafe have been pulled from the market.

- Provided that copies of the medical records are stored at a secure off-site location, they are not lost in the event of a natural disaster, such as a hurricane, or an intentional attack, such as a terrorist bombing.

- Information is communicated in a timely manner in the event of an act of bioterrorism or the widespread outbreak of disease.

QUALITY

A 2001 report by the Institute of Medicine titled *Crossing the Quality Chasm: A New Health System for the 21st Century* found that only 55 percent of Americans receive recommended medical care that is consistent with guidelines based on scientific knowledge. Electronic health records make it possible for providers to deliver more effective care to patients based on a complete picture of their past and present conditions. The report defines effective care as "providing services based on scientific knowledge to those who could benefit and at the same time refraining from providing services to those not likely to benefit."

With EHRs, physicians have access to evidence-based guidelines for diagnosing and treating conditions and to the latest clinical research and best practice guidelines. **Evidence-based medicine** refers to the use of the latest and most accurate clinical research in medical decision making and patient care.

evidence-based medicine
medical care based on the latest and most accurate clinical research

Electronic health records also enhance the quality of health care in the following ways:

- Patients are contacted with reminders about preventive care screenings.

- Patients suffering from chronic diseases, such as diabetes, are able to monitor their conditions at home and report results via the Internet, saving them numerous visits to the doctor.

- Health care consumers can review data about the quality and performance of providers and facilities when deciding on where to obtain health care.

EFFICIENCY

The retrieval of information from an EHR is immediate, which greatly improves efficiency and can be critical in emergency situations. Compared to sorting through papers in a folder, an electronic search saves critical time when vital patient information is needed.

Electronic health records also save valuable time for health care providers by reducing the time needed to enter information about patients. Currently, physicians spend almost 40 percent of their time writing progress notes. With EHRs, physicians are finished entering notes when the patient leaves the examination room or shortly after. Nurses and medical assistants record information directly into the computer, so there is no need to copy information to a paper chart.

In regard to the efficiency of health care, electronic health records also

- Improve the overall efficiency of the workflow in the physician practice or hospital

- Speed the delivery of diagnostic test results to the physician and the patient through electronic transmission

- Allow two or more people to work with a patient's record at the same time

- Eliminate the need to search for a misplaced or lost patient chart

- Permit physicians to review a summary of the patient's health information at a glance instead of flipping through pages

- Eliminate the need to manually enter diagnosis and procedure codes from a paper-based encounter form

- Reduce the time it takes to refill a prescription through electronic prescribing

- Organize all information in one place, including in-house messages, telephone messages, requests for information, and referral letters

- Enable physicians to receive payment for services more quickly because patient encounter information is automatically transferred to the billing software

Health Information Technology for Economic and Clinical Health Act (HITECH) part of the American Recovery and Reinvestment Act of 2009 that provides financial incentives to physicians and hospitals to adopt EHRs and strengthens HIPAA privacy and security regulations

Recognizing the potential benefits of EHRs to physicians and hospitals, Congress passed the **Health Information Technology for Economic and Clinical Health Act (HITECH),** part of the American Recovery and Reinvestment Act of 2009 (ARRA). The HITECH Act is intended to promote the use of EHRs in physician practices and hospitals through the use of financial incentives. Under the HITECH Act, physicians who adopt and use EHRs are eligible for annual incentive payments from Medicare and Medicaid. Physicians who derive at least 30 percent or more of their income from Medicaid are also eligible for financial incentives, and those who practice in underserved areas are eligible for an extra 10 percent from Medicare. It is important to note that a provider must do more than simply purchase an EHR; to be eligible for the financial incentives, providers must demonstrate "meaningful use" of the technology. For example, the EHR must be capable of sharing patient records with physicians outside the physician's own medical group and of transmitting electronic prescriptions to pharmacies.

Even with financial incentives, successful implementation of EHRs is not expected to be quick or easy. Small practices, where most primary care is delivered, may lack the expertise and resources required to purchase, install, and use information technology. The transition from paper records to EHRs also represents a fundamental change in the way a physician office operates and interacts with patients. Everyone who works in the office, whether in a clinical or an administrative position, in the front office or the back office, will have to learn a new way of doing things.

2.4 THE IMPACT OF HIT ON DOCUMENTATION AND CODING

Every service submitted for payment—including medical care, diagnostic tests, consultations, and surgeries—must be documented in the patient's medical record. Documentation is directly linked to the financial health of the practice. If a treatment is given to a patient and the provider fails to document it, the service will not be reimbursed. Incomplete or inaccurate records may result in claim denials or even in an investigation as part of the federal government's effort to identify and reduce fraud in the Medicare program.

Before the use of EHRs, physicians documented patient visits using dictation. The dictated notes were transcribed into word-processing files and printed. Coders then reviewed the documentation and assigned diagnosis and procedure codes to each encounter. These codes were recorded on a paper encounter form, which was forwarded to the billing staff for posting in the PMP.

When an EHR is implemented, the process of documenting and coding changes. Offices that use a PMP and an EHR that are integrated—capable of exchanging data with each other—can implement a fully electronic workflow. **Workflow** is simply a set of activities designed to produce a specific outcome. In this instance, the workflow consists of the activities required for the physician to receive reimbursement for services.

workflow a set of activities designed to produce a specific outcome

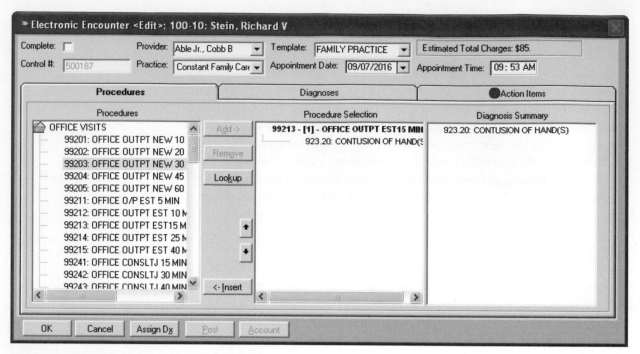

Figure 2-7 An Electronic Encounter Form in an Electronic Health Record

Electronic health records contain tools that make documenting patient encounters more efficient for providers. While these tools vary from one program to another, most EHRs offer a variety of options, such as entering notes by typing or using voice recognition software, or choosing commonly used clinical words, phrases, and symptoms from templates. With a template, the physician responds to prompts on the computer during the patient examination. The EHR then uses these responses to create a progress note and to assign preliminary diagnosis and procedure codes. These codes appear on an electronic encounter form (EEF) (see Figure 2-7).

computer-assisted coding
assigning preliminary diagnosis and procedure codes using computer software

The process of assigning preliminary diagnosis and procedure codes with a computer is known as **computer-assisted coding.** Computer-assisted coding works in a variety of ways. Some programs assign codes based on keywords that are included in the template the provider uses when documenting the visit in the EHR. Other programs analyze words, phrases, and sentences in the electronic documentation to determine the appropriate codes. In either case, the codes assigned by the software are merely suggestions. They should never be accepted and used without review by a professional coder. If the coder wants to review the documentation before finalizing the codes, the EHR provides fast access to the patient's chart. Once the codes are finalized, the EEF is transmitted to the PMP for posting. Most EHRs offer the option of autoposting.

Not all providers use a fully electronic workflow; some use a combination of paper and electronic methods. This may be by choice, or it may be because they have implemented an EHR program that cannot

TABLE 2-2	Documentation and Coding in a Paper-Based Office
The provider writes or dictates notes either during or after examination of the patient.	
↓	
Written notes are filed in the patient's chart; dictated notes must be transcribed and then reviewed for accuracy by the provider.	
↓	
A coder reviews the provider's documentation and assigns codes for the patient's diagnosis and for the services that were provided on an encounter form.	
↓	
The forms are forwarded to the billing department, where a billing staff member manually enters the information into the practice management program.	
↓	
Using the PMP, the billing staff member generates claims and electronically transmits them to payers for reimbursement.	

share data with the PMP. Most practices that purchase an EHR program today already have a PMP in place, since they have been required to file Medicare claims electronically since 2005. In many cases, the EHR software is not produced by the same software vendor that created the PMP software. Additional programming is required for the two programs to exchange meaningful data.

In an office that uses paper and electronic processes, the coder reviews the electronic encounter form and physician documentation in the EHR, and then prints the encounter form. The paper form is forwarded to the billing department, where a staff member manually enters the diagnosis and procedure codes into the PMP.

Tables 2-2 and 2-3 illustrate the documentation and coding process in a paper-based and in an electronic workflow.

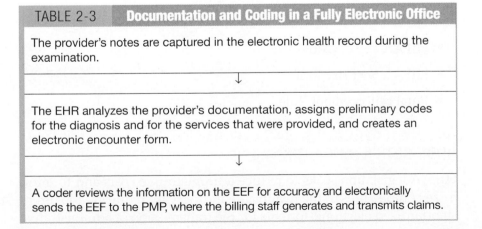

TABLE 2-3	Documentation and Coding in a Fully Electronic Office
The provider's notes are captured in the electronic health record during the examination.	
↓	
The EHR analyzes the provider's documentation, assigns preliminary codes for the diagnosis and for the services that were provided, and creates an electronic encounter form.	
↓	
A coder reviews the information on the EEF for accuracy and electronically sends the EEF to the PMP, where the billing staff generates and transmits claims.	

Even a partially electronic workflow is more efficient than a paper-based workflow. In a paper-based workflow, the coding and billing process normally takes anywhere from three to fourteen days. As a result, there is an extended lag between the time the service was provided and the time the provider receives reimbursement. Also, it has been estimated that physicians lose as much as 10 percent of potential revenue as a result of forgetting to bill for services, losing patients' paperwork, making errors when preparing claims, and other reasons.

In an office with a fully electronic workflow, the coding and billing process can be reduced to as little as twenty-four hours. In addition, having electronic documentation on which to assign codes ensures that documentation exists for all services billed. Electronic workflow also reduces the number of unbilled procedures due to lost or forgotten procedures. Finally, electronic workflow is more efficient: codes can be automatically posted to patient accounts in the PMP, and the time between the patient visit and the submission of the claim for payment is shortened, leading to more timely reimbursement.

2.5 HIPAA LEGISLATION AND ITS IMPACT ON PHYSICIAN PRACTICES

Health Insurance Portability and Accountability Act of 1996 (HIPAA) federal act that set forth guidelines for standardizing the electronic data interchange of administrative and financial transactions, exposing fraud and abuse in government programs, and protecting the security and privacy of health information

In 1996, Congress passed the **Health Insurance Portability and Accountability Act of 1996 (HIPAA).** The legislation was designed to

- Ensure the portability of insurance coverage when employees move from job to job

- Increase accountability and decrease fraud and abuse in health care

- Improve the efficiency of health care transactions and mandate standards for health information

- Ensure the security and privacy of health information

One section of the legislation, known as HIPAA Administrative Simplification, focuses on mandating nationwide standards for health information and protecting its security and privacy. This legislation contains a number of rules, including the

- HIPAA Electronic Transaction and Code Sets standards

- HIPAA Privacy Rule

- HIPAA Security Rule

- Final Enforcement Rule

HIPAA ELECTRONIC TRANSACTION AND CODE SETS STANDARDS

HIPAA legislation seeks to reduce administrative costs and to minimize complexities in the health care industry by requiring the use of standardized electronic formats for the transmission of administrative and financial data. The **HIPAA Electronic Transaction and Code Sets standards** describe a particular electronic format that providers and health plans must use to send and receive health care transactions. The Centers for Medicare and Medicaid Services (CMS) is responsible for enforcing the Electronic Transaction and Code Sets standards.

The electronic transmission of data—called **electronic data interchange (EDI)**—involves sending information from computer to computer. Many different EDI systems have been used in health care, causing a confusing array of software programs required to decipher messages. To address this situation, the HIPAA legislation standardized EDI formats and requires any practice working with electronic transactions to use them to send and receive data. The electronic formats are based on EDI standards called ASC X12, after the initials of the national committee that developed them, and a number has been assigned to each standard transaction.

The HIPAA standards cover electronic transactions that are frequently exchanged between medical offices and health plans and that contain patient-identifiable health-related administrative information, including health claims, health plan eligibility, enrollment and disenrollment, payments for care and health plan premiums, claim status, first injury reports, coordination of benefits, and others. The following are the required electronic formats:

- **X12-270/271 Health Care Eligibility Benefit Inquiry and Response** Questions and answers about whether patients' health plans cover planned treatments and procedures

- **X12-276/277 Health Care Claim Status Request and Response** Questions and answers between providers—such as medical offices and hospitals—and payers about claims that are due to be paid

- **X12-278 Health Care Services Review—Request for Review and Response** Questions and answers between patients, or providers on their behalf, and managed care organizations for approval to see medical specialists

- **X12-835 Claims Payment and Remittance Advice** The payment and RA are sent from the payer to the provider; the payment may be via **electronic funds transfer (EFT)** from the payer directly to the provider's bank, similar to an ATM transaction

- **X12-837 Health Care Claim or Encounter** Data about the billing provider who requests payment, the patient, the diagnoses, and the procedures sent by a provider to a payer

Most physician practices are required to use the HIPAA-standard electronic claim format called **X12-837 Health Care Claim**, or 837P. This claim is called the professional claim because it is used to bill for a physician's services. A hospital's claim is called an institutional claim, and there are also HIPAA dental claims and drug claims.

HIPAA Electronic Transaction and Code Sets standards regulations requiring electronic transactions such as claim transmission to use standardized formats

electronic data interchange (EDI) the exchange of routine business transactions from one computer to another using publicly available communications protocols

electronic funds transfer (EFT) the electronic routing of funds between banks

X12-837 Health Care Claim (837P) HIPAA standard format for electronic transmission of a professional claim from a provider to a health plan

CMS-1500 (08/05) the mandated paper insurance claim form

Exempt practices use the **CMS-1500 (08/05)** paper claim, which is the currently mandated paper claim form.

In addition to standards for electronic transactions for claims, the Administrative Simplification legislation establishes standard medical code sets for use in health care transactions. For example, ICD-9-CM codes are required for diagnoses and CPT codes are mandated for procedures.

National Provider Identifier (NPI) a standard identifier for health care providers consisting of ten numbers

HIPAA legislation also requires the use of a national standard identifier for all health care providers. The **National Provider Identifier (NPI)** is a ten-position identifier consisting of all numbers. The numbers do not contain any information about health care providers, such as the state in which they practice or their provider type or specialization. Under HIPAA legislation, any individual or organization that provides health care services must obtain an NPI. The NPI replaces all previous identification numbers.

HIPAA PRIVACY REQUIREMENTS

HIPAA Privacy Rule regulations for protecting individually identifiable information about a patient's health and payment for health care that is created or received by a health care provider

protected health information (PHI) information about a patient's health or payment for health care that can be used to identify the person

As part of the Administrative Simplification provisions, the **HIPAA Privacy Rule** protects individually identifiable health information. Health information is information about a patient's past, present, or future physical or mental health or payment for health care. If this information can be used to find out the person's identification, it is referred to as **protected health information (PHI).** Except for treatment, payment, and health care operations (TPO), the Privacy Rule limits the release of protected health information without the patient's consent. The Final Enforcement Rule mandates that the HIPAA Privacy Rule is enforced by the Office for Civil Rights.

The HIPAA Privacy Rule must be followed by all covered entities—health plans, health care clearinghouses, and health care providers—and their business associates. The rules mandate that a covered entity must

- Adopt a set of privacy practices that are appropriate for its health care services

- Notify patients about their privacy rights and how their information can be used or disclosed

- Train employees so that they understand the privacy practices

- Appoint a staff member to be the privacy official responsible for seeing that the privacy practices are adopted and followed

- Secure patient records containing individually identifiable health information so that they are not readily available to those who do not need them

Under the HIPAA Privacy Rule, medical practices must have a written Notice of Privacy Practices (see Figure 2-8). This document describes the medical office's system for using and disclosing PHI. It also

NOTICE OF PRIVACY PRACTICES

OUR COMMITMENT TO YOUR PRIVACY

Our practice is dedicated to maintaining the privacy of your protected health information (PHI). In conducting our business, we will create records regarding you and the treatment and services we provide to you. We are required by law to maintain the confidentiality of health information that identifies you. We also are required by law to provide you with this notice of our legal duties and the privacy practices that we maintain in our practice concerning your PHI. By federal and state law, we must follow the terms of the notice of privacy practices that we have in effect at the time.

We realize that these laws are complicated, but we must provide you with the following important information:
- How we may use and disclose your PHI
- Your privacy rights in your PHI
- Our obligations concerning the use and disclosure of your PHI

The terms of this notice apply to all records containing your PHI that are created or retained by our practice. We reserve the right to revise or amend this Notice of Privacy Practices. Any revision or amendment to this notice will be effective for all of your records that our practice has created or maintained in the past, and for any of your records that we may create or maintain in the future. Our practice will post a copy of our current Notice in our offices in a visible location at all times, and you may request a copy of our most current Notice at any time.

WE MAY USE AND DISCLOSE YOUR PROTECTED HEALTH INFORMATION (PHI) IN THE FOLLOWING WAYS:

The following categories describe the different ways in which we may use and disclose your PHI.

1. Treatment. Our practice may use your PHI to treat you. For example, we may ask you to have laboratory tests (such as blood or urine tests), and we may use the results to help us reach a diagnosis. We might use your PHI in order to write a prescription for you, or we might disclose your PHI to a pharmacy when we order a prescription for you. Many of the people who work for our practice — including, but not limited to, our doctors and nurses — may use or disclose your PHI in order to treat you or to assist others in your treatment. Additionally, we may disclose your PHI to others who may assist in your care, such as your spouse, children or parents. Finally, we may also disclose your PHI to other health care providers for purposes related to your treatment.

2. Payment. Our practice may use and disclose your PHI in order to bill and collect payment for the services and items you may receive from us. For example, we may contact your health insurer to certify that you are eligible for benefits (and for what range of benefits), and we may provide your insurer with details regarding your treatment to determine if your insurer will cover, or pay for, your treatment. We also may use and disclose your PHI to obtain payment from third parties that may be responsible for such costs, such as family members. Also, we may use your PHI to bill you directly for services and items. We may disclose your PHI to other health care providers and entities to assist in their billing and collection efforts.

Figure 2-8 Excerpt from a Notice of Privacy Practices

establishes the office's privacy complaint procedures, explains that disclosure is limited to the minimum necessary information, and discusses how consent for other types of information release is obtained. Medical practices are required to display the Notice of Privacy Practices in a prominent place in the office. The office must make a good-faith effort to obtain a patient's written acknowledgment of having received and read the Notice of Privacy Practices in the form of a signed Acknowledgment of Receipt of Notice of Privacy Practices (see Figure 2-9).

Acknowledgment of Receipt of Privacy Practices Notice

PART A: The Patient.

Name: _____

Address: _____

Telephone: _____ E-mail: _____

Patient Number: _____ Social Security Number: _____

PART B: Acknowledgment of Receipt of Privacy Practices Notice.

I, _____ , acknowledge that I have received a Notice of Privacy Practices.

Signature: _____ Date: _____
If a personal representative signs this authorization on behalf of the individual, complete the following:

Personal Representative's Name: _____

Relationship to Individual: _____

PART C: Good-Faith Effort to Obtain Acknowledgment of Receipt.

Describe your good-faith effort to obtain the individual's signature on this form: _____
_____
_____

Describe the reason why the indvidual would not sign this form. _____
_____
_____

SIGNATURE.
I attest that the above information is correct.

Signature: _____ Date: _____

Print Name: _____ Title: _____
Include this acknowledgment of receipt in the individual's records.

Figure 2-9 Acknowledgement of Receipt of Privacy Practices Form

HIPAA SECURITY REQUIREMENTS

The **HIPAA Security Rule** outlines safeguards to protect the confidentiality, integrity, and availability of health information that is stored on a computer system or transmitted across computer networks, including the Internet. While the HIPAA Privacy Rule applies to all forms of protected health information, whether electronic, paper, or oral, the HIPAA Security Rule covers only PHI that is created, received, maintained, or transmitted in electronic form. The security standards are divided into three categories: administrative, physical, and technical safeguards.

Administrative safeguards are administrative policies and procedures designed to protect electronic health information. The management of security is assigned to one individual, who conducts an assessment of the current level of data security. Once that assessment is complete, security policies and procedures are developed or modified to meet current needs. Security training is provided to educate staff members about the policies and to raise awareness of security and privacy issues.

Physical safeguards are the mechanisms required to protect electronic systems, equipment, and data from threats, environmental hazards, and unauthorized intrusion. Threats include computer hackers, disgruntled employees, or angry patients. Health information stored on computers can be at risk from physical threats, such as unplanned system outages or storage media failures. Electronic information is also at risk from environmental hazards, such as fire, flood, or earthquake.

For these reasons, medical practices create regular backups of computerized information. Many practices back up their files at the end of each day. The backup files are stored at a remote physical location to minimize the likelihood of data loss in a large-scale disaster. In the event of a major disaster, data from the remote site can easily be recovered.

Unauthorized intrusion is access by individuals who do not have a "need to know." For example, individuals who are not working with confidential patient information should not be able to view this type of information on an office computer monitor. To prevent intrusion, offices limit physical access to computers. Security measures can be as simple as a lock on the door or as advanced as an electronic device that requires fingerprint authentication to gain access.

Technical safeguards are the automated processes used to protect data and control access to data. Access to information is granted on an as-needed basis. For example, the individual responsible for scheduling may not need access to billing data. Examples of technical safeguards include computer passwords, antivirus and firewall software, and secure transmission systems for sending patient data from one computer to another.

HIPAA Security Rule regulations outlining the minimum administrative, technical, and physical safeguards required to prevent unauthorized access to protected health care information

administrative safeguards policies and procedures designed to protect electronic health information outlined by the HIPAA Security Rule

physical safeguards mechanisms required to protect electronic systems, equipment, and data from threats, environmental hazards, and unauthorized intrusion

technical safeguards automated processes used to protect data and control access to data

As an additional security measure, computer programs can keep track of data entry and create an **audit trail**—a report that shows who has accessed information and when. When new data are entered or existing data are changed, a log records the time and date of the entry as well as the name of the computer operator. The practice manager reviews the log on a regular basis to detect irregularities. If an error has been made, the program lists the name of the person and the date the information was entered.

HIPAA IN THE AGE OF HEALTH INFORMATION TECHNOLOGY

Since HIPAA was enacted in 1996, the field of health information technology has changed dramatically. The increased use of information technology in health care to cut costs, improve patient safety, and provide the best possible care places large amounts of protected health information at greater risk. A greater volume of confidential clinical patient information is available in electronic form. While the proliferation of health information networks provides many points of access to patient information, it also increases the possibility of unauthorized access. In addition, increased use of portable computing and storage devices means that health information can be moved from place to place with ease. This increases the possibility of data being lost or devices being stolen.

In the past, health records could be viewed by only one person at a time. If the medical assistant was updating a patient's chart, the physician was not able to use it at the same time. In addition, files did not commonly leave a physician office or hospital facility. Desktop computers, bulky paper files, and large backup tapes made it difficult to move data from one place to another. In large part, the locks on office doors were safeguards against intruders. So while paper records restrict the ability to exchange information with other health care professionals, privacy and confidentiality may be easier to maintain in a paper-based office. However, to realize the many benefits that electronic health records have to offer, information must be computerized and exchanged among providers and facilities.

The challenges facing the health care field today are to protect electronic health information exchanged over computer networks and to convince the public to trust the electronic system, just as they have trusted their physicians with protected health information. Consumer attitudes and behaviors are influenced by reports in the media of stolen credit card numbers, Internet fraud, and identity theft. Because of the size and scope of today's computer networks, a breach puts thousands of people's records at risk. A **breach** is the acquisition, access, use, or disclosure of unsecured PHI in a manner not permitted under the HIPAA Privacy Rule, thus compromising the security or privacy of the PHI. Recent examples are:

- In May 2009, Connecticut-based insurer Health Net discovered that a portable computer disk drive disappeared from the company's office. The disk drive contained protected health information, Social Security numbers, and bank account numbers for almost 500,000 past and present subscribers.

- In October 2009, hard drives were stolen from a Blue Cross and Blue Shield of Tennessee training facility. The hard drives contained files with identifying information for up to 500,000 members, including their Social Security numbers and other private health data.

2.6 THE HITECH ACT'S IMPACT ON PRIVACY AND SECURITY

Recognizing that existing HIPAA laws did not provide adequate protection in an increasingly electronic health care environment, Congress included additional privacy and security regulations in the HITECH Act of 2009.

BREACH NOTIFICATION

To prevent breaches of health information, the HITECH Act requires patients' protected health information to be made secure by using specified technologies and methods that will make the PHI "unusable, unreadable, or indecipherable to unauthorized individuals." The Department of Health and Human Services (HHS) has released guidance on specific technologies and methods, such as encryption, that can be used to secure PHI. If a breach of unsecured health information occurs, HITECH requires health care providers, health plans, and other entities covered by HIPAA to notify patients, the federal government, and the media of the breach.

MONETARY PENALTIES

The Act also calls for stiffer penalties for privacy and security violations. For example, facilities that have privacy breaches will pay fines ranging from $100 to $50,000 per violation, depending on whether the facility could have reasonably avoided the breach.

ENFORCEMENT

Under HITECH, the Office for Civil Rights is required to conduct audits to ensure compliance with HIPAA rules. An audit is a formal examination or review undertaken to determine whether a health care organization's staff members comply with regulations. An audit does not involve reviewing every document. Instead, a representative sample of the whole is studied to review whether erroneous or fraudulent behavior exists. Previously, audits were permissible, but not required.

2.1 Describe the functions of practice management programs. Pages 28–32	Scheduling - Keep track of patients' appointments and physicians' schedules. Claims and billing - Create and transmit claims to insurance carriers for payment. - Create and print statements that are mailed to patients for payment. Reimbursement - Post payments from insurance carriers. - Record payments from patients and print walkout statements.
2.2 Identify the core functions of an electronic health record program. Pages 32–38	- Health information and data elements - Results management - Order management - Decision support - Electronic communication and connectivity - Patient support - Administrative support - Population reporting and management
2.3 Discuss the advantages of electronic health records. Pages 39–41	Safety - Errors due to illegible handwriting are eliminated. - Electronic alerts warn physicians of allergies, drug conflicts, and medications taken off the market. - Records are not lost in the event of a disaster, since a backup can be stored offsite. - Response to public health events is more rapid. Quality - Physicians have access to the latest evidence-based guidelines for treatment. - Preventive care screenings are tracked and reminders sent. - Physicians can monitor care remotely using the Internet. - Consumers can review quality information about providers and facilities.

	Efficiency - Information is accessed immediately. - Electronic search saves time. - Time required for writing progress notes is reduced. - The delivery of test results is speeded. - The time from the patient encounter until the physician is paid is reduced.
2.4 Describe the impact of health information technology on documentation and coding. Pages 41–44	In an electronic workflow, preliminary codes are assigned by the EHR, reviewed by the coder, and automatically posted in the PMP. Not all offices use a fully electronic workflow. In these offices, paper encounter forms may be printed from the EHR and the codes manually entered in the PMP.
2.5 Discuss how the HIPAA Privacy Rule and Security Rule protect patient health information. Pages 44–51	- The HIPAA Privacy Rule regulates the use and disclosure of patients' protected health information (PHI). To release PHI for other than treatment, payment, or health care operations, an authorization must be signed by the patient. The authorization document must be in plain language and have a description of the information to be used, who can disclose it and for what purpose, who will receive it, an authorization date, and the patient's signature. - The HIPAA Security Rule requires covered entities to establish three types of safeguards to protect the confidentiality, integrity, and availability of electronic PHI: administrative safeguards (office policies and procedures designed to protect PHI); physical safeguards (mechanisms to protect electronic systems, equipment, and data from threats, environmental hazards, and unauthorized intrusion); and technical safeguards (the technology and related policies and procedures used to protect electronic data and control access to it, such as firewalls and antivirus software).
2.6 Explain how the measures put in place by the HITECH Act strengthen HIPAA privacy and security requirements. Page 51	- The HITECH Act requires PHI to be made secure by using specified technologies and methods to make it "unusable, unreadable, or indecipherable to unauthorized individuals." - If a breach occurs, HITECH requires health care providers, health plans, and other entities covered by HIPAA to notify patients, the federal government, and the media of the breach. - Fines for privacy and security violations have been increased. - The Office for Civil Rights (OCR) must conduct audits to ensure compliance with HIPAA rules; previously, audits were not mandatory.

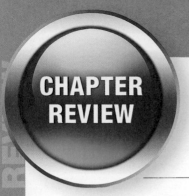

USING TERMINOLOGY

Match the terms on the left with the definitions on the right.

_____ **1.** *[LO 2.1]* audit/edit report

_____ **2.** *[LO 2.5]* protected health information (PHI)

_____ **3.** *[LO 2.1]* clearinghouse

_____ **4.** *[LO 2.2]* electronic prescribing

_____ **5.** *[LO 2.5]* National Provider Identifier (NPI)

_____ **6.** *[LO 2.5]* electronic data interchange (EDI)

_____ **7.** *[LO 2.2]* personal health record (PHR)

_____ **8.** *[LO 2.5]* HIPAA Security Rule

_____ **9.** *[LO 2.5]* HIPAA Electronic Transaction and Code Sets standards

_____ **10.** *[LO 2.2]* electronic medical record (EMR)

_____ **11.** *[LO 2.1]* walkout statement

_____ **12.** *[LO 2.5]* X12-837 Health Care Claim (837P)

a. Regulations that require electronic transactions to use standardized formats.

b. A computerized record of one physician's encounters with a patient over time, including medical history, diagnosis, treatment, and prognosis.

c. A document listing charges and payments that is given to a patient after an office visit.

d. A national standard identifier for all health care providers consisting of ten numbers.

e. A comprehensive record of health information that is created and maintained by an individual over time.

f. The electronic format of the claim used by physician offices to bill for services.

g. The use of computers and handheld devices to write and transmit prescriptions to a pharmacy in a secure digital format.

h. A report that lists errors in a claim.

i. An organization that receives claims from a provider, checks and prepares them for processing, and transmits them to insurance carriers in a standardized format.

j. The transfer of business transactions from one computer to another using communications protocols.

k. Information about a patient's past, present, or future physical or mental health or payment for health care that can be used to identify the person.

l. Regulations outlining the minimum safeguards required to prevent unauthorized access to electronic health care information.

CHECKING YOUR UNDERSTANDING

Write "T" or "F" in the blank to indicate whether you think the statement is true or false.

1. *[LO 2.5]* The HIPAA Electronic Transaction and Code Sets standards specify standard medical code sets, such as ICD-9-CM and CPT-4. _____

2. *[LO 2.2]* Electronic prescribing is a core function of an electronic health record. _____

3. *[LO 2.5]* Computer programs use audit trails to help ensure the privacy and confidentiality of patient health care information. _____

4. *[LO 2.5]* All medical offices, regardless of size, must use the HIPAA-standard X12-837 claim. _____

5. *[LO 2.2]* Clinical and administrative job functions in a physician practice are altered when an EHR is implemented. _____

6. *[LO 2.1]* The HIPAA standards require a practice that uses a clearinghouse to have a contract that states the procedures that must be followed to ensure HIPAA compliance. _____

7. *[LO 2.3]* Electronic health records are less prone to privacy and security issues than are paper-based records. _____

Choose the best answer.

1. *[LO 2.5]* The HIPAA Security Rule specifies the _____, technical, and physical safeguards required to prevent unauthorized access to health care information.

   a. administrative

   b. clinical

   c. legal

2. *[LO 2.2]* Electronic health records are used to record data such as physicians' reports of examinations, surgical procedures, tests results, and

   a. billing codes

   b. X-rays

   c. insurance claims

3. *[LO 2.5]* Many medical offices assign _____ to individuals who have access to computer data as a security measure.

   a. identification numbers

   b. private offices

   c. passwords

4. *[LO 2.5]* The HIPAA standard electronic format for the exchange of payment and remittance advice is the

   a. X12-835

   b. X12-278

   c. X12-271

5. *[LO 2.4]* An electronic workflow requires _____ and an electronic health record program that are capable of exchanging data.

   a. a clearinghouse

   b. an electronic data interchange

   c. a practice management program

6. *[LO 2.1]* Which reports are designed to provide payers with clean claims, thus reducing the number of claim rejections due to missing or incorrect data?

   a. clearinghouse

   b. electronic data interchange

   c. audit/edit

APPLYING YOUR KNOWLEDGE

Answer the question below in the space provided.

2.1. *[LO 2.5]* Why are paper medical records more secure than electronic health records?

_____

_____

THINKING ABOUT IT

Answer the questions below in the space provided.

2.1. *[LO 2.4]* Why does a medical insurance specialist need to learn about electronic health records?

_____

_____

2.2. *[LO 2.5]* What might happen in an office in which HIPAA privacy and security guidelines were not followed? What would the consequences be?

_____

_____

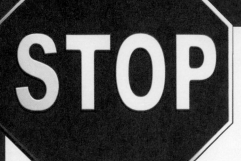

STOP! Before you proceed on your CiMO adventure, read these important tips! You need to make sure that Medisoft® Advanced Version 16 and the "CIMO7e" Student Data File are loaded on your computer!

STEP A. Make Sure Medisoft Advanced Version 16 Is Installed On Your School's Computer.

It is possible that Medisoft Advanced Version 16 (the actual software program) has already been installed on the computer you are using. If this is the case, you do not need to install it again. However, you still may need to load the Student Data File (the patient database needed to complete the exercises); if so, you can skip ahead to Step C.

How do I know if Medisoft Version 16 is installed?

1. Click the **Start** button, select **All Programs,** and look for the Medisoft folder. If you find a Medisoft folder, click Medisoft Advanced to launch the program.

2. To determine which version of Medisoft is installed, click **Help** on the menu bar, and then click **About Medisoft.** Look in the Window that appears, which lists the version number of the program.

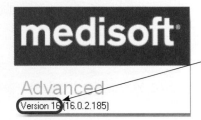

3. If you see Version 16, skip to Step C.

STEP B. Install Medisoft Version 16 If Your School's Computer Does Not Have It.
(*Please skip ahead to Step C if the Medisoft software is already loaded.)

If you are working on a school computer, please check with your instructor.

***Instructors, if you need help, please request a copy of *The McGraw-Hill Guide to Success for Medisoft Advanced Version 16* from your sales representative. You can find more information about this guide at the book's online learning center website at www.mhhe.com/cimo7e.

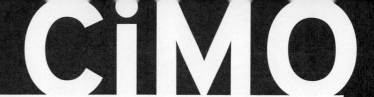

REMINDER! Make sure the Student Data File is loaded so that you can complete your work in Chapter 3 and the chapters that follow!

STEP C. Check To See If The "CIMO7e" Student Data File Is Installed.

1. Start Medisoft Advanced Version 16 by double-clicking on the desktop icon.
2. Look at the title bar that contains the words "Medisoft Advanced". If the "CIMO7e" Student Data File has already been installed, you should see "CIMO7e" to the right of "Medisoft Advanced".

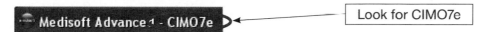

Medisoft Advanced - CIMO7e ◄────── Look for CIMO7e

STEP D. Load The "CiMO7e" Student Data File If Your Computer Does Not Have It.

1. Go to the book's website at www.mhhe.com/cimo7e.
2. On the opening screen, you will see this statement: Students, click here for help if you need to load **Medisoft or the Student Data File.**
3. This will take you directly to the <u>Medisoft Student Resources</u> page in the student center with the "CIMO7e" Student Data File.
4. Click the link labeled <u>CIMO7e Student Data File Instructions.pdf</u> and download the file. When it has finished downloading, open the file on your computer and print it.
5. Click on the link for the <u>CIMO7e.zip</u> file and download the file to your computer desktop. This installer provides the patient database you will use to complete the Medisoft exercises in the textbook.
6. Follow the instructions in the <u>CIMO7e Student Data File Instructions.pdf</u> document to extract the zip file and install the "CIMO7e" Student Data File on the computer.
7. Do not try to open the "CIMO7e" Student Data File until you have opened Medisoft first!

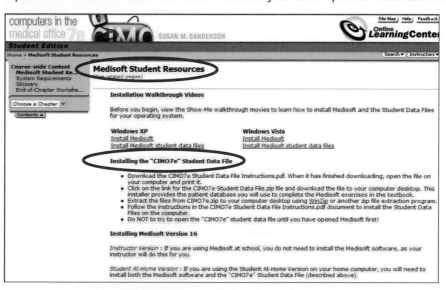

Need help? Contact the Digital Care Support Team.

Visit our Digital CARE Support website at www.mhhe.com/support. Browse our FAQs (Frequently Asked Questions), product documentation, and/or contact a CARE support representative. The Digital CARE Support Team is available Sunday through Friday.

Homework Version of Medisoft: An OPTIONAL Student At-Home Version of Medisoft is available for purchase.
To purchase a copy of the Medisoft Advanced Version 16 Student At-Home CD, check with your instructor.

How to Install the Medisoft Advanced Version 16 Demo from the Student At-Home CD
If you are working on your home computer and need to install Medisoft, follow these steps *before* loading the "CiMO7e" Student Data File. The Student At-Home CD contains a fully functional limited version of the Medisoft Advanced Version 16 program. *You will need this CD before you can proceed.* If your instructor did not require you to purchase the Student-At Home CD packaged with your textbook, or as a separate CD purchase, SKIP this part.

1. Go to the book's website at www.mhhe.com/cimo7e.
2. On the opening screen, you will see this statement: Students, click here for help if you need to load **Medisoft or the Student Data File.**
3. This will take you directly <u>to</u> the <u>Medisoft Student Resources</u> page in the student center with the instruction to load Medisoft.
4. Download and print the <u>Medisoft 16 Student At-Home CD Installation Instructions.pdf</u> document.
5. Place the Student At-Home CD in your CD drive.
6. Follow the instructions in the PDF document to install the software.
7. Go to STEP D on page 59 to follow the instructions to download the "CIMO7e" Student Data File if needed.

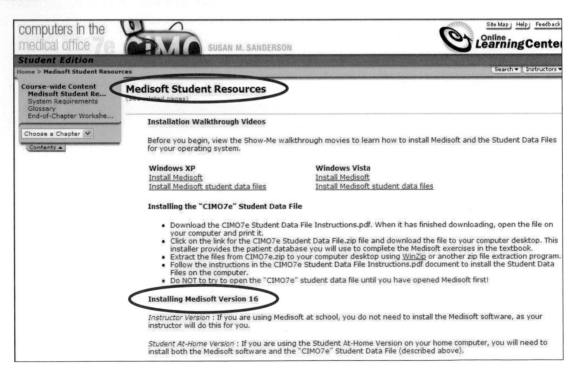

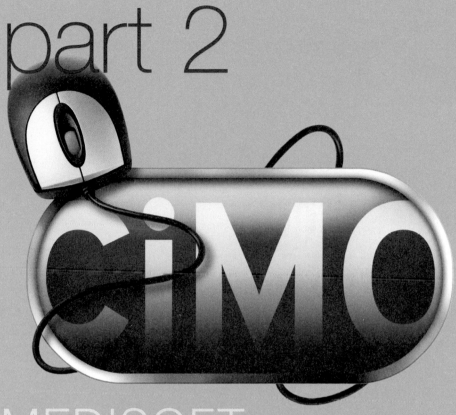

part 2

MEDISOFT ADVANCED TRAINING

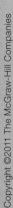

Introduction to Medisoft

key terms

access rights

Auto Log Off

backup data

database

knowledge base

Medisoft Program Date

MMDDCCYY format

packing data

purging data

rebuilding indexes

recalculating balances

restoring data

learning outcomes

When you finish this chapter, you will be able to:

3.1 List the six databases Medisoft uses to store information.

3.2 List the menus in Medisoft.

3.3 Explain the function of the Medisoft toolbar.

3.4 Explain how to enter, edit, save, and delete data in Medisoft.

3.5 Describe how to change the Medisoft Program Date.

3.6 Discuss three types of help available in Medisoft.

3.7 Explain how to create and restore backup files in Medisoft.

3.8 Describe the functions of the file maintenance utilities in Medisoft.

3.9 Describe the Medisoft security features used to ensure compliance with HIPAA and HITECH regulations.

what you need to know

To use this chapter, you need to know how to:

- Start your computer and Microsoft Windows.
- Use the keyboard and mouse.

Medisoft® is a practice management program (PMP). This is also referred to as a practice management system (PMS). Information on patients, providers, insurance carriers, and patient and insurance billing is stored and processed by the system. Medisoft is widely used by medical practices throughout the United States. It is typically used to accomplish the following daily work in a medical practice:

- Enter information on new patients and change information on established patients as needed
- Enter transactions, such as charges, to patients' accounts
- Submit insurance claims to payers
- Record payments and adjustments from patients and insurance companies
- Print walkout statements and remainder statements for patients
- Monitor collections activities
- Print standard reports and create custom reports
- Schedule appointments

Many of the general working concepts used in operating Medisoft are similar to those in other practice management programs. Thus, you should be able to transfer many skills taught in this text/workbook to other programs.

3.1 THE MEDISOFT DATABASES

database a collection of related bits of information

Information entered into Medisoft is stored in databases. A **database** is a collection of related pieces of information. Medisoft stores six major types of data:

1. **Provider data** The provider database has information about the physicians as well as the practice, such as name, address, phone number, and tax and provider identification numbers.

2. **Patient data** Each patient information form is stored in the patient database. The patient's unique chart number and personal information—name, address, phone number, e-mail address, birth date, Social Security number, gender, marital status, and employer—are examples of information stored in this database.

3. **Insurance carriers** The insurance carrier database contains the name, address, and other data about each insurance carrier used by patients, such as the type of plan. Usually, this database also contains information on each carrier's electronic claim submission requirements.

4. **Diagnosis codes** The diagnosis code database contains the *International Classification of Diseases*, Ninth Revision, *Clinical Modification* (ICD-9-CM) codes that indicate the reason a

service is provided. The codes entered in this database are those most frequently used by the practice. The practice's encounter form or superbill often serves as a source document when the Medisoft system is first set up.

5. **Procedure codes** The procedure code database contains the data needed to create charges. The *Current Procedural Terminology* (CPT) codes most often used by the practice are selected for this database. The practice's encounter form is often a good source document for the codes. Other claim data elements, such as place of service (POS) and the charge for each procedure, are also stored in the procedure code database.

6. **Transactions** The transaction database stores information about each patient's visits, diagnoses, and procedures, as well as received and outstanding payments. Transactions in the form of charges, payments, and adjustments are also stored in the transaction database.

Within Medisoft, each database is linked, or related, to each of the others by having at least one fact in common. For example, information entered in the patient database is shared with the transaction database, linking the two. Information is entered only once; Medisoft selects the data from each database as needed.

Before a medical office begins using Medisoft, basic information about the practice and its patients must be entered in the computer. The author has created a database—the Student Data File—that you will use to complete the exercises in this book. Check with your instructor to determine whether the Student Data File has already been loaded on your computer. If your instructor has not already loaded the data, go to the Online Learning Center at www.mhhe.com/cimo7e, and download the Student Data File. You will need to load the database before you do the exercises in this chapter.

3.2 THE MEDISOFT MENUS

Medisoft offers choices of actions through a series of menus. Commands are issued by clicking options on the menus or by clicking shortcut buttons on the toolbar. The menu bar lists the names of the menus in Medisoft: File, Edit, Activities, Lists, Reports, Tools, Window, and Help (see Figure 3-1). Beneath each menu name is a pull-down menu with one or more options.

FILE MENU

The File menu is used to open an existing practice or create a new practice. It is also used to back up data and restore data, set program and security options, change the program date, and perform file maintenance activities (see Figure 3-2).

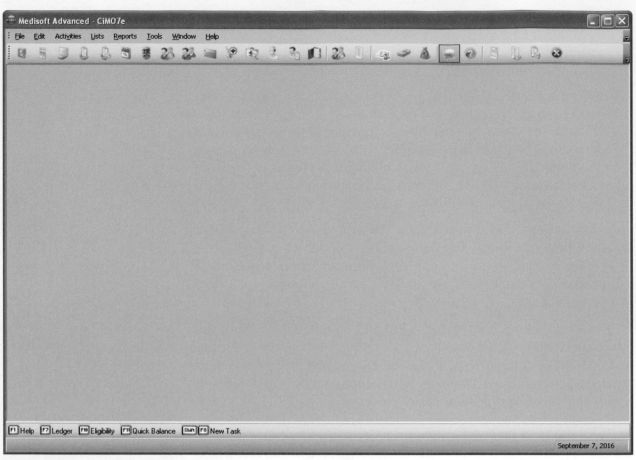

Figure 3-1   Main Medisoft Window

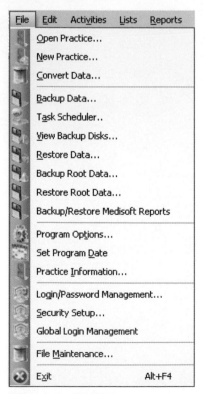

Figure 3-2   File Menu

EDIT MENU

The Edit menu contains the basic commands needed to move, change, or delete information (see Figure 3-3). These commands are Cut, Copy, Paste, and Delete.

ACTIVITIES MENU

Most medical office data collected on a day-to-day basis are entered through options on the Activities menu (see Figure 3-4). This menu is used to perform most billing tasks in a medical practice, including

- Entering financial transactions
- Creating insurance claims
- Creating patient statements
- Entering deposits
- Viewing unprocessed transactions coming from an electronic health record (EHR)
- Viewing summaries of patient account information
- Calculating billing charges

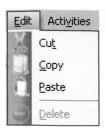

Figure 3-3
Edit Menu

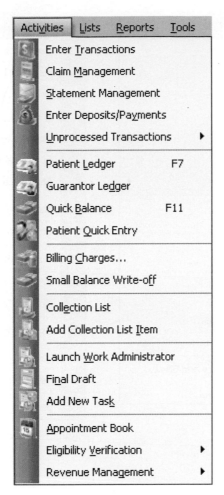

Figure 3-4   **Activities Menu**

Figure 3-5   **Lists Menu**

- Writing off small account balances
- Performing collections activities
- Launching the Work Administrator
- Opening the appointment scheduler

The Activities menu also contains options for verifying patient eligibility with insurance carriers (Eligibility Verification) and for launching the Revenue Management functions.

LISTS MENU

Information on new patients, such as name, address, and employer, is entered through the Lists menu (see Figure 3-5). If information needs to be changed on an established patient, it is also updated through this menu. The Lists menu provides access to lists of procedure and diagnosis codes, insurance carriers, electronic data receivers, referring providers, facilities, providers, billing codes, contacts, claim rejection messages, and payment plans. Information on any of these lists may be updated and printed when necessary.

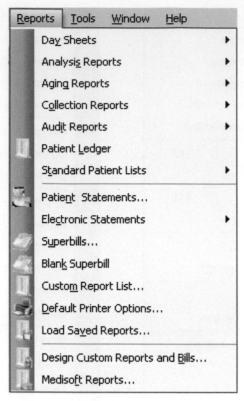

Figure 3-6 Reports Menu

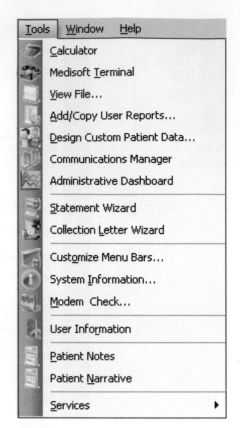

Figure 3-7 Tools Menu

REPORTS MENU

The Reports menu is used to print reports about patients' accounts and other reports about the practice (see Figure 3-6). Medisoft comes with a number of standard report formats, such as day sheets, aging reports, and patient ledgers. Version 16 also contains several hundred new reports, which are accessed by selecting the Medisoft Reports option at the bottom of the Reports menu. Practices may create their own report formats using the Design Custom Reports and Bills option.

TOOLS MENU

The Tools menu provides access to a number of utilities that are built into Medisoft, such as a calculator. It is also used to customize various components of the program to meet the needs of the individual practice. Custom collection letters and patient statements can be easily created by using one of the available wizards. The Communications Manager, which allows Medisoft to exchange information with an electronic health record (EHR) such as Medisoft Clinical, is also found on the Tools menu. The Tools menu is displayed in Figure 3-7.

WINDOW MENU

Using the Window menu, it is possible to switch back and forth between several open windows. For example, if the Patient List dialog box and the Transaction Entry dialog box were both open, the Window

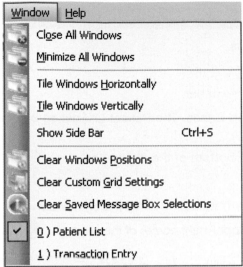

Figure 3-8 Window Menu

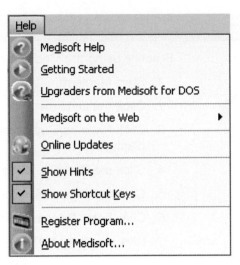

Figure 3-9 Help Menu

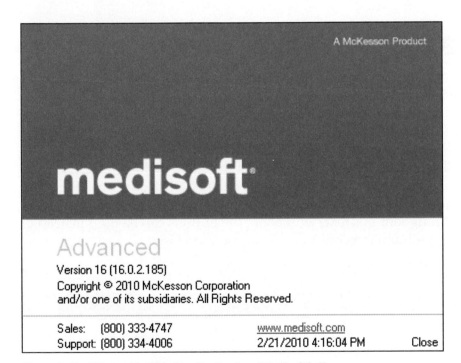

Figure 3-10 Window That Displays the Version of Medisoft in Use

menu would look like the menu in Figure 3-8. The Window menu also has other selections, such as an option to close all windows.

HELP MENU

The Help menu, shown in Figure 3-9, is used to access Medisoft's built-in help feature and provides a link to Medisoft support on the World Wide Web. The help menu also contains an option for identifying the version of the program in use (About Medisoft). For the exercises in this text/workbook to work successfully, you must be using Version 16 of Medisoft (see Figure 3-10).

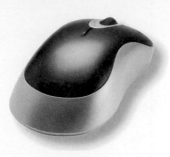

Practice using the Medisoft menus.

1. Start Medisoft.

2. Click the Lists menu on the menu bar.

3. Click Patients/Guarantors and Cases. The Patient List dialog box is displayed.

4. Click the Close button at the bottom of the dialog box.

5. Click the Activities menu.

6. Click Enter Transactions. The Transaction Entry dialog box appears.

7. Click the Close button in the upper-right corner of the window.

 You have completed Exercise 3-1.

3.3 THE MEDISOFT TOOLBAR

Located below the menu bar, the toolbar contains twenty-six buttons with icons that represent the most common activities performed in Medisoft (see Figure 3-11 and Table 3-1). These buttons are shortcuts for frequently used menu commands. When you click a button, the corresponding Medisoft dialog box opens. For example, clicking the Claim Management button opens the same dialog box as selecting the Claim Management option on the Activities menu. When you move your cursor over an icon, a description of the icon is displayed. Throughout this text/workbook, the buttons can be used instead of the pull-down menus to perform common tasks.

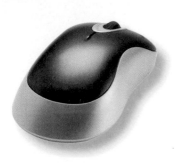

Practice using buttons on the toolbar. *Note:* You will need to look at Table 3-1 on pages 71–72 to complete this exercise.

1. Click the Provider List button. The Provider List dialog box opens.

2. Close the dialog box by clicking the X in the upper-right corner of the window.

3. Click the Procedure Code List button. The Procedure/Payment/ Adjustment List dialog box is displayed.

4. Close the dialog box by clicking the Close button in the lower-right section of the window.

 You have completed Exercise 3-2.

Figure 3-11   Medisoft Toolbar

TABLE 3-1	Medisoft Toolbar Buttons		
Button	Button Name	Opens	Activity
	Transaction Entry	Transaction Entry dialog box	Enter, edit, or delete transactions
	Claim Management	Claim Management dialog box	Create and transmit insurance claims
	Statement Management	Statement Management dialog box	Create statements
	Collection List	Collection List dialog box	View, add, edit, or delete items on collection list
	Add Collection List Item	Add Collection List Item dialog box	Add items to the collection list
	Appointment Book	Office Hours	Schedule appointments
	View Eligibility Verification Results (F10)	Eligibility Verification Results dialog box	Review results of eligibility verification inquiries
	Patient Quick Entry	Patient Quick Entry dialog box	Use predefined templates to enter new patients
	Patient List	Patient List dialog box	Enter patient information
	Insurance Carrier List	Insurance Carrier List dialog box	Enter insurance carriers
	Procedure Code List	Procedure/Payment/Adjustment Code List dialog box	Enter procedure codes
	Diagnosis Code List	Diagnosis List dialog box	Enter diagnosis codes
	Provider List	Provider List dialog box	Enter providers
	Referring Provider List	Referring Provider List dialog box	Enter referring providers
	Address List	Address List dialog box	Enter addresses
	Patient Recall Entry	Patient Recall dialog box	Enter Patient Recall data
	Custom Reports List	Open Report dialog box	Open a custom report

(continued)

TABLE 3-1   *Continued*

Button	Button Name	Opens	Activity
	Quick Ledger	Quick Ledger dialog box	View a patient's ledger
	Quick Balance	Quick Balance dialog box	View a patient's balance
	Enter Deposits and Apply Payments	Deposit List dialog box	Enter deposits and payments
	Show/Hide Hints	Show or Hide Hints	Turn the Hints feature on and off
	Medisoft Help	Medisoft Help	Access Medisoft's built-in help feature
	Edit Patient Notes in Final Draft	Final Draft untitled document	Use built-in word processor to create and edit patient notes
	Launch Medisoft Reports	Medisoft Reports window	Provides access to additional reports
	Launch Work Administrator	Assignment List	Assign tasks to practice staff
	Exit Program	Exit Program	Exit the Medisoft program

3.4 ENTERING, EDITING, SAVING, AND DELETING DATA IN MEDISOFT

The process of entering, editing, saving, and deleting data in Medisoft is similar to the way these functions are done in other Windows programs. If you know how to use a word-processing program, for example, the techniques used to manipulate data in Medisoft should be familiar to you.

ENTERING DATA

All data, whether patients' addresses or treatment procedures, are entered into Medisoft through the menus on the menu bar or through the buttons on the toolbar. Selecting an option from the menus or toolbar opens a dialog box. The Tab key is used to move between text boxes within a dialog box. Some information, such as a patient's name, is entered by keying data into a text box. At other times, selections are made from a list of choices already present, such as when making a selection from the drop-down list of providers already in the database.

EDITING DATA

If information already entered needs to be changed, the correction is made by following the steps originally used to enter the data.

For example, if a patient's phone number has changed, you enter the new number by entering it in the phone number field, right over the old number. Once saved, the newly entered information takes the place of the older data.

Edit a procedure code in a charge transaction.

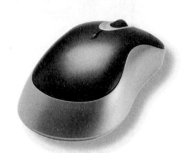

1. Click the Activities menu.

2. Click Enter Transactions.

3. Click the drop-down arrow in the Chart box. The Chart drop-down list is opened (see Figure 3-12).

4. To select James Smith, key the first two letters of his chart number (SMITHJA0): **SM.** Notice that the system goes to the entry for the first patient whose chart number begins with *SM,* in this case James Smith (see Figure 3-13).

5. Press the Tab key. James Smith's information is displayed (see Figure 3-14).

6. To edit a transaction, click in the field that needs to be changed. In this case, in the Procedure field, click the entry 92516. Notice that the entry in the field becomes highlighted.

7. Click again in the Procedure field. A pop-up list of procedure codes is displayed.

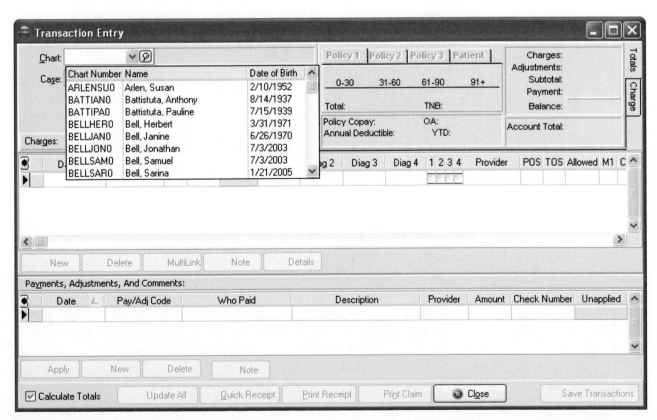

Figure 3-12 Transaction Entry Chart Drop-down List

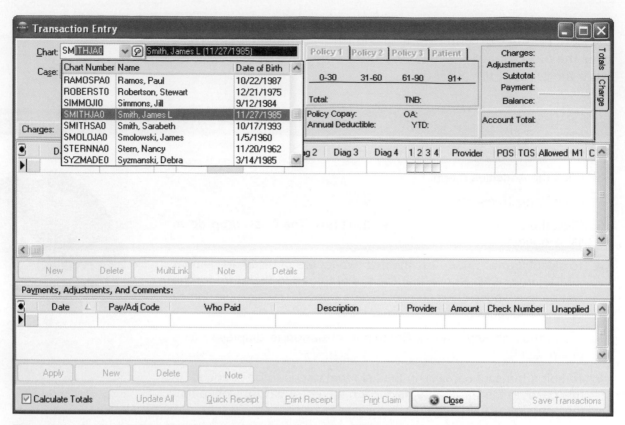

Figure 3-13 Transaction Entry Chart Drop-down List After the Letters *SM* Are Keyed

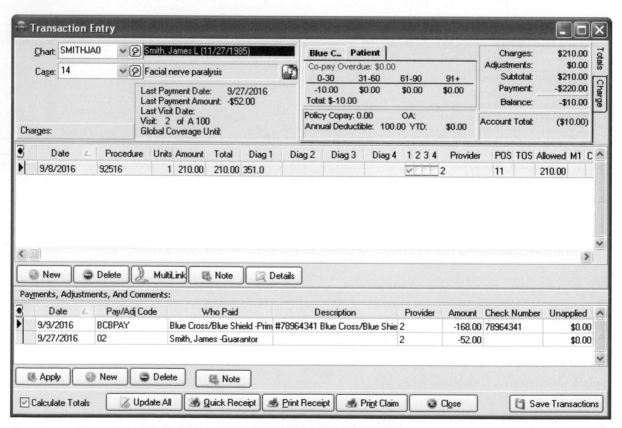

Figure 3-14 Transaction Entry Dialog Box with James Smith's Information Displayed

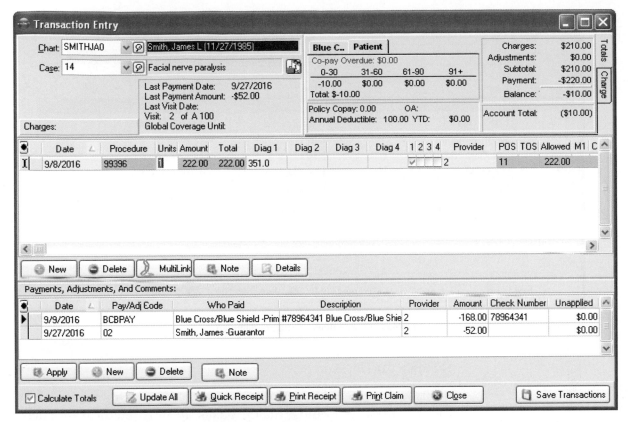

Figure 3-15 Transaction Entry Dialog Box After Code 99396 Is Entered

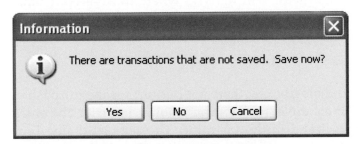

Figure 3-16 Transaction Entry Save Warning Dialog Box

8. Select a new code from the list by clicking it. Scroll down the pop-up list of codes, and click 99396. Notice that the new code is displayed in the Procedure field, but the entry in the Amount field has not changed. This does not happen until the Tab key is pressed. Press the Tab key now, and watch the entry in the Amount field change (see Figure 3-15).

9. Press the Tab key repeatedly, and watch as the cursor moves from box to box.

10. Exit the Transaction Entry dialog box by clicking the Close button or by clicking the close icon in the upper-right corner of the dialog box. An Information box is displayed, asking whether the changes should be saved (see Figure 3-16). In this case, click the No button. The changes are not saved, and the Transaction Entry window closes. **CiMC**

 You have completed Exercise 3-3.

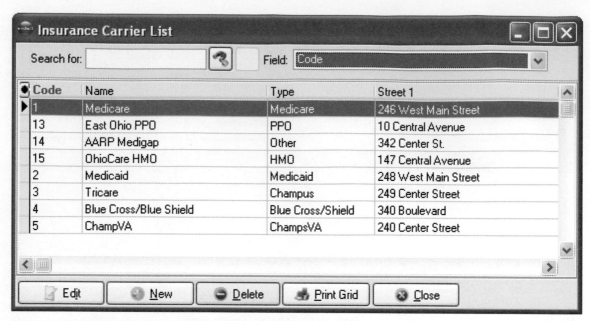

Figure 3-17 Insurance Carrier List Dialog Box with Delete Button Highlighted

SAVING DATA

Information entered into Medisoft is saved by clicking the Save button that appears in most dialog boxes. In most medical practices, data are saved to the network drive. For the purposes of this text/workbook, your instructor will tell you where to save your data. This may be a hard drive, a directory on a network drive, a flash drive, or some other type of storage device.

DELETING DATA

In some Medisoft dialog boxes, there are buttons for the purpose of deleting data. For example, to delete an insurance carrier, the entry for the carrier is clicked in the Insurance Carrier List dialog box. Then, the Delete button is clicked (see Figure 3-17). Medisoft will ask for a confirmation before deleting the data.

In other dialog boxes, there is no button for deleting data. In this situation, select the text that is to be deleted, and click either the Delete key on the keyboard or the right mouse button. A shortcut menu is displayed that contains an option to delete the entry (see Figure 3-18).

3.5 CHANGING THE MEDISOFT PROGRAM DATE

Medisoft Program Date date the program uses to record when a transaction occurred

Medisoft is a date-sensitive program. When transactions are entered in the program, if the dates are not accurate, they will be of little value to the practice. Many times, date-sensitive information is not entered into Medisoft on the same day that the event or transaction occurred. For example, Friday afternoon's office visits may not be entered into the program until Monday. If the **Medisoft Program Date**—the date the

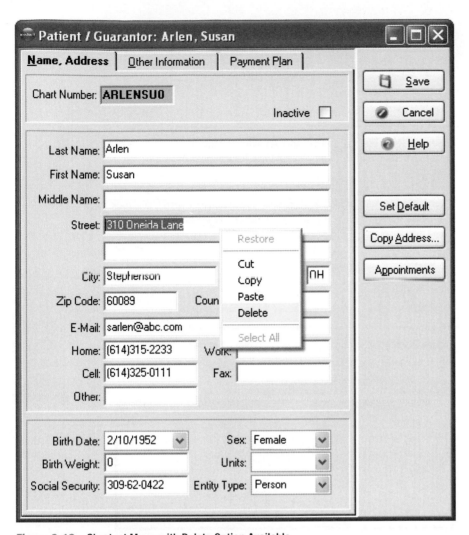

Figure 3-18   Shortcut Menu with Delete Option Available

program uses to record when a transaction occurred—is not changed to Friday's date before entering the data, all the information entered on Monday will be stored as Monday's transactions. For this reason, it is important to know how to change the Medisoft Program Date.

For the exercises in this text/workbook, you will need to change the Medisoft Program Date to the date specified at the beginning of each exercise. Most of the exercises take place in the year 2016. When a date is entered that is in the future (relative to the actual date on which the entry is made), the program displays one of several dialog boxes (see Figures 3-19a, b, c, and d). For example, if the exercise date is September 10, 2016, but the data are actually being entered on February 9, 2011, the program recognizes that a future date has been entered.

Depending on where in the program the date is entered, the dialog box will vary. If a change is made to the pop-up calendar, the dialog box in

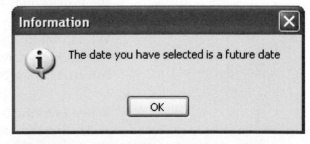

Figure 3-19a   Dialog Box That Appears When a Future Date Is Entered

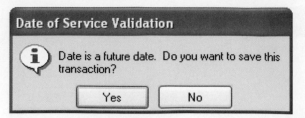

Figure 3-19b   Dialog Box That Appears When a Future
Date Is Entered While Entering Patient Visit Transactions

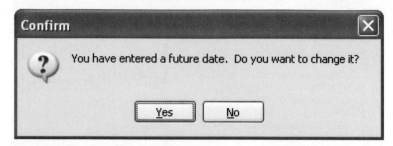

Figure 3-19c   Dialog Box That Appears When a Future Date Is Entered While
Entering Deposits

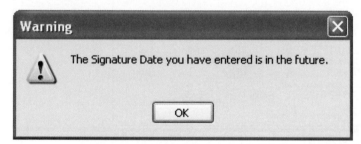

Figure 3-19d   Warning Box That Appears When a Future Date Is
Entered as the Patient's Signature Date

Figure 3-19a appears as a notification that the date selected is in the future. To keep the future date, click the OK button.

When entering patient office visit transactions, the Date of Service Validation window appears and asks whether the transaction should be saved (see Figure 3-19b). To keep the future date and save the transaction, it is necessary to click the Yes button.

When entering deposits, a Confirm dialog box appears and asks whether the date should be changed (see Figure 3-19c). To keep the future date, the No button must be clicked.

When entering a signature date for a patient, a Warning dialog box states that the date you entered is in the future (see Figure 3-19d). To continue, the OK button is clicked.

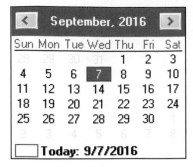

Figure 3-20   Medisoft Pop-up Calendar

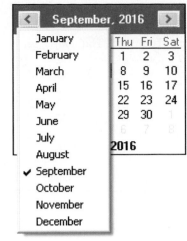

Figure 3-21   Calendar Month Pop-up List

Slightly different procedures for changing the program date are used in Windows XP, Windows Vista, and Windows 7. Follow the instructions for your computer's operating system.

WINDOWS XP

The following steps are used to change the Medisoft Program Date in Windows XP:

1. Click Set Program Date on the File menu. A pop-up calendar is displayed (see Figure 3-20). *Note:* You can also directly click the date that is displayed in the lower-right corner of the window.

2. To change the month, click the word displayed for the current month, and a pop-up list of months appears. Click the desired month on the pop-up list (see Figure 3-21).

3. To change the year, follow the same procedure. Click the current year, and select the desired year from the pop-up list (see Figure 3-22).

4. Select the desired day of the month by clicking that date in the calendar. If the date you have selected is in the future, a pop-up message appears to remind you that you have selected a future date. To continue with the date change, click the OK button. The calendar closes, and the desired date is displayed on the status bar.

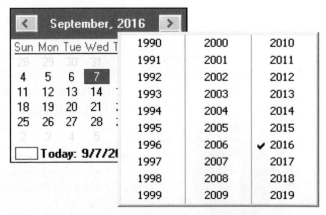

Figure 3-22   Calendar Year Pop-up List

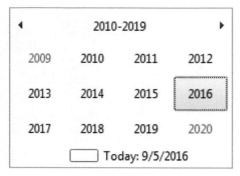

Figure 3-23　Medisoft Pop-Up Calendar

Figure 3-24　Calendar Month Window

WINDOWS VISTA AND WINDOWS 7

The following steps are used to change the Medisoft Program Date in Windows Vista and Windows 7:

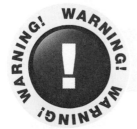

Figure 3-25　Calendar Year Window

1. Click Set Program Date on the File menu. A pop-up calendar is displayed in the lower-right corner of the window (see Figure 3-23). *Note:* You can also click directly on the date that is displayed in the lower-right corner of the window.

2. To change the month, click the word displayed for the current month, and the abbreviations for the months appear in the calendar window. Click the desired month (see Figure 3-24).

3. To change the year, follow the same procedure. Click the current year, and select the desired year from the years that appear in the window (see Figure 3-25).

4. Select the desired day of the month by clicking that date in the calendar. If the date you have selected is in the future, a pop-up message appears to remind you that you have selected a future date. To continue with the date change, click the OK button. The calendar closes, and the desired date is displayed on the status bar.

MMDDCCYY format the way dates must be keyed in Medisoft, in which *MM* stands for the month, *DD* stands for the day, *CC* represents the century, and *YY* stands for the year

In most Medisoft dialog boxes, if a pop-up calendar is not used, dates must be entered manually in the MMDDCCYY format. In the **MMDDCCYY format,** *MM* stands for the month, *DD* stands for the day, *CC* represents the century, and *YY* stands for the year. Each day, month, century, and year entry must contain two digits, and no punctuation can be used. For example, February 1, 2016, would be keyed *02012016.*

Dates are very important! If incorrect dates are used when entering data, the information in reports will be inaccurate. Be sure to change the Medisoft Program Date as specified at the beginning of each exercise.

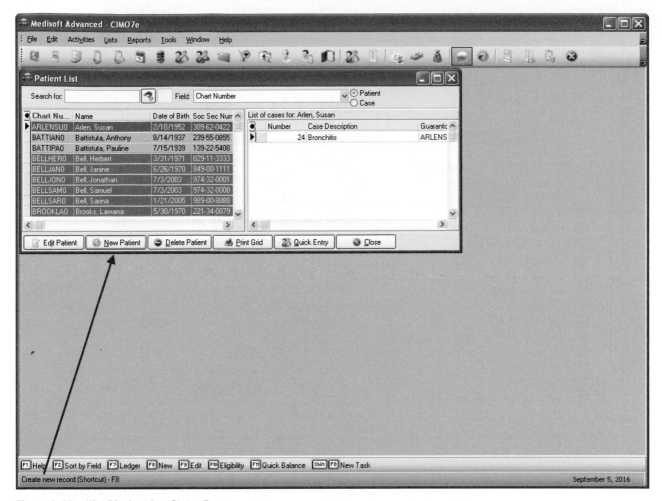

Figure 3-26   Hint Displayed on Status Bar

3.6 USING MEDISOFT HELP

Medisoft offers users three different types of help.

HINTS

As the cursor moves over certain fields, hints appear on the status bar at the bottom of the screen. For example, when the cursor is over the New Patient button, a related hint is displayed (see Figure 3-26). The Hint feature can be turned on or off by clicking Show Hints on the Help menu.

BUILT-IN

For more detailed help, Medisoft has an extensive help feature built into the program itself, which is accessed by selecting Medisoft Help on the Help menu (see Figure 3-27).

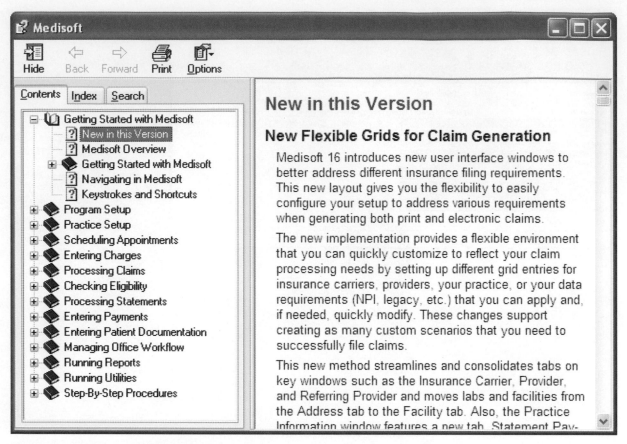

Figure 3-27   Medisoft Built-in Help Feature

ONLINE

The Help menu also provides access to Medisoft help available on the Medisoft corporate website at http://www.Medisoft.com (see Figure 3-28). The website contains a searchable **knowledge base,** which is a collection of up-to-date technical information about Medisoft products.

knowledge base a collection of up-to-date technical information

---

EXERCISE 3-4   **USING BUILT-IN HELP**

Practice using Medisoft's built-in help.

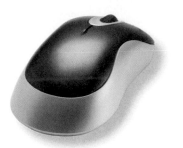

1. Click the Help menu.
2. Click Medisoft Help. Medisoft displays a list of topics for which help is available.
3. In the left column, select the Index tab.
4. Scroll down to locate Diagnosis Entry in the list of terms. Double click Diagnosis Entry. Information on entering diagnosis codes is displayed on the right side of the window. *Note:* You can also locate information by entering the word diagnosis in the blank box below the Index label.
5. Click the Close box in the upper-right corner to close the Help window.

 You have completed Exercise 3-4.

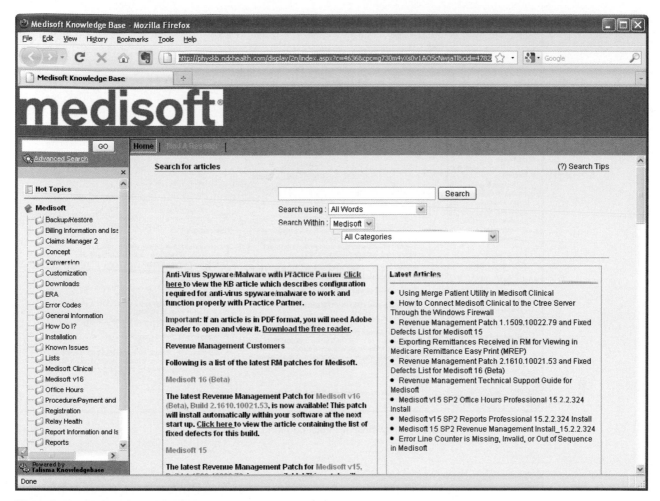

Figure 3-28   Medisoft Knowledge Base

Practice using Medisoft's online help.

1. Access the Internet. On the Medisoft Help menu, select Medisoft on the Web > Knowledge Base.

2. Enter **transactions** in the search box.

3. Accept the entries in Search using: (All Words) and in Search Within: (Medisoft) (All Categories). Your screen should look like Figure 3-29, on the next page.

4. Click the Search button. Your screen should look like Figure 3-30, on the next page.

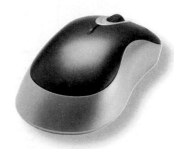

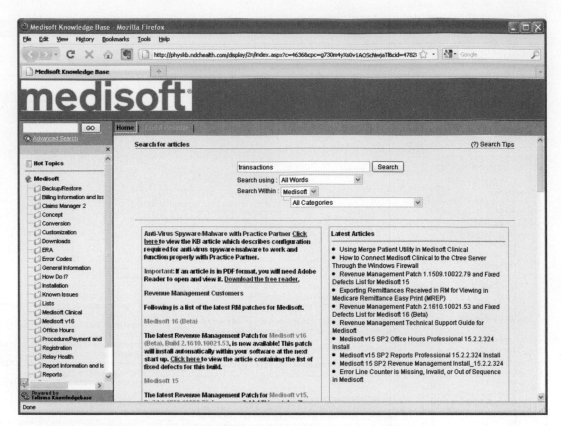

Figure 3-29   Medisoft Knowledge Base with Search Term Entered

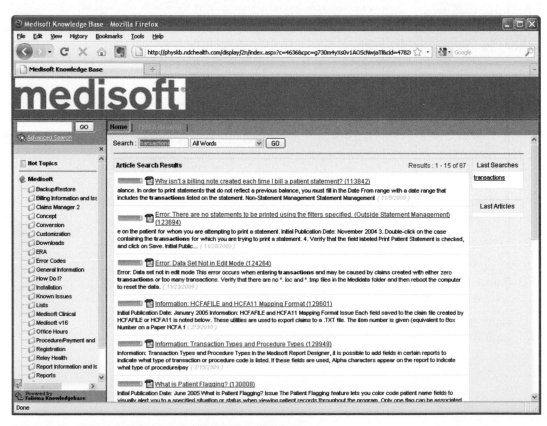

Figure 3-30   Search Results in the Medisoft Knowledge Base

5. Click the title of one of the articles to read it.

6. Click the Close box to exit the Medisoft Knowledge Base. Terminate your Internet connection, if appropriate. **CiMC**

 You have completed Exercise 3-5.

3.7 CREATING AND RESTORING BACKUP FILES

Medisoft is exited by clicking Exit on the File menu or by clicking the Close box. To avoid the inconvenience of exiting and restarting Medisoft many times a day when the computer is needed for a different program, Medisoft can be made temporarily inactive by using the Minimize button, the first of the three small buttons in the upper-right corner of the window. Medisoft can be reactivated at any time by clicking the Medisoft button on the Windows taskbar.

CREATING A BACKUP FILE WHILE EXITING MEDISOFT

Data are periodically saved on removable media, such as flash drives, through a process known as backing up. The extra copy of data files made at a specific point in time is known as **backup data.** Backup data can be used to restore data to the system in the event the data in the system are accidentally lost or destroyed. Backups are performed on a regular schedule, determined by the practice. Many practices back up data at the end of each day. A copy of backup data is usually stored at a location other than the office, in case of a natural or man-made disaster at the office facility.

backup data a copy of data files made at a specific point in time that can be used to restore data

In a school setting, files are also backed up regularly to store each student's work securely and separately. If you are a student using this book in a school environment, it is important to make a backup copy of your work after each Medisoft session. This ensures that you can restore your work during the next session and be able to use your own data even if another student uses the computer after you or if, for any reason, the data on the school computer are changed or corrupted.

In Medisoft, the Backup Data option on the File menu can be used to make a backup copy of the active database at any time. By default, Medisoft also displays a Backup Reminder dialog box every time the program is exited. The Backup Reminder dialog box gives you the opportunity to back up your work every time you exit Medisoft (see Figure 3-31). To perform the backup, click the Back Up Data Now button. A Backup Warning dialog box may appear, indicating that if others are using the same practice data, they should exit Medisoft before the

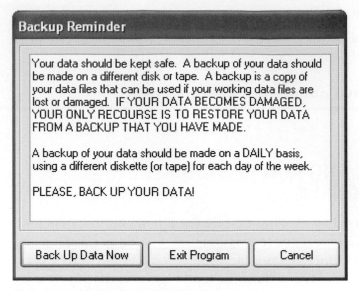

Figure 3-31   Backup Reminder Dialog Box

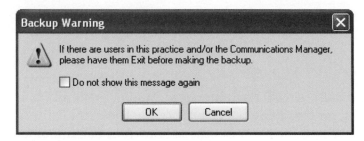

Figure 3-32   Backup Warning Dialog Box

backup is made (see Figure 3-32). To continue to exit the program without making a backup, click the Exit Program button in the Backup Reminder dialog box. The following exercise provides practice.

EXERCISE 3-6   BACKING UP

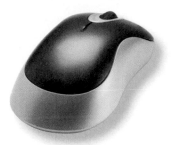

Practice backing up your work on exiting Medisoft.

1. To exit Medisoft, click Exit on the File menu, or click the Exit button on the toolbar.

2. The Backup Reminder dialog box appears, displaying three options: Back Up Data Now, Exit Program, and Cancel. For the purposes of this text, it is recommended that you back up your work each time you exit the program. Your instructor will tell you where to save your backup.

3. Click the Back Up Data Now button. If a Backup Warning dialog box appears, click the OK button.

4. The Medisoft Backup dialog box is displayed (see Figure 3-33). Depending on the last time the dialog box was accessed, the Destination File Path and Name box may already contain an entry. Your instructor will tell you what to enter in this field.

5. Medisoft automatically displays the location of the database files to be backed up in the Source Path box in the lower half of the dialog box.

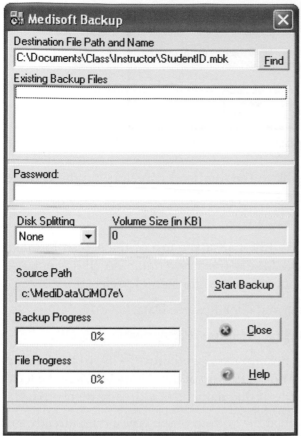

Figure 3-33 Backup Dialog Box

Figure 3-34 Backup Complete Message

6. Click the Start Backup button.

7. The program backs up the latest database files and displays an Information dialog box indicating that the backup is complete (see Figure 3-34). Click OK.

8. Close the Medisoft Backup dialog box by clicking the Close button.

9. The Medisoft Backup dialog box disappears, and the Medisoft program closes. **CiMO**

✓ **You have completed Exercise 3-6.**

RESTORING THE BACKUP FILE

The process of retrieving data from backup storage devices is referred to as **restoring data.** Whenever a new Medisoft session begins, the following steps can be used to restore the backup file, if required. If you share a computer in an instructional environment, it is recommended that you perform a restore before each new session to be sure you are working with your own data.

restoring data the process of retrieving data from backup storage devices

In this example, backups are stored on the C drive, and the Medisoft program files are located on the C drive.

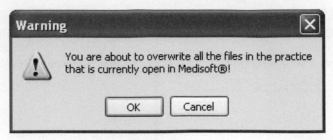

Figure 3-35   Restore Warning Box

To restore StudentID.mbk to the Medisoft directory on the C drive (C:\MediData\CiMO7e):

1. Start Medisoft.

2. Check the program's title bar at the top of the screen to make sure the CiMO7e database is the active database. (If it is not, use the Open Practice option on the File menu to select it.)

3. Open the File menu, and click Restore Data.

4. When the Warning box in Figure 3-35 appears, click OK.

5. The Restore dialog box appears (see Figure 3-36). In the Backup File Path and Name box at the top of the dialog box, key the location of the backup file, if this name is not already displayed.

6. The Destination Path at the bottom of the box should already say c:\MediData\CiMO7e.

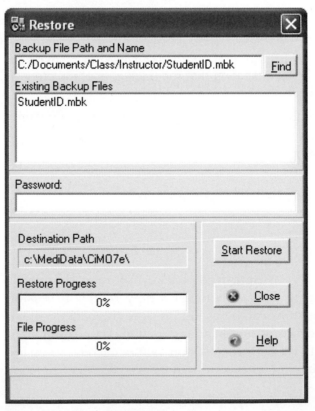

Figure 3-36   Restore Dialog Box

7. Click the Start Restore button.

8. When the Confirm box appears, click OK.

9. An Information dialog box appears indicating that the restore is complete. Click OK to continue.

10. Click the Close button to close the Restore dialog box. The Restore dialog box disappears. You are ready to begin the next session.

3.8 MEDISOFT'S FILE MAINTENANCE UTILITIES

In addition to the backup and restore features, Medisoft provides four features to assist in maintaining data files stored in a system. These four features are found on tabs in the File Maintenance dialog box (see Figure 3-37).

1. Rebuild Indexes

2. Pack Data

3. Purge Data

4. Recalculate Balances

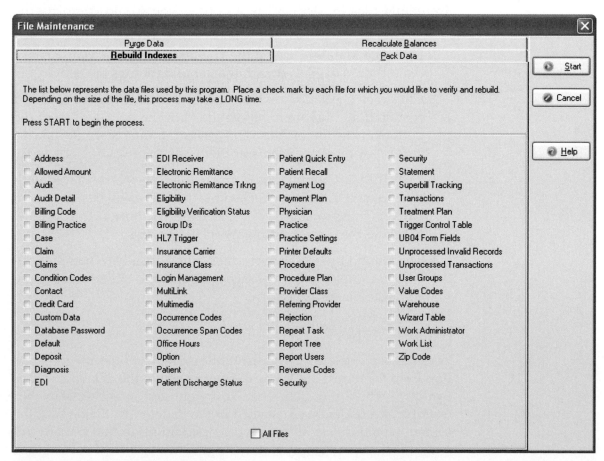

Figure 3-37 File Maintenance Dialog Box

The dialog box is accessed by clicking File Maintenance on the File menu. If the medical office's database is large, Medisoft's utilities may take a long time to finish. For this reason, it is usually a good idea to use the utility functions at the end of the day or when the system will not be needed for a while.

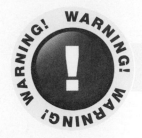

rebuilding indexes a process that checks and verifies data and corrects any internal problems with the data

> Do not attempt to perform the utility functions listed in this chapter unless told to do so by your instructor. Loss of data could occur.

REBUILDING INDEXES

Rebuilding indexes is a process that checks and verifies data and corrects any internal data problems. The rebuild does not check or verify the content of the data; it does not change the content of any data files. For example, the system will not check whether John Fitzwilliams paid $50 on his last visit.

To keep files working efficiently, files should be rebuilt about once a month. Files to be rebuilt are selected from the list of files in the Rebuild Indexes tab (refer back to Figure 3-37). If the database is large, rebuilding indexes can take a long time.

To rebuild files in Medisoft in an office, you would complete the following steps:

1. Click File Maintenance on the File menu. The File Maintenance dialog box is displayed with the Rebuild Indexes tab active.

2. Click each check box next to the files that are to be verified and rebuilt. If all files are to be rebuilt, click the All Files box at the bottom of the list of files. This saves the time it would take to click a box for every Medisoft file.

3. Click the Start button. The Confirm dialog box is displayed with the message "All of the checked file processes will be performed. Do you want to continue?" Click the OK button to continue. (Clicking the Cancel button aborts the process.)

4. The rebuild process is performed automatically. When the process is complete, the message "All checked file processes are complete." is displayed.

PACKING DATA

When data are deleted in Medisoft, the system empties the information from the record but keeps the empty slot in the database so it is available when new data need to be entered in the system. For example, if a patient were deleted in the Patient List dialog box, the system would delete all the records pertaining to that patient but would maintain an empty slot in the patient database. The next time a new patient was entered, the data for the new patient would

| Purge Data | Recalculate Balances |
| Rebuild Indexes | **Pack Data** |

The list below represents the data files used by this program. Place a check mark by each file for which you would like to verify and rebuild. Depending on the size of the file, this process may take a LONG time.

Press START to begin the process.

Address	EDI Receiver	Patient Quick Entry	Security
Allowed Amount	Electronic Remittance	Patient Recall	Statement
Audit	Electronic Remittance Trkng	Payment Log	Superbill Tracking
Audit Detail	Eligibility	Payment Plan	Transactions
Billing Code	Eligibility Verification Status	Physician	Treatment Plan
Billing Practice	Group IDs	Practice	Trigger Control Table
Case	HL7 Trigger	Practice Settings	UB04 Form Fields
Claim	Insurance Carrier	Printer Defaults	Unprocessed Invalid Records
Claims	Insurance Class	Procedure	Unprocessed Transactions
Condition Codes	Login Management	Procedure Plan	User Groups
Contact	MultiLink	Provider Class	Value Codes
Credit Card	Multimedia	Referring Provider	Warehouse
Custom Data	Occurrence Codes	Rejection	Wizard Table
Database Password	Occurrence Span Codes	Repeat Task	Work Administrator
Default	Office Hours	Report Tree	Work List
Deposit	Option	Report Users	Zip Code
Diagnosis	Patient	Revenue Codes	
EDI	Patient Discharge Status	Security	

☐ All Files

Figure 3-38 Pack Data Tab

occupy the vacant slot in the database. When there is not much space on the hard disk, it may be desirable to delete the vacant slots to make more disk space available. The deletion of vacant slots from the database is known as **packing data.** Data for packing can be selected from the list of files in the Pack Data tab (see Figure 3-38). (Only transaction files with zero balances can be deleted.) If the database is large, packing data can take a long time.

packing data the deletion of vacant slots from the database

To pack files in an office situation, you would complete the following steps:

1. Click File Maintenance on the File menu. The File Maintenance dialog box is displayed with the Rebuild Indexes tab active. Make the Pack Data tab active.

2. Click each check box next to the files that are to be packed.

3. If all files are to be packed, click the All Files box at the bottom of the list of files.

4. Click the Start button. The Confirm dialog box is displayed with the message "All of the checked file processes will be performed. Do you want to continue?" Click the OK button to continue. (Clicking the Cancel button aborts the process.)

5. The pack process is performed automatically. When the process is complete, the message "All checked file processes are complete." is displayed.

PURGING DATA

purging data the process of deleting files of patients who are no longer seen by a provider in a practice

The process of deleting files of patients who are no longer seen by a provider in a practice is called **purging data.** Purging data frees space on the computer and permits the system to run more efficiently. However, purging should be done with great caution. Once data are purged from the system, they cannot be retrieved, except from a backup file. As a safety precaution, always perform a backup before purging.

The Purge Data tab offers several options (see Figure 3-39). Data can be purged for appointments, claims, statements, recalls, closed cases,

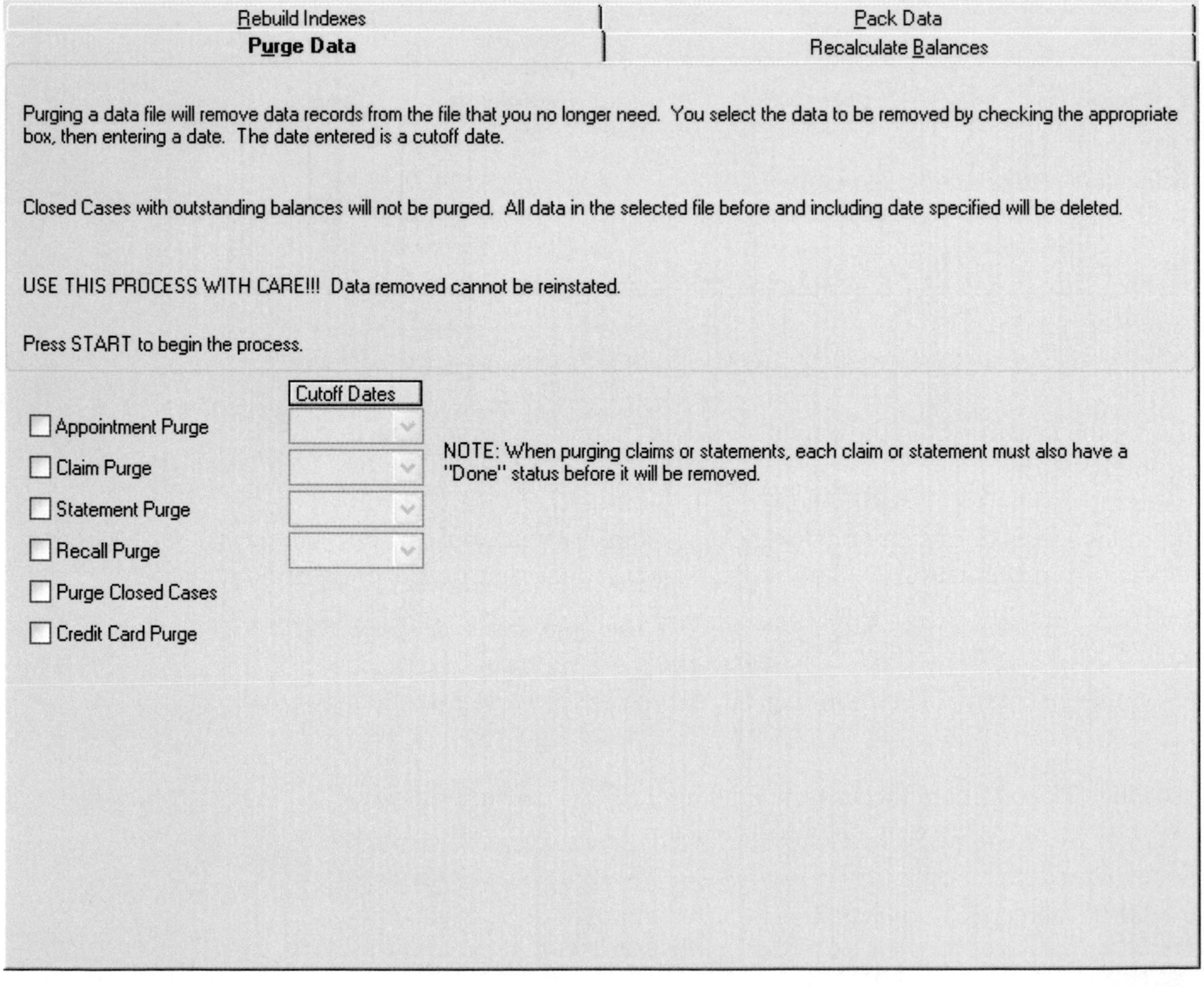

Figure 3-39 Purge Data Tab

and credit card entries. All options except Purge Closed Cases and Credit Card Purge are purged by date. A cutoff date is entered, and Medisoft deletes all data up to that date. For example, if all the data entered prior to December 31, 2010, are to be purged, that date would be entered as the cutoff date. Data entered in cases that have been closed are purged by clicking the check box labeled Purge Closed Cases.

To purge data in an office situation, you would complete the following steps:

1. Click File Maintenance on the File menu. The File Maintenance dialog box is displayed with the Rebuild Indexes tab active. Make the Purge Data tab active.

2. Click each check box next to the files that are to be purged. Enter a cutoff date in the Cutoff Dates box.

3. Click the Start button. The Confirm dialog box is displayed with the message "All of the checked file processes will be performed. Do you want to continue?" Click the OK button to continue. (Clicking the Cancel button aborts the process.)

4. The purge process is performed automatically. When the process is complete, the message "All checked file processes are complete." is displayed.

RECALCULATING PATIENT BALANCES

As transaction entries are changed or deleted, there are times when the balance listed on the screen is not accurate. **Recalculating balances** refers to the process of updating balances to reflect the most recent changes made to the data. This feature is accessed through the Recalculate Balances tab on the File Maintenance dialog box (see Figure 3-40).

recalculating balances the process of updating balances to reflect the most recent changes made to the data

When balances are recalculated, the system reviews every patient's data and recalculates the balances. The process can be time-consuming. Individual patient balances can be recalculated in the Transaction Entry dialog box by clicking the Account Total column.

To recalculate balances in an office situation, you would complete the following steps:

1. Click File Maintenance on the File menu. The File Maintenance dialog box is displayed with the Rebuild Indexes tab active. Make the Recalculate Balances tab active.

2. Click to place a check mark in the appropriate box(es).

3. Click the Start button. The Confirm dialog box is displayed with the message "All of the checked file processes will be performed.

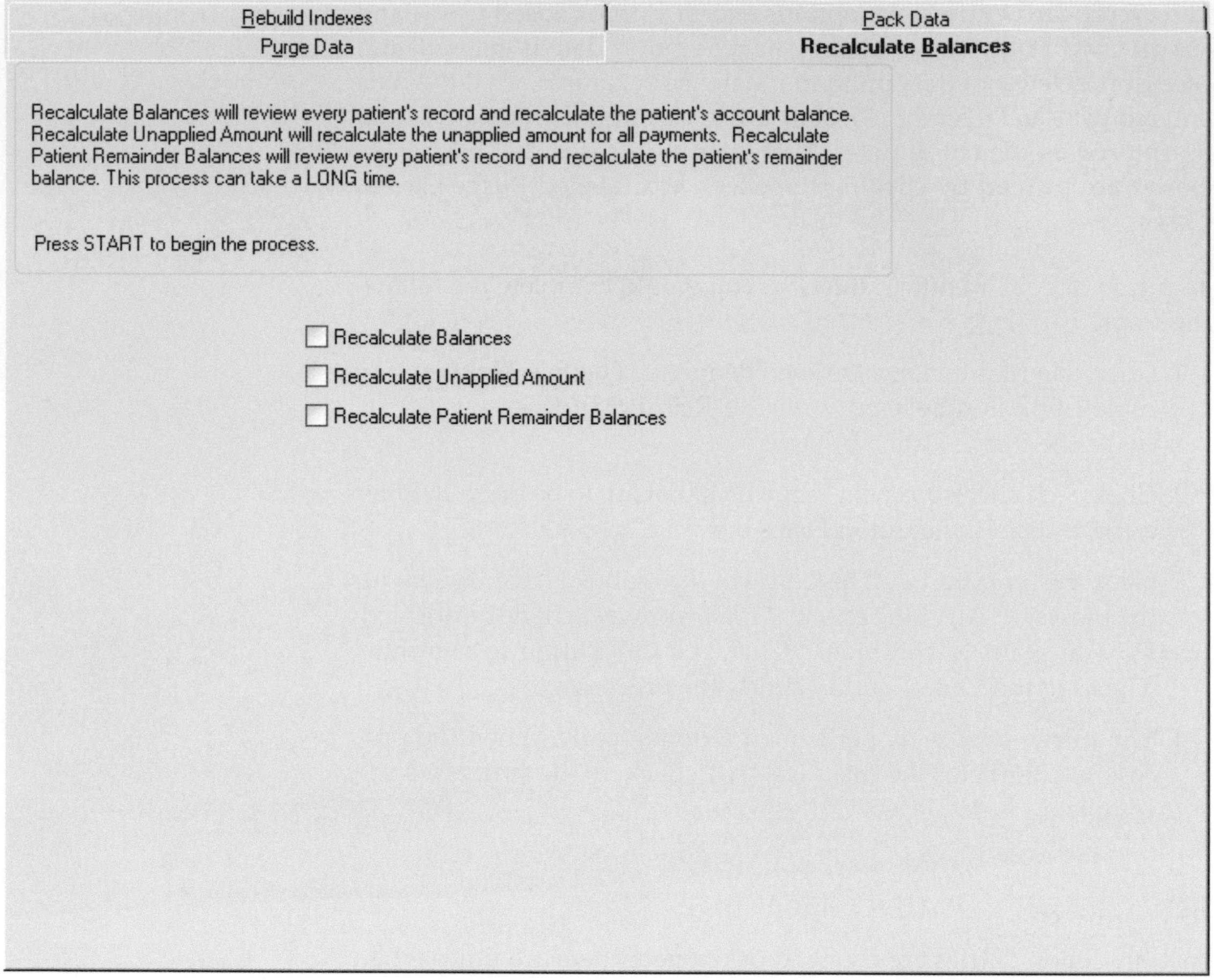

| Rebuild Indexes | Pack Data |
| Purge Data | **Recalculate Balances** |

Recalculate Balances will review every patient's record and recalculate the patient's account balance. Recalculate Unapplied Amount will recalculate the unapplied amount for all payments. Recalculate Patient Remainder Balances will review every patient's record and recalculate the patient's remainder balance. This process can take a LONG time.

Press START to begin the process.

☐ Recalculate Balances
☐ Recalculate Unapplied Amount
☐ Recalculate Patient Remainder Balances

Figure 3-40   Recalculate Balances Tab

Do you want to continue?" Click the OK button to continue. (Clicking the Cancel button aborts the process.)

4. The recalculate process is performed automatically. When the process is complete, the message "All checked file processes are complete." is displayed.

3.9 USING MEDISOFT SECURITY FEATURES TO ENSURE HIPAA AND HITECH COMPLIANCE

Medisoft offers a number of features to protect the privacy and security of patients' protected health information in accordance with HIPAA and HITECH regulations. Security is set up in Medisoft by first assigning the administrative function to an individual in the practice, usually the office manager. The administrator has unlimited access to the program. The Security Setup option on the File menu is used to set up the administrator. The administrator can

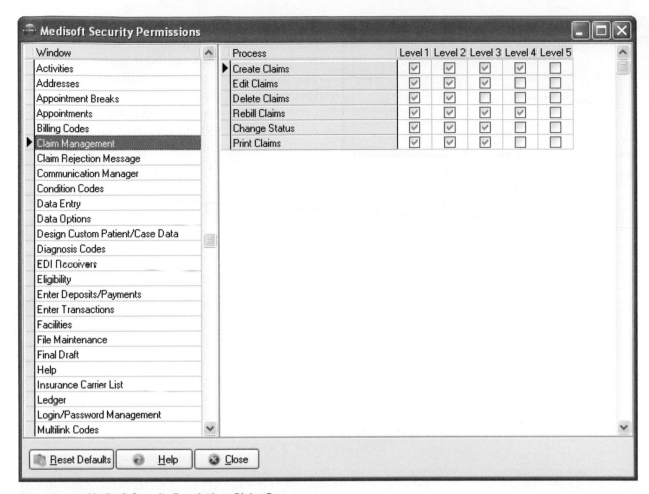

Figure 3-41 Medisoft Security Permissions Dialog Box

assign access rights to each level of security by clicking the Permissions option on the File menu. (*Note:* The Permissions option does not appear in the File menu until the security administrator has been set up in the Security Setup window.) **Access rights** determine which areas of the program a particular user can access, and whether that user can only view data or has rights to enter or edit data.

access rights security option that determines the areas of the program a user can access, and whether the user has rights to enter or edit data

When the Permissions option is selected on the File menu, the Medisoft Security Permissions dialog box appears. Each function within the program is listed alphabetically in the left side of the dialog box (see Figure 3-41). The right side of the dialog box displays security level assignments. A check mark under a level heading means that anyone with that level of security has the ability to perform that task or has access to that portion of the program.

Medisoft security consists of five levels of program access, with level 1 having the most access rights and level 5 the fewest. Level 1 is for unlimited access and is designed to be used exclusively by the administrator. Levels 2, 3, 4, and 5 are set up to meet the needs of the practice. Generally, the administrator decides what staff roles and tasks belong in what level and assigns users accordingly.

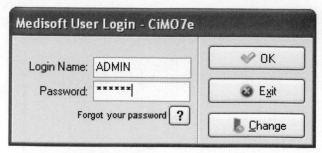

Figure 3-42 Medisoft User Login Dialog Box

In the Medisoft Security Permissions dialog box illustrated in Figure 3-41, the permissions for the Claim Management features are displayed. Notice that users with access levels 1 through 4 can create claims; only level 5 users cannot create claims. Permission for editing claims is restricted to users in levels 1 through 3, while deleting claims is limited to users in levels 1 and 2.

USER LOGINS AND AUDIT CONTROLS

Once security has been set up in Medisoft, users are assigned user names and passwords, and they must log in to access the program (see Figure 3-42).

Requiring users to log in limits access to the program to those who have been assigned logins, and also allows tracking the actions of users within the program though an audit report. The audit function can be used to track changes made in the program, as well as who made the changes. Options for the audit report are selected in the Audit tab of the Program Options dialog box, accessed via the File menu (see Figure 3-43). For database tables to be audited, check marks must appear in the boxes in the Update and/or Delete

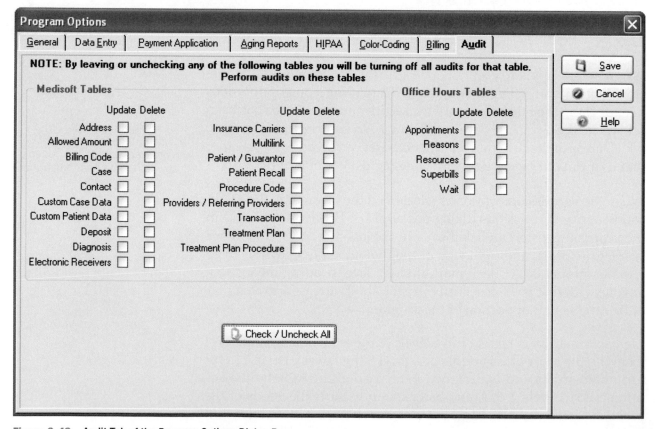

Figure 3-43 Audit Tab of the Program Options Dialog Box

columns. If the Update box is checked, the program tracks changes to the table; if the Delete box is checked, the program tracks deletions of data from the table.

AUTO LOG OFF AND UNAPPROVED CODES

Another tab in the Program Options dialog box allows practice administrators to select options to help protect patient information from unauthorized access. The HIPAA tab (see Figure 3-44) contains an Auto Log Off option and a Warn on Unapproved Codes option. The **Auto Log Off** feature is designed to protect data files from unauthorized access by logging a user off after detecting no activity for a specified number of minutes. If a user steps away from his or her desk without first logging off, information in the Medisoft program can be viewed by anyone who uses the computer. This feature automatically logs the user off, preventing access to the program. The Auto Log Off field can be set for up to 59 minutes.

Auto Log Off feature of Medisoft that automatically logs a user out of the program after a period of inactivity

The Warn on Unapproved Codes box, when checked, is used to trigger a warning box to pop up every time a transaction is saved with a code that has not been marked HIPAA compliant. Codes are marked as compliant by checking the HIPAA Approved box in the Procedure/Payment/Adjustment dialog box for each procedure code, and in the HIPAA Approved box in the Diagnosis dialog box for each diagnosis code.

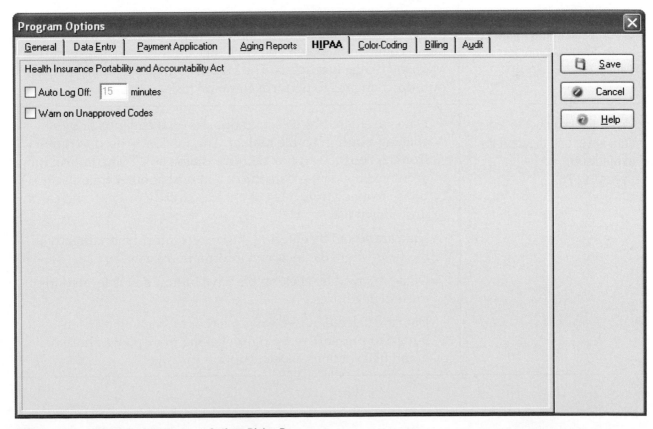

Figure 3-44   HIPAA Tab of the Program Options Dialog Box

3.1 List the six databases Medisoft uses to store information. Pages 64–65	- Provider data - Patient data - Insurance carriers - Diagnosis codes - Procedure codes - Transactions
3.2 List the menus in Medisoft. Pages 65–70	- File - Edit - Activities - Lists - Reports - Tools - Window - Help
3.3 Explain the function of the Medisoft toolbar. Pages 70–72	The toolbar contains buttons that are shortcuts for frequently used menu commands. When you click on a button, the corresponding Medisoft dialog box opens. The buttons can be used instead of the pull-down menus to perform common tasks.
3.4 Explain how to enter, edit, save, and delete data in Medisoft. Pages 72–76	- Data are entered by selecting options on the menus or by clicking a button on the toolbar. The Tab key is used to move from text box to text box within a dialog box. Some information is entered by keying data into a text box; at other times, selections are made from a list of choices already present, such as a drop-down list. - Data are edited by entering the correct information directly in the field where the incorrect information exists. - Data are saved by clicking the Save button that is located in most dialog boxes. - Data are deleted in two ways—either by clicking a Delete button (if present), or by right-clicking to display a shortcut menu that contains a Delete option.

3.5 Describe how to change the Program Date in Medisoft. Pages 76–80	Windows XP 1. Click Set Program Date on the File menu, or click the date displayed in the lower-right corner of the Medisoft window. 2. To change the month, click the word displayed for the current month, and a pop-up list of months appears. Click the desired month on the pop-up list. 3. To change the year, click the current year, and select the desired year from the pop-up list. 4. Select the desired day of the month by clicking that date in the calendar. Vista or Windows 7 1. Click Set Program Date on the File menu, or click the date displayed in the lower-right corner of the Medisoft window. 2. To change the month, click the word displayed for the current month, and the abbreviations for the months appear in the calendar window. Click the desired month. 3. To change the year, click the current year, and select the desired year from the years that appear in the window. 4. Select the desired day of the month by clicking that date in the calendar.
3.6 Discuss three types of help available in Medisoft. Pages 81–85	- Hints appear on the status bar at the bottom of the screen as the cursor moves over certain fields. - Medisoft's extensive built-in help feature is accessed by selecting Medisoft Help on the Help menu. - Help is also available online at http://www.Medisoft.com, which can be accessed by selecting Medisoft on the Web on the Help menu. The website contains a searchable knowledge base, which is a collection of up-to-date technical information about Medisoft products.
3.7 Explain how to create and restore backup files in Medisoft. Pages 85–89	Creating a Backup File 1. To exit Medisoft and create a backup file, click Exit on the File menu, or click the Exit button on the toolbar. 2. The Backup Reminder dialog box appears. 3. Click the Back Up Data Now button. If a Backup Warning dialog box appears, click the OK button. 4. The Medisoft Backup dialog box is displayed. Your instructor will tell you what to enter in the top field. 5. Click the Start Backup button.

6. The program backs up the latest database files and displays an Information dialog box indicating that the backup is complete. Click OK.

7. Close the Medisoft Backup dialog box by clicking the Close button.

Restoring a Backup File

1. Check the program's title bar at the top of the screen to make sure the CiMO7e database is the active database. (If it is not, use the Open Practice option on the File menu to select it.)

2. Open the File menu, and click Restore Data.

3. When the Warning box appears, click OK.

4. The Restore dialog box appears. In the Backup File Path and Name box at the top of the dialog box, key the location of the backup file, if this name is not already displayed.

5. Click the Start Restore button.

6. When the Confirm box appears, click OK.

7. An Information dialog box appears indicating that the restore is complete. Click OK to continue.

8. Click the Close button to close the Restore dialog box. The Restore dialog box disappears. You are ready to begin the next session.

3.8 Describe the functions of the file maintenance utilities in Medisoft.
Pages 89–94

- Rebuilding indexes checks and verifies data and corrects any internal problems with the data.

- Packing data deletes vacant slots in the database that remain after data have been deleted from the program.

- Purging data deletes all data as of a user-specified date.

- Recalculating balances updates balances to reflect the most recent changes made to the data.

3.9 Describe the Medisoft security features used to ensure compliance with HIPAA and HITECH regulations.
Pages 94–97

- The ability to view and alter data in different areas of the program is restricted by assigning access rights to each user.

- Users are assigned logins and passwords to limit access to the program and to track their activities within the program.

- The Auto Log Off feature automatically logs a user out of Medisoft after a specified number of minutes pass without any activity, preventing access to the program by unauthorized users.

- The Warn on Unapproved Codes feature sends a warning message when a transaction is saved with a code that is not HIPAA approved.

USING TERMINOLOGY

Match the terms on the left with the definitions on the right.

_____ **1.** *[LO 3.9]* access rights

_____ **2.** *[LO 3.9]* Auto Log Off

_____ **3.** *[LO 3.7]* backup data

_____ **4.** *[LO 3.6]* knowledge base

_____ **5.** *[LO 3.5]* MMDDCCYY format

_____ **6.** *[LO 3.8]* packing data

_____ **7.** *[LO 3.1]* database

_____ **8.** *[LO 3.8]* purging data

_____ **9.** *[LO 3.8]* rebuilding indexes

_____ **10.** *[LO 3.8]* recalculating balances

_____ **11.** *[LO 3.7]* restoring data

a. The process of retrieving data from backup storage devices.

b. A searchable collection of up-to-date technical information.

c. A collection of related pieces of information.

d. A feature that automatically logs a user out of the program after a specified number of minutes of inactivity.

e. The process of updating balances to reflect the most recent changes made to the data.

f. The process of deleting files of patients who are no longer seen by a provider in a practice.

g. The way dates must be keyed.

h. An option that determines which areas of the program a user can access, and whether the user can only view data or has rights to enter or edit data.

i. A copy of data files made at a specific point in time that can be used to restore data to the system.

j. A process that checks and verifies data and corrects any internal problems with the data.

k. The deletion of vacant slots from the database.

CHECKING YOUR UNDERSTANDING

Answer the questions below in the space provided.

1. *[LO 3.2]* Describe two ways of issuing a command in Medisoft.

   _____

   _____

2. *[LO 3.4]* What are two ways data are entered in a box?

   _____

   _____

3. *[LO 3.6]* What three types of Medisoft help are available?

   _____

   _____

4. *[LO 3.2]* Which menu provides access to Office Hours, Medisoft's scheduling feature?

   _____

   _____

5. *[LO 3.5]* What is the format for entering dates in Medisoft?

   _____

   _____

6. *[LO 3.7]* Describe two ways of exiting Medisoft.

   _____

   _____

7. *[LO 3.7]* Why is it important to back up data regularly?

   _____

   _____

8. *[LO 3.8]* Why is extra caution required when purging data?

   _____

   _____

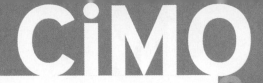

9. *[LO 3.7]* When is a data restore performed?

_____

_____

10. *[LO 3.9]* Give an example of how Medisoft's Auto Log Off feature protects patient data.

_____

_____

11. *[LO 3.9]* Give two reasons why it is important to assign each user a login ID and password.

_____

_____

APPLYING YOUR KNOWLEDGE

Answer the questions below in the space provided.

3.1. *[LO 3.6]* Use Medisoft's built-in help feature to look up information on the following topics:

   a. How to enter diagnosis codes

   b. How to print procedure code lists from the Medisoft database

3.2. *[LO 3.7]* You come to work on a Monday morning and find that the office computer is not working. The system manager informs everyone that the computer's hard disk crashed and that all data that were not backed up are lost. What do you do?

THINKING ABOUT IT

Answer the questions below in the space provided.

3.1. *[LO 3.5]* Why is it important to know how to change dates in Medisoft? What could happen if dates are entered incorrectly?

_____

_____

3.2. *[LO 3.7]* Why is it important to know how to back up and restore Medisoft database files?

_____

_____

AT THE COMPUTER

Answer the following questions at the computer.

3.1. *[LO 3.2]* How many options are there in the Reports menu?

_____

_____

3.2. *[LO 3.2]* What is the first choice on the Lists menu?

_____

_____

3.3. *[LO 3.2]* List the options on the Activities menu.

_____

_____

3.4. *[LO 3.5, 3.7]* Set the Medisoft Program Date to December 1, 2016, and then exit Medisoft.

_____

_____

Entering Patient Information

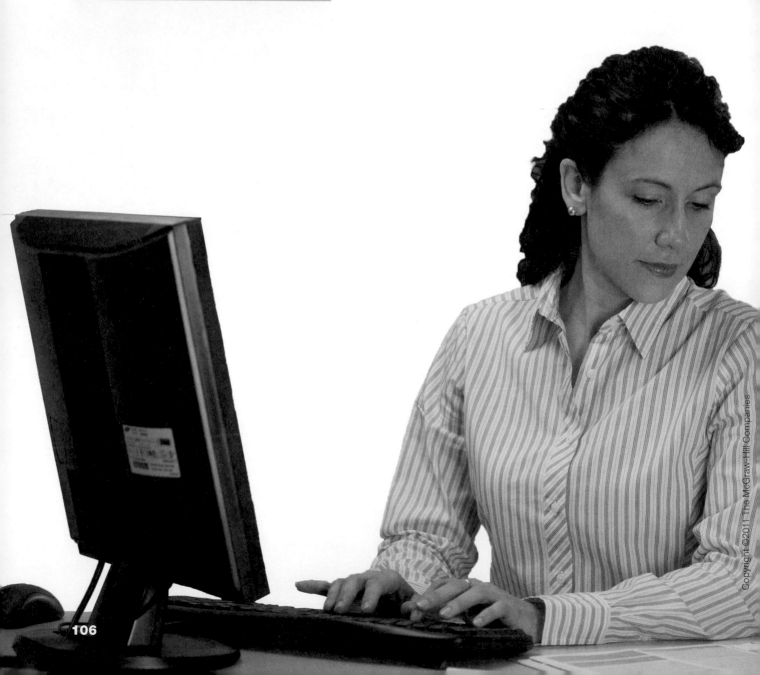

key terms

chart number
established patient
guarantor
new patient

learning outcomes

When you finish this chapter, you will be able to:

4.1 Explain how patient information is organized in Medisoft.

4.2 Discuss how a new patient is added in Medisoft.

4.3 Describe how to search for a patient in Medisoft.

4.4 Describe how patient information is edited in Medisoft.

what you need to know

To use this chapter, you need to know how to:

- Start Medisoft.
- Move around the Medisoft menus.
- Use the Medisoft toolbar.
- Enter and edit data in Medisoft.
- Exit Medisoft.

4.1 HOW PATIENT INFORMATION IS ORGANIZED IN MEDISOFT®

Figure 4-1
Patient List
Shortcut Button

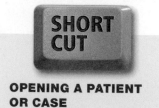

OPENING A PATIENT OR CASE

The quickest way to open a patient or case is to double click on the line associated with a patient or case.

Patient information is accessed through the Patient List dialog box. The Patient List dialog box is displayed when Patients/ Guarantors and Cases is clicked on the Lists menu or when the corresponding shortcut button is clicked on the toolbar (see Figure 4-1).

The Patient List dialog box (see Figure 4-2) is divided into two primary sections. The left side of the window displays information about patients, and the right side of the window contains information about cases. Cases are covered in Chapter 5.

On the upper-right side of the Patient List dialog box, there are two radio buttons: Patient and Case. When the Patient radio button is clicked, the left side of the window becomes active. Correspondingly, when the Case radio button is clicked, the right side of the window becomes active. The command buttons at the bottom of the dialog box vary, depending on which side of the window is active. When the Patient window is active, the command buttons at the bottom of the screen include Edit Patient, New Patient, Delete Patient, Print Grid, Quick Entry, and Close.

The Patient window contains the following fields: Chart Number, Name, Date of Birth, Social Security Number, Patient ID #2, Patient Type, Phone 1, Provider, Last Name, Billing Code, and Patient Indicator. There is not enough room in the Patient window to display all this information, so only a portion is visible at one time. The additional patient information can be viewed by using the scroll bar, maximizing the dialog box, or resizing the Patient area of the dialog box (see Figure 4-3).

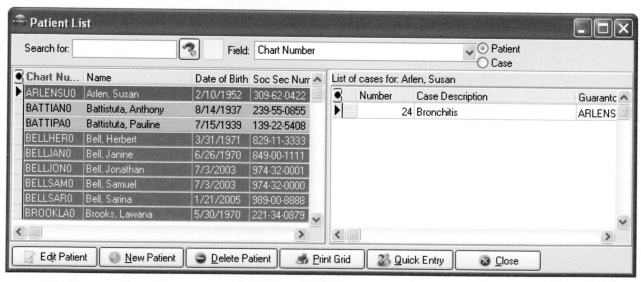

Figure 4-2   Patient List Dialog Box

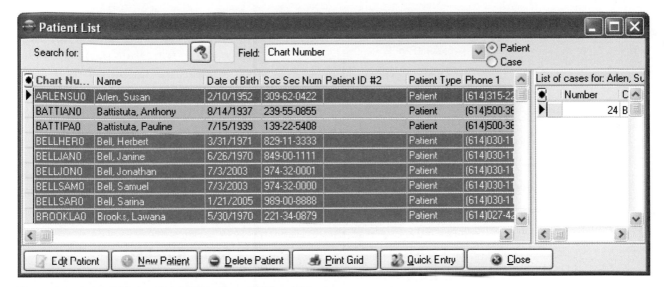

Figure 4-3　Patient Window Expanded to Show Additional Columns

Information in the Patient window is color-coded. In the exercises in this text/workbook, the patient identification color codes shown in Figure 4-4 are assigned to represent the patient's insurance carrier.

4.2 ENTERING NEW PATIENT INFORMATION

A **new patient** is a patient who has not received services from the same provider or a provider of the same specialty within the same practice for a period of three years. An **established patient** is a patient who has been seen by a provider in the practice in the same specialty within three years.

Information on a new patient is entered in Medisoft by clicking the New Patient button at the bottom of the Patient List dialog box (see Figure 4-5). This action opens the Patient/Guarantor dialog box (see Figure 4-6). The Patient/Guarantor dialog box contains three tabs: the Name, Address tab, the Other Information tab, and the Payment Plan tab.

Several buttons are located on the right side of the Patient/Guarantor dialog box. These buttons include:

Save　Saves the information entered in the dialog box.

Cancel　Closes the dialog box and discards any information entered.

Help　Displays the Medisoft help window for Patient/Guarantor Entry.

Set Default　Sets the information in this window as the default for all new patients. (To undo, hold the CTRL key down, and this button changes to Remove Default.)

Copy Address　Copies demographic information from another patient or guarantor entry.

new patient a patient who has not received services from the same provider or a provider of the same specialty within the same practice for a period of three years

established patient a patient who has been seen by a provider in the practice in the same specialty within three years

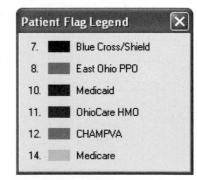

Figure 4-4　Color Legend for Patient List Window

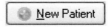

Figure 4-5　New Patient Button

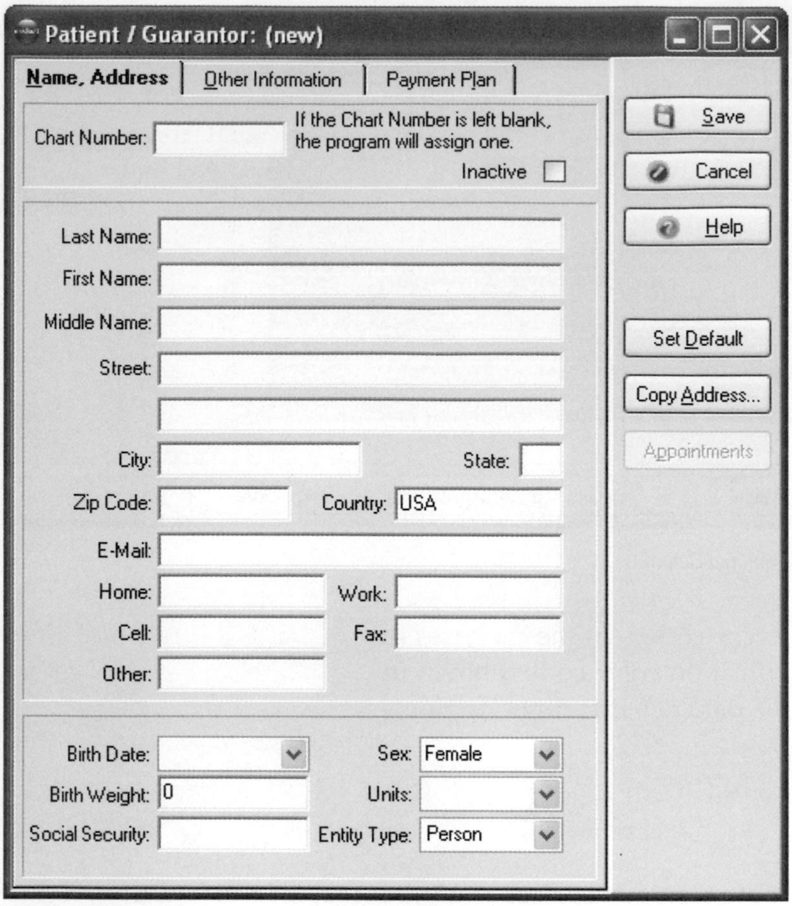

Figure 4-6 Patient/Guarantor Dialog Box with Name, Address Tab Active

Appointments Opens a window with a list of scheduled appointments for the patient. (The Appointments button is grayed and cannot be selected if a patient has no appointments scheduled.)

NAME, ADDRESS TAB

The Name, Address tab is where basic patient information is entered (see Figure 4-6).

Chart Number

The **chart number** is a unique number that identifies a patient. In Medisoft, a chart number links together all the information about a patient that is stored in the different databases, such as name, address, charges, and insurance claims. Each patient is assigned an eight-character chart number. If the Chart Number box for a patient is left blank, the system will assign a number.

chart number a unique number that identifies a patient

Medical practices may use different methods for assigning chart numbers, although these general guidelines must be followed:

- No special characters, such as hyphens, periods, or spaces, are allowed.

- No two chart numbers can be the same.

For the purposes of this text/workbook, the following method is used to assign chart numbers:

- The first five characters of the chart number are the first five letters of a patient's last name. If the patient's last name has fewer than five characters, add the beginning letters of the patient's first name.

- The next two characters are the first two letters of a patient's first name. (If the first two letters of the first name were used to complete the first five letters, the next two letters of the patient's first name are used.)

- The last character is always a zero, displayed in this text/workbook with the symbol "Ø."

For example, the chart number for John Fitzwilliams would begin with the first five letters of his last name (FITZW), followed by the first two characters of his first name (JO), followed by a zero (Ø). John's complete chart number would be FITZWJOØ. Following the same rules, John's daughter Sarah would have a chart number of FITZWSAØ.

CHART NUMBERS   EXERCISE 4-1

Create a chart number for each of these patients, and write it in the space provided.

Albert Wong _____

Jessica Sypkowski _____

John James _____

 You have completed Exercise 4-1.

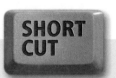

Personal Data

In addition to the chart number, personal information about a patient is entered in the Name, Address tab.

Name, Address, Phone Numbers, E-Mail   Medisoft provides fields for name and address as well as a number of fields for contact methods. There are boxes for e-mail address, home phone, work phone, cell phone, fax, and other. Phone and fax numbers must be entered without parentheses or hyphens.

Birth Date   The patient's birth date is entered in the Birth Date box using the MMDDCCYY format.

Sex   This drop-down list contains choices for the patient's gender: male or female.

Birth Weight   If the patient is a newborn, the birth weight is entered in this field.

Units   This field indicates whether the birth weight is listed in pounds or grams.

Social Security   The nine-digit Social Security number is entered without hyphens; Medisoft automatically adds hyphens.

Entity Type   This field is used for the direct transmission of electronic claims to an insurance carrier. The options in this field are person and non-person.

OTHER INFORMATION TAB

The Other Information tab within the Patient/Guarantor dialog box contains facts about a patient's employment and other miscellaneous information (see Figure 4-7).

SHORT CUT

USING COPY ADDRESS

The Copy Address button saves time when entering patients with the same address, such as family members. Clicking on the Copy Address button provides an option to copy demographic information from a patient already in the database.

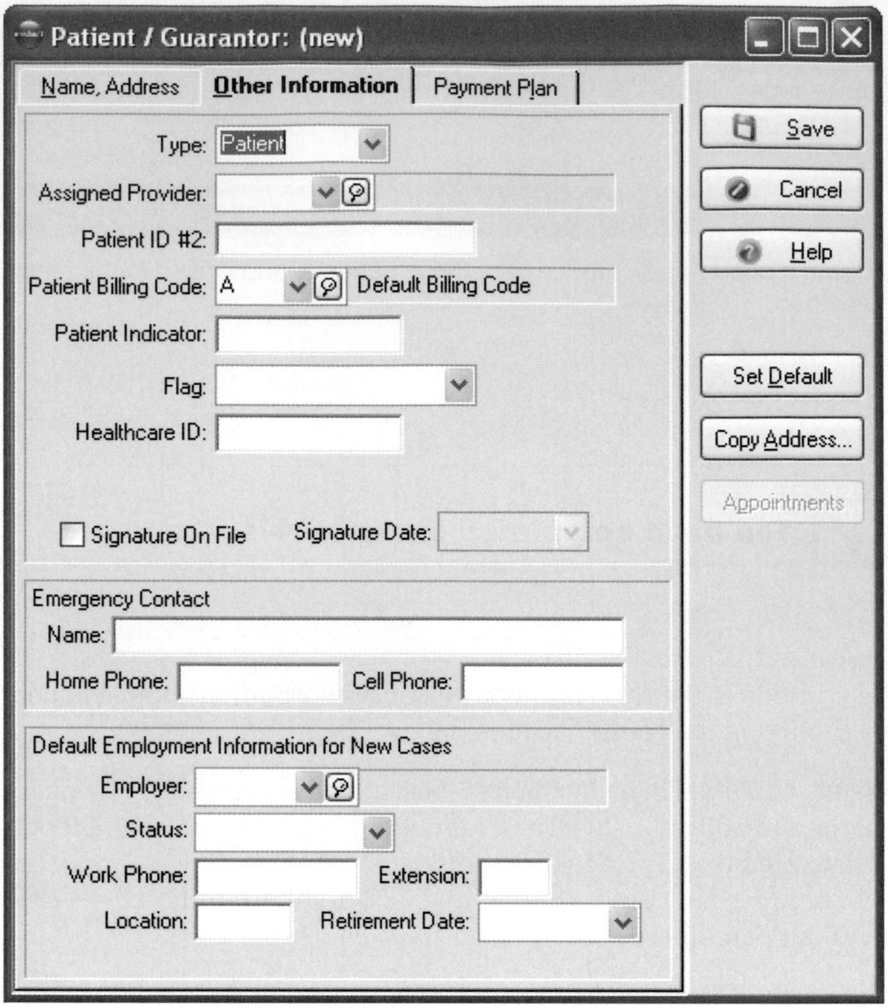

Figure 4-7   Other Information Tab

Type   The Type drop-down list is used for billing purposes to designate whether an individual is a patient or guarantor. A patient is an individual who is a patient of the practice, whether or not he or she is also the insurance policyholder. The term **guarantor** refers to an individual who may not be a patient of the practice but who is financially responsible for a patient account. For example, if the insurance policy of a parent who is not a patient provides coverage for a child who is a patient, the parent is the guarantor. In this case, the guarantor (the parent) is entered in Medisoft first, and then the patient (the child) is entered.

Information about the patient is always entered in Medisoft in the Name/Address tab. When the patient is not the policyholder, information about the guarantor must also be entered in the Medisoft database for insurance claims to be processed. This information is collected from the patient information or patient update form.

Assigned Provider   The Assigned Provider drop-down list contains codes assigned to the doctors in the practice (see Figure 4-8). The code for the specific doctor who provides care to this patient is selected.

guarantor an individual who may not be a patient of the practice, but who is financially responsible for a patient account

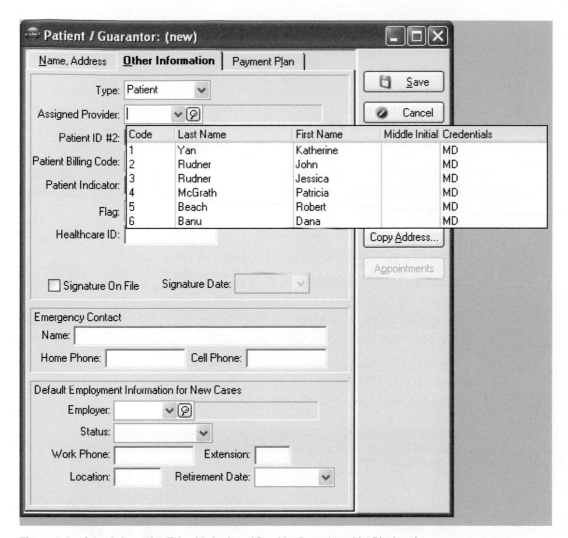

Figure 4-8 Other Information Tab with Assigned Provider Drop-down List Displayed

Patient ID #2 The Patient ID #2 box is used by some medical practices as a second identification system in addition to chart numbers.

Patient Billing Code The Patient Billing Code is an optional field used to categorize patients according to the billing codes that the practice has set up in Medisoft. For example, Billing Code A might be for patients with insurance coverage, B for cash patients, and so on. Some practices use billing codes to classify patients according to a billing cycle—patients with Billing Code A are billed on the first of the month, and those with Billing Code B on the fifteenth of the month.

Patient Indicator The Patient Indicator is an optional field that practices can use to classify types of patients, such as workers' compensation patients, cash patients, and diabetic patients.

Flag This field can be used to organize patients into groups and assign a color code to each group. In this text/workbook, the flag is assigned to patients' insurance plans.

Healthcare ID The Healthcare ID is not used at present; it is included for future implementation of the HIPAA legislation.

Signature on File A check mark in the Signature on File check box means that the patient's signature is on file for the purpose of submitting insurance claims. This box must be completed. If it is not, the insurance carrier will not accept and process insurance claims. The signature is usually found on the patient information form.

Signature Date The date keyed in the Signature Date box is the date the patient signed the insurance release form. The date is also found on the patient information form.

Emergency Contact Information about how to contact someone in case of a patient emergency is entered in these fields.

Employer The code for the patient's employer is selected from the drop-down list of employers in the database (see Figure 4-9). If the patient's employer is not in the database, this information must be entered before the code can be selected. (This process is described later in the chapter.)

Status The Status drop-down list displays the following choices for the patient's employment status: Not employed, Full time, Part time, Retired, and Unknown.

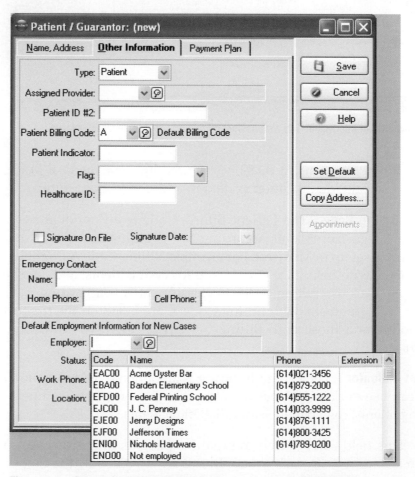

Figure 4-9 Other Information Tab with Employer Drop-down List Displayed

Work Phone and Extension   Work phone numbers should be entered without parentheses or hyphens.

Location   Some companies have multiple locations. If the patient supplies information on the specific company location, it is entered in this box.

Retirement Date   The Retirement Date box is filled in only if the patient is already retired. Retirement dates should be entered in the MMDDCCYY format.

When all of the fields in the Name, Address tab and the Other Information tab have been filled in, entries should be checked for accuracy. If any information needs to be corrected, it can easily be changed. Once the information has been checked and necessary corrections made, it is saved by clicking the Save button.

PAYMENT PLAN TAB

The Payment Plan tab is used when a patient's account is overdue and a payment plan has been created to pay down the remaining balance (see Figure 4-10).

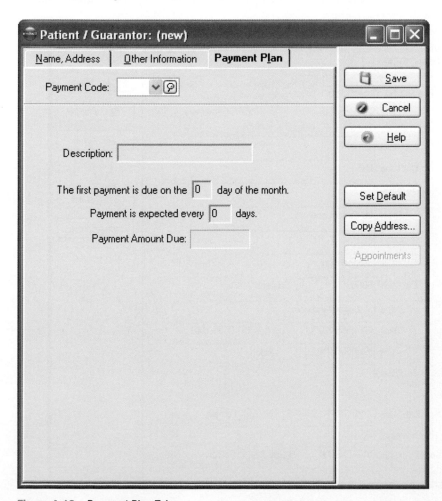

Figure 4-10   Payment Plan Tab

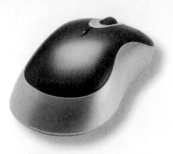

Using Source Document 1 (located in Part 4 of this book), complete the Patient/Guarantor dialog box for Hiro Tanaka, a new patient of Dr. Yan.

1. Start Medisoft by clicking the Start button and selecting All Programs, Medisoft, Medisoft Advanced.

2. On the Lists menu, click Patients/Guarantors and Cases, or click the corresponding shortcut button on the toolbar.

3. Scroll down the list of patients to make sure Hiro Tanaka is not already in the patient database.

4. Click the New Patient button.

5. Create a chart number for this patient. Remember, in this text/workbook, the chart number should be the first five letters of the patient's last name, followed by the first two letters of the patient's first name, followed by a Ø. Click the Chart Number box, and enter the chart number. *Note:* You do not need to enter the chart number in capital letters; the program automatically capitalizes your entry. Press the Tab key twice to advance to the Last Name field.

6. Enter the patient's last name, first name, etc. Fill in the rest of the boxes for which you have data on the Name, Address tab, pressing the Tab key to move from box to box. Check your work against Figure 4-11.

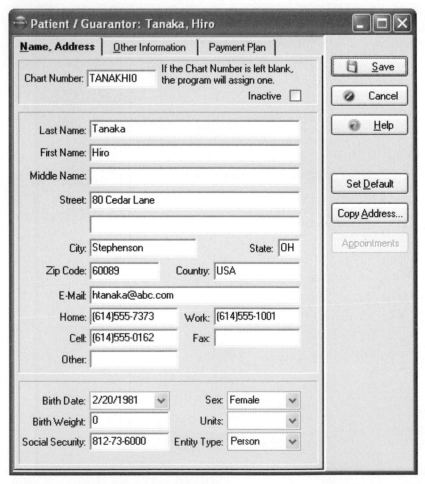

Figure 4-11   Name, Address Tab Completed

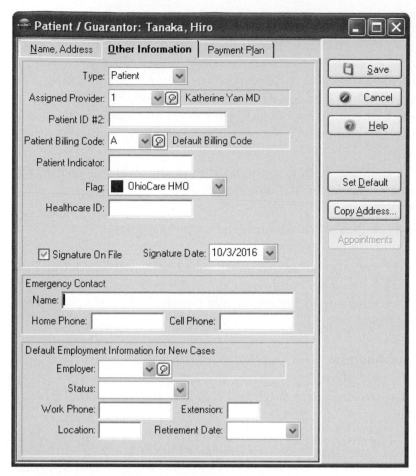

Figure 4-12 Other Information Tab Completed

7. Click the Other Information tab. Be sure to select an Assigned Provider (Dr. Yan is Tanaka's assigned provider) so the exercises in this chapter will work.

8. Select Tanaka's insurance carrier in the Flag field.

9. Make no entries in the following boxes: Patient ID #2, Patient Indicator, Healthcare ID, and Emergency Contact boxes. Accept the default entry in the Patient Billing Code box. Click the Signature on File box and enter **10/03/2016** as the Signature Date. A Confirm box appears, stating that you have entered a future date and asking whether you want to change it. Click No. A Warning box is displayed, stating that the date entered is in the future. Click OK.

10. Since Tanaka's employer is not in the database, leave the employer boxes blank for now.

11. Check your entries against Figure 4-12, and make corrections if necessary.

12. Click the Save button to save the data on Tanaka.

13. Verify that Tanaka has been added to the list in the Patient List dialog box.

14. Close the Patient List dialog box. **ᴄiMᴏ**

✓ **You have completed Exercise 4-2.**

ADDING AN EMPLOYER TO THE ADDRESS LIST

If the patient's employer does not appear on the Employer drop-down list in the Other Information tab, it must be entered using the Address feature. Addresses are entered by clicking the Addresses command on the Lists menu, which displays the Address List dialog box (see Figure 4-13) and clicking the New button.

Clicking the New button at the bottom of the Address List dialog box displays the Address dialog box (see Figure 4-14).

The Address dialog box contains the following boxes.

Code The code for an employer should begin with the letter *E* to indicate that this is an employer. Codes can be a combination of letters and numbers up to a maximum of five characters. If a code is not assigned, the system will assign one.

Name and Address The employer's name is entered in the Name box. This field allows up to thirty characters. The employer's street, city, state (two characters only), and ZIP code are entered in the boxes provided.

Type The Type drop-down list displays a list of kinds of addresses: Attorney, Employer, Miscellaneous, and Referral Source. For example, when the address being entered is that of an employer, "Employer" is selected.

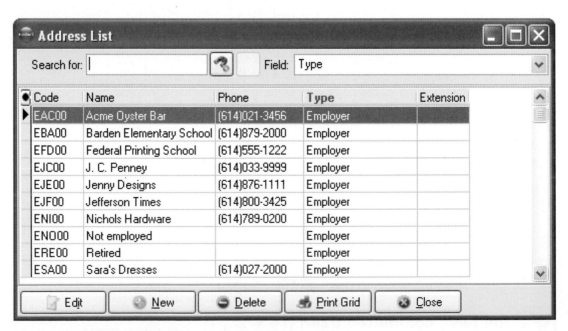

Figure 4-13 Address List Dialog Box

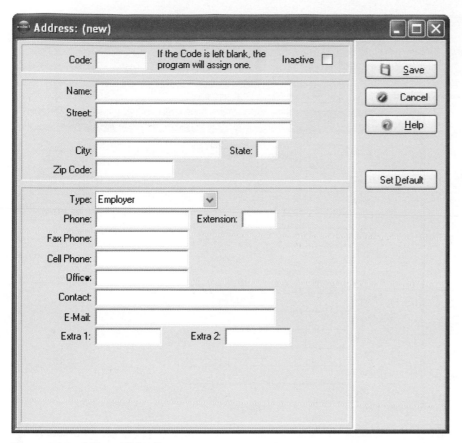

Figure 4-14　Address Dialog Box

Phone, Extension, Fax Phone, Cell Phone　In the Phone box, the employer's phone number is entered, without parentheses or hyphens. If there is an extension, it is entered in the Extension box. If there is a cell phone, it is entered in the Cell Phone box. The employer's fax number is entered in the Fax Phone box.

Office　This field can be used to note a particular office within an organization.

Contact　The Contact box is used to enter the name of an individual at the place of employment. If there is no contact person, the box is left blank.

E-Mail　This box provides a field for the employer's e-mail address.

Extra 1, Extra 2　The Extra 1 and Extra 2 boxes are available to keep track of additional information that needs to be recorded and stored for future reference.

When all the information on the employer has been entered, it is saved by clicking the Save button.

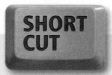

ENTERING DATA WITH F8

Throughout Medisoft, the F8 function key serves as a shortcut for entering data. For example, clicking once in the Employer box on the Other Information tab and then pressing F8 brings up the Address dialog box, in which a new employer can be entered. The F8 key shortcut enables users to enter data in Medisoft in another part of the program without leaving the current dialog box. Once the F8 key is pressed, the dialog box used to enter new addresses is opened, with the Patient List and Patient/Guarantor dialog boxes still open in the background (see Figure 4-15).

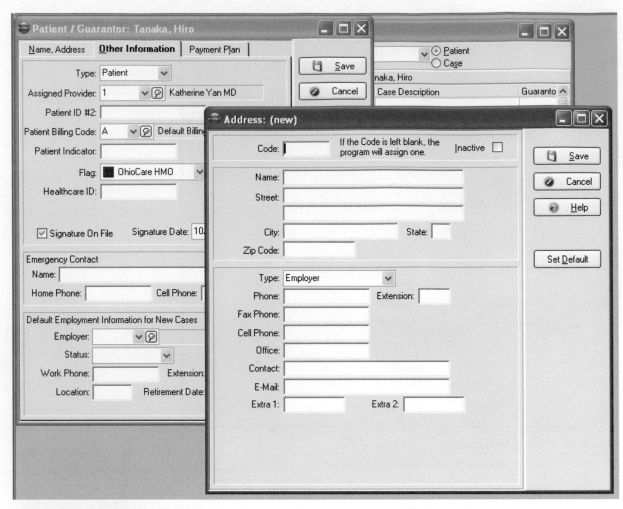

Figure 4-15 Address Dialog Box with Patient List and Patient/Guarantor Boxes Visible in Background

---

EXERCISE 4-3   ADDING AN EMPLOYER

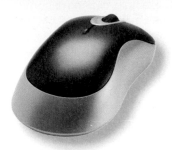

Practice entering information about an employer.

1. Click Addresses on the Lists menu. The Address List dialog box is displayed.

2. Click the New button at the bottom of the dialog box. The Address dialog box is displayed.

3. In the Code box, key **EMCØØ** for McCray Manufacturing, Inc. (**E** for employer, followed by the first two letters of the employer's name, followed by two zeros). Press the Tab key twice.

4. Key **McCray Manufacturing Inc.** in the Name box. Press the Tab key.

5. In the Street box, key **1311 Kings Highway**. Press the Tab key twice.

6. Key **Stephenson** in the City box. Press the Tab key.

7. Key **OH** in the State box. Press the Tab key.

8. Key **60089** in the Zip Code box. Press the Tab key.

9. Verify that Employer is displayed in the Type box. If it is not, click Employer in the drop-down list, and press the Tab key.

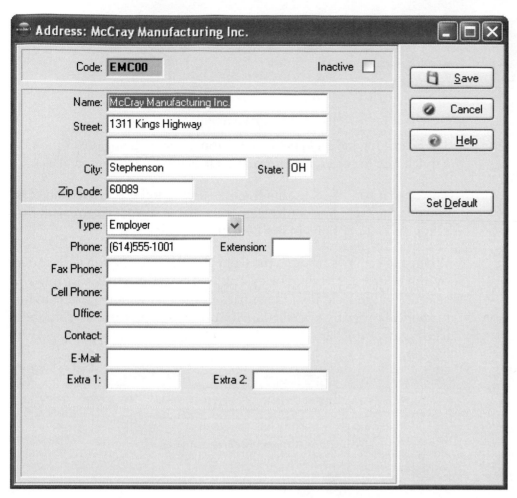

Figure 4-16 Address Tab Completed

10. Key **6145551001** in the Phone box. Press the Tab key.

11. Leave the remaining boxes blank. Check your work against Figure 4-16.

12. Click the Save button to store the information you have entered.

13. Click the Close button to exit the Address List dialog box.

✓ **You have completed Exercise 4-3.**

4.3 SEARCHING FOR PATIENT INFORMATION

A patient who comes to a medical practice for the first time fills out a patient information form. The information on this form needs to be entered into the Medisoft patient/guarantor database before insurance claims can be submitted. However, before information on a patient is entered into the system, it is important to search the database to be certain that the patient does not already exist there.

Medisoft provides two options for conducting searches: Search for and Field boxes and Locate buttons.

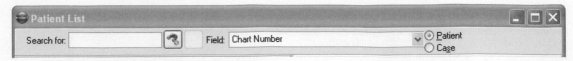

Figure 4-17 Search for and Field Boxes

SEARCH FOR AND FIELD OPTION

The Search for and Field boxes at the top of many dialog boxes provide a quick way to search for information in Medisoft (see Figure 4-17).

The Search for box contains the text that is to be searched on. The entry in the Field box controls how the list is sorted. Figure 4-18 displays the Field options in the Patient List dialog box.

When a selection is made in the Field box, the information is re-sorted by the selected criteria. For example, if Social Security Number is selected in the Field box, the entries in the List window are listed in numerical order by Social Security number, from lowest to highest (see Figure 4-19).

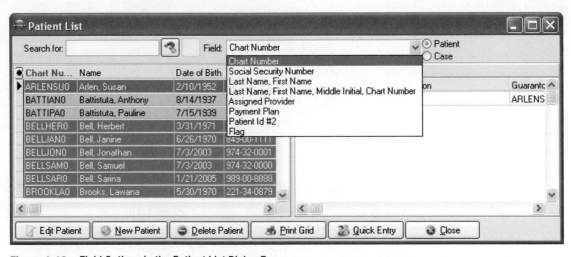

Figure 4-18 Field Options in the Patient List Dialog Box

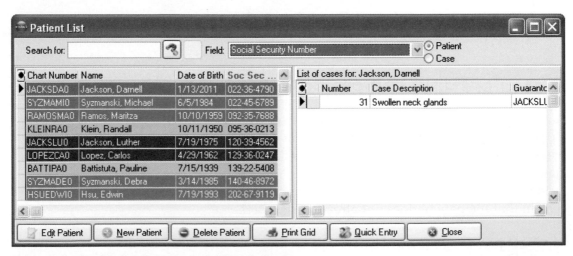

Figure 4-19 List Window Sorted by Social Security Number

TABLE 4-1	Field Options for Medisoft Searches
List Window	**Field Options**
Patient List	Chart Number; Social Security Number; Last Name, First Name; Last Name, First Name, Middle Initial, Chart Number; Assigned Provider; Payment Plan; Patient ID #2; Flag
Insurance Carrier List	Code, Name
Procedure/Payment/ Adjustment List	Type, Description, Code 1
Diagnosis Code List	Description, Code 1
Address List	Type, Code, Name
Provider List	Code; Last Name, First Name
Referring Provider List	Code; Last Name, First Name

The Search for and Field feature is used in the following Medisoft dialog boxes: Patient List, Insurance Carrier List, Procedure/ Payment/Adjustment List, Diagnosis Code List, Address List, Provider List, and Referring Provider List. Table 4-1 displays the Field box options for each of these Medisoft dialog boxes.

After an entry is made in the Field box, the search criteria are entered in the Search field. As each letter or number is entered, the list automatically filters out records that do not match. For example, if the Field box is set to Last Name, First Name in the Patient List dialog box and *S* is entered in the Search field, the program eliminates all data from the list except patients whose last names begin with *S* (see Figure 4-20).

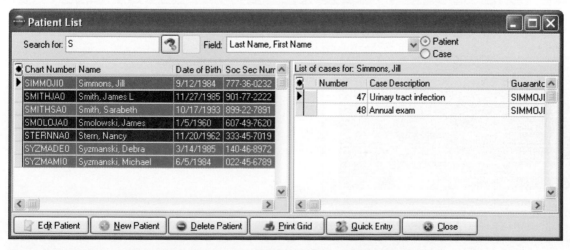

Figure 4-20   Patient List Dialog Box with Search for Patients Whose Last Names Begin with *S*

To restore the Patient list to its default setting (all patients listed), delete the entry in the Search for box.

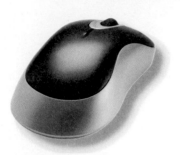

EXERCISE 4-4	SEARCH USING FIELD BOX

Use the Search feature to locate information on James Smolowski.

1. On the Lists menu, click Patients/Guarantors and Cases, or click the corresponding shortcut button. The Patient List dialog box is displayed, and the cursor is blinking in the Search for box. Confirm that the entry in the Field box is Last Name, First Name.

2. Enter the first letter of the patient's last name. Notice that when you keyed *S*, the list window filtered the data so that only patients whose last names begin with *S* are listed. Now enter the second letter of his last name, **m**. The list now displays only those patients whose last names begin with the letters *Sm*. Now enter the third letter, **o**. Smolowski is the only patient whose name begins with the letters *Smo,* so he is the only patient listed.

3. To restore the Patient window so that all patients are listed, delete the letters entered in the Search for box.

4. Click the Close button to exit the Patient List dialog box. **CiMO**

 You have completed Exercise 4-4.

LOCATE BUTTONS OPTION

Another option for finding information in Medisoft is to use the Locate buttons (see Figure 4-21).

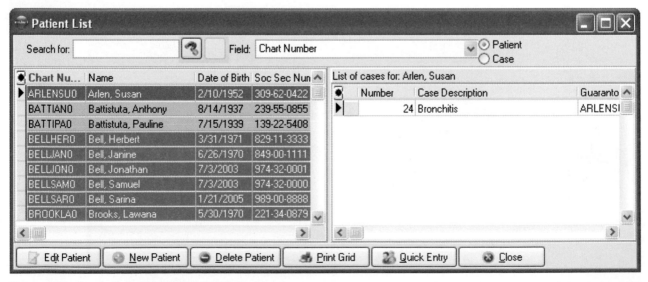

Figure 4-21   Locate Button Highlighted in Yellow

When a Locate button is clicked, a Locate dialog box is displayed. Figure 4-22 shows the Locate Patient dialog box.

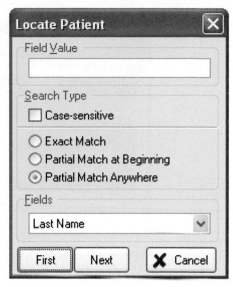

Field Value

The information entered in the Field Value box at the top of the window can be part of a name, birth date, payment date or amount, or assigned provider. Any combination of numbers and letters can be used.

Search Type

Case-Sensitive Use to make the search sensitive to uppercase or lowercase letters.

Exact Match Use when an entry in the Field Value box is exactly as entered in the program.

Figure 4-22 Locate Patient Dialog Box

Partial Match at Beginning Use when unsure of the correct spelling or entry at the end of the word.

Partial Match Anywhere Use when unsure of the correct spelling or entry.

Fields

The Fields box provides a drop-down list from which to choose the field that contains the information that is being matched. For example, if searching for a patient by last name, select the Last Name field. The available fields are determined by the type of information you are working with. For example, if you are looking for a particular chart number, you have nineteen fields from which to choose as the basis of your search. Searching for cases gives access to up to ninety-one fields.

Once the criteria are selected, clicking the First button starts a search for the first match to the criteria. If a match is found, the Locate window is closed, and the search result is highlighted in the Search window. If a match is not found, a message is displayed.

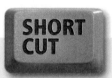

SEARCHING WITH LOCATE WINDOW

To make searching easier, right-click a column heading in a window that contains several columns. From the shortcut menu that appears, select Locate, or press CTRL + L. This opens a Locate window that defaults the Fields selection to the column you selected.

| SEARCH USING LOCATE BUTTON | EXERCISE 4-5 |

Practice searching for and editing information on Hiro Tanaka.

1. Open the Patient List dialog box.

2. Click the Locate button to the right of the Search for field. The Locate Patient dialog box appears.

3. Enter **TANAKA** in the Field Value box.

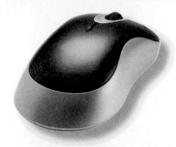

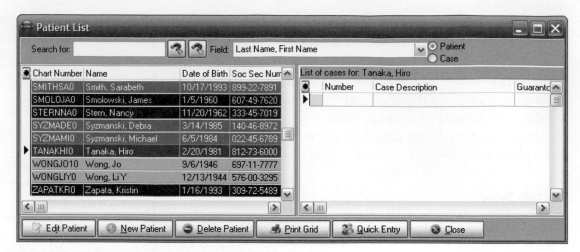

Figure 4-23 Selection Triangle Pointing to Hiro Tanaka

4. The Case-sensitive field should not be checked.

5. The Partial Match Anywhere button should be selected.

6. The Field drop-down list should be set to Last Name.

7. Click the First button. In the left side of the Patient List dialog box, the selection triangle should be pointing at Tanaka, Hiro (see Figure 4-23).

8. Keep this Patient List window open, since you will use it to edit Hiro Tanaka's information in Exercise 4-6. **ciMc**

 You have completed Exercise 4-5.

4.4 EDITING PATIENT INFORMATION

From time to time, patients notify the practice that they have moved, changed jobs or insurance carriers, and so on. When this happens, information needs to be updated in Medisoft's patient/guarantor database.

The process of changing information about a patient is similar to that of entering information for a new patient. The Patients/Guarantors and Cases command is selected from the Lists menu. A search is usually performed to locate the chart number of the patient whose record needs to be updated. Clicking the Edit button displays the Patient/Guarantor dialog box, where changes can be made. Clicking the Save button stores the changes.

Practice searching for and editing information on Hiro Tanaka.

1. With the Patient List window still open to Hiro Tanaka, click the Edit Patient button.

2. Click the Other Information tab.

3. Click the down arrow button in the Employer box. Click McCray Manufacturing Inc. on the drop-down list. Notice that the program automatically enters the phone number in the Work Phone box.

4. Select Full time from the Status drop-down list.

5. Click the Save button to store the information you have entered.

6. Close the Patient List dialog box.

 You have completed Exercise 4-6.

APPLYING YOUR SKILLS

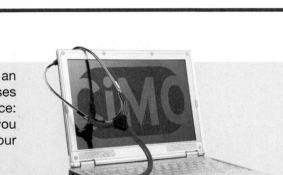

At the end of each chapter, you will apply what you have learned in an Applying Your Skills exercise. This exercise is similar to the exercises you completed throughout the chapter, with one important difference: step-by-step instructions are not provided. You must rely on what you learned and practiced in the chapter to complete the Applying Your Skills exercise.

1: ENTERING A NEW PATIENT

Lisa Wright is a new patient who has just arrived for her office visit with her primary care provider, Dr. Jessica Rudner. Using Source Document 2, complete the Name, Address tab and the Other Information tab in the Patient/Guarantor dialog box. (*Note:* Not all text boxes will have entries.)

Remember to create a backup of your work before exiting Medisoft! To help you keep track of your work, name the backup file after the chapter you are working on, for example, StudentID-c4.mbk.

ELECTRONIC HEALTH RECORD EXCHANGE

Transferring Patient Information

Some practice management programs and electronic health record programs are able to exchange patient information. This saves time and reduces errors, since patient information is entered in one program and then transferred to the other, eliminating the need to enter the information twice.

Patient information in Medisoft, such as that displayed in the illustration below, is transferred to an electronic health record program.

(continued)

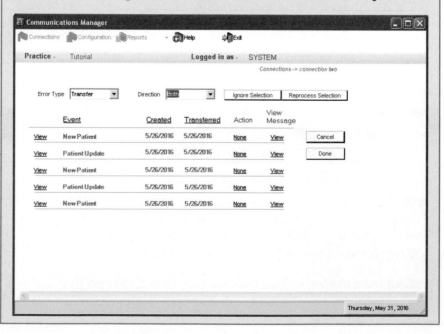

The next illustration shows a list of patient information that has been received by Medisoft from an electronic health record program. As you can see, the list includes information on new patients as well as updated information about established patients.

Name: _____ Date: _____

After completing all the exercises in the chapter, answer the following questions in the spaces provided.

1. What is entered in the Chart Number field for Hiro Tanaka (Name, Address tab)?

_____

2. Which patient is found as a result of the search in Exercise 4-4?

_____

3. Which patient is found as a result of the search in Exercise 4-5?

_____

4. What is the entry in the Employer field for Hiro Tanaka (Other Information tab)?

_____

5. What is the entry in the Signature Date box for Hiro Tanaka (Other Information tab)?

_____

6. What is entered in the Chart Number field for Lisa Wright (Name, Address tab)?

_____

7. What is entered in the Flag field for Lisa Wright (Other Information tab)?

_____

8. What is entered in the Work Phone field for Hiro Tanaka (Other Information tab)?

_____

9. What is entered in the Status field for Lisa Wright (Other Information tab)?

_____

10. What is entered in the Birth Date field for Lisa Wright (Name, Address tab)?

_____

cIMO
chapter summary

4.1 Explain how patient information is organized in Medisoft. Pages 108–109	Patient information is accessed through the Patient List dialog box. This box is displayed when the Patients/Guarantors and Cases option is clicked on the Lists menu or when the shortcut button is clicked on the toolbar.
	
	The Patient List dialog box has two primary sections:
	- Patient
	   The left side of the window displays information about patients.
	- Cases
	   The right side of the window contains information about cases.

4.2 Discuss how a new patient is added in Medisoft. Pages 109–121	1. Click Patients/Guarantors and Cases on the Lists menu. 2. Click the New Patient button. 3. Complete the Name, Address and Other Information tabs. 4. Click the Save button.
4.3 Describe how to search for a patient in Medisoft. Pages 121–126	There are two ways of searching for a patient in Medisoft. 1. In the Patient List dialog box, enter a search term in the Search for box and make a corresponding selection in the Field box. 2. In the Patient List dialog box, click the Locate button. In the Locate Patient box that appears, enter a search term or number in the Field Value field, and make appropriate selections in the remaining fields. When finished making selections, click the First button to display the first record that matches the search.
4.4 Describe how patient information is edited in Medisoft. Pages 126–127	Information about a patient is edited in the same way it is entered. To edit patient information, select Patients/Guarantors and Cases on the Lists menu. A search is usually performed to locate the chart number of the patient whose record needs to be updated. Clicking the Edit button displays the Patient/Guarantor dialog box, where changes can be made. Clicking the Save button stores the changes.

USING TERMINOLOGY

Define the terms in the space provided.

1. *[LO 4.2]* chart number

2. *[LO 4.2]* established patient

3. *[LO 4.2]* guarantor

4. *[LO 4.2]* new patient

CHECKING YOUR UNDERSTANDING

Answer the questions below in the space provided.

1. *[LO 4.3]* To search for Paul Ramos, can you key either "Paul" or "Ramos"? Explain.

2. *[LO 4.2]* Create a chart number for a patient named William Burroughs.

3. *[LO 4.2]* Sam Wu has no insurance of his own but is covered by his wife's insurance policy. How would you indicate this in the Patient/Guarantor dialog box?

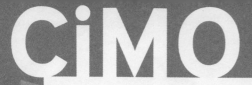

4. *[LO 4.4]* A patient's phone number has changed. How would you replace the existing phone number in Medisoft?

_____

_____

5. *[LO 4.2]* How would you enter the Social Security number 123-45-6789?

_____

_____

APPLYING YOUR KNOWLEDGE

Answer the following question in the space provided.

4.1. *[LO 4.2, 4.3]* Jane Taylor-Burke comes to the office. She thinks she saw Dr. Yan a few years ago for a flu shot, but she is not sure. You need to decide whether to enter Ms. Taylor-Burke as a new patient in the Medisoft database. What should you do?

_____

_____

THINKING ABOUT IT

Answer the questions below in the space provided.

4.1. *[LO 4.1]* Why does each patient need to be assigned a chart number?

_____

_____

4.2. *[LO 4.1]* Why are guarantors entered in Medisoft when they are not patients of the practice?

_____

_____

AT THE COMPUTER

Answer the following questions at the computer.

4.1. *[LO 4.3]* How many patients in the database have the last name of Smith?

_____

_____

4.2. *[LO 4.3]* What is the name of the patient who is found when you search for the letters *JO*?

_____

_____

4.3. *[LO 4.2, 4.3]* What is Li Y. Wong's chart number?

_____

_____

4.4. *[LO 4.3]* In the Patient List dialog box, search for information on Leila Patterson. What steps did you take to find the information?

_____

_____

chapter
5

Working with Cases

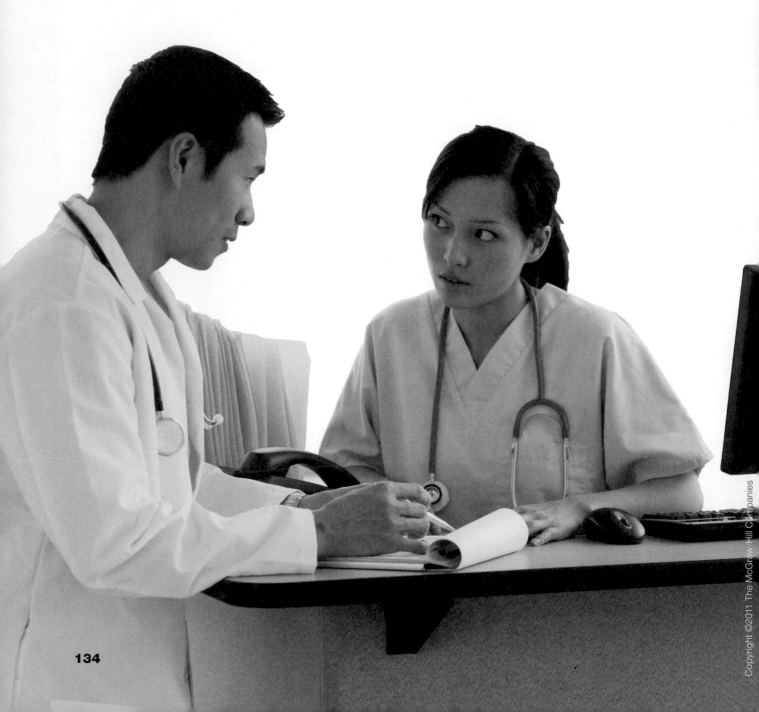

key terms

capitated plan

case

chart

primary insurance carrier

record of treatment and
 progress

referring provider

sponsor

learning outcomes

When you finish this chapter, you will be able to:

5.1 Describe when it is necessary to create a new case in Medisoft.

5.2 List the eleven tabs in the Case dialog box.

5.3 Review the information contained in the Personal tab and the Account tab.

5.4 Discuss the information recorded in the Policy 1, 2, 3, and Medicaid and Tricare tabs in Medisoft.

5.5 Describe the information contained in the Diagnosis tab and the Condition tab in Medisoft.

5.6 Review the purpose of the Miscellaneous, Comment, and EDI tabs in Medisoft.

5.7 Describe how to edit information in a case.

what you need to know

To use this chapter you need to know how to:

- Use the Medisoft Search feature.
- Enter patient information in Medisoft.
- Locate and change information about an established patient.

5.1 UNDERSTANDING CASES

case a grouping of transactions that share a common element

Each time a physician treats a patient, a record is made of the encounter. The information in the record is used to document the patient's medical condition, and also to bill for services. In Medisoft®, this information is entered and stored in a **case,** which is a grouping of transactions that share a common element. These transactions represent the services and treatments that the physician provided to the patient during the visit. To receive payment, the office must transmit these transactions to the patient's insurance carrier in the form of an insurance claim.

WHEN TO SET UP A NEW CASE

Most often, transactions are grouped into cases based on the medical condition for which a patient seeks treatment. For example, if a patient has a chronic condition such as diabetes, charges for all visits related to diabetes are stored in one case. If the same patient also has hypertension, all visits for treatment of hypertension are stored in another case. Patients with chronic conditions often have many transactions in a single case.

On the other hand, a patient may require more than one case per office visit if treatment is provided for two or more unrelated conditions. For example, a patient who visits the physician complaining of migraine headaches may also ask for an influenza vaccination. Since the two conditions are unrelated, two cases would need to be created: one for the migraine headaches, and one for the vaccination. In contrast, a patient who is treated for shortness of breath and chest pain during exertion would require one case if the physician determines that the two complaints are related to the same diagnosis.

In these examples just described, it is the patient's medical condition that determines whether more than one case is needed, since each different medical condition requires its own case. There are other instances when a separate case must be created, such as a change in insurance. When a patient changes insurance plans, a new case is set up, even if the same condition is being treated. This makes it easier to submit insurance claims to the appropriate carrier. Transactions that took place while the previous policy was in effect must be submitted under that policy. Transactions that occur after the change in policies must be submitted to the new carrier. By opening a new case, transactions for the two insurance carriers can be kept separate. The information needed to submit claims to the previous carrier is still intact, while information for claims under the new policy is current.

Similarly, when a patient is injured at work and is treated under workers' compensation insurance, a new case must be created so that the claims are billed to the workers' compensation plan, not to the patient's personal policy.

CASE EXAMPLES

The following scenarios provide examples of when new cases are—and are not—required.

Example 1

Among Dr. Yan's patients today is Josephine Tremblay, a Medicare patient. Josephine has a number of chronic health conditions, including diabetes, arthritis, hypertension, and asthma. She has four cases already set up in Medisoft, one for each of her chronic conditions. Today she is seeing Dr. Yan because she is experiencing lower back pain. From this information alone, we cannot determine whether to create a new case, since the back pain may be due to one of her existing conditions. When the billing assistant reviews the electronic encounter form, she sees that Dr. Yan has diagnosed Mrs. Tremblay with lower back pain due to arthritis. Since arthritis is one of Mrs. Tremblay's existing cases, no new case is needed.

Example 2

Dr. Jessica Rudner has just finished examining Kimberly DeJong. Ms. DeJong is a twenty-five-year-old woman who has an existing case for rosacea, a chronic skin condition. Today, Ms. DeJong received an antimalarial prescription in preparation for her travel to India. Since this visit is not related to her existing case for rosacea, a new case will be created.

Example 3

Jose Gonzales has been a patient of Dr. John Rudner for three months. During that time, he was diagnosed with hypertension and started on medication. He has come in today for a follow-up visit, to see how well the medication is working. The front desk staff asks him if any information has changed since his last visit, and he indicates that he changed jobs and has a new health plan. Even though he is being treated for the same condition (hypertension), claims for today's visit must be sent to the new insurance carrier. To ensure that today's charges are submitted to the new carrier, a new case must be created.

Example 4

David Weber is the seven-year-old son of Marcia and Ronald Weber, who are divorced. David has not been seen by Dr. Yan except for routine immunizations each year before school starts. David has been covered by his father's insurance plan since the divorce. David's father recently lost his job, and David is now covered by his mother's health plan. Today, David's father has brought him in for his annual immunizations. A new case must be created even though David has an existing case for annual immunizations, because he is covered by a different insurance plan. If a new case were not created, the charges would be submitted to the insurance plan listed in the existing case, and the claim would be rejected.

5.2 NAVIGATING CASES IN MEDISOFT

In Chapter 4, you learned that certain patient information is stored in the Patient/Guarantor dialog box. The data stored in the Patient/Guarantor dialog box is primarily demographic, including a patient's name, address, date of birth, Social Security number, employer, and so on.

The information about a patient's medical conditions and treatments—including the diagnosis, procedures, provider, and insurance plan—is stored in the Case dialog box. The same Patient List dialog box that you worked with in Chapter 4 is used to access the Case dialog box. It is accessed by choosing Patients/Guarantors and Cases from the Lists menu.

CASE COMMAND BUTTONS

When the Case radio button in the Patient List dialog box is clicked, the following command buttons appear at the bottom of the Patient List dialog box: Edit Case, New Case, Delete Case, Copy Case, Print Grid, Quick Entry, and Close (see Figure 5-1).

Edit Case   The Edit Case button is used to add, delete, or change information in an existing case. When the Edit Case button is clicked, the Case dialog box is displayed. Case information to be updated is contained in eleven different tabs. For example, if a patient gets married, information needs to be updated in the Personal tab. The only item in the Case dialog box that cannot be changed is the case number. All other boxes are edited by moving the cursor to the box and making the change, whether this involves rekeying, selecting and deselecting check boxes, or clicking a different option on a drop-down list.

New Case   The New Case button creates a new case.

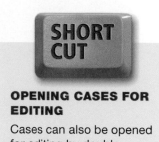

OPENING CASES FOR EDITING

Cases can also be opened for editing by double clicking on the case number/description in the Case window within the Patient List dialog box.

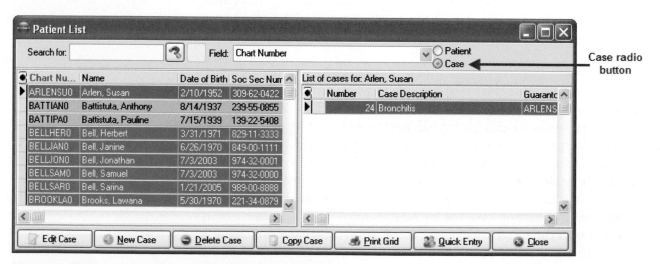

Figure 5-1   Patient List Dialog Box with Case Radio Button Selected

Delete Case   The Delete Case button deletes a case from the system if the case has no open transactions. Open transactions are charges that have not been fully paid by the insurance carrier or the policyholder. The Delete Case button should be used with caution; once deleted, information cannot be retrieved. Cases should be deleted only when it is definite that the patient's records will never be needed again. Medical offices usually have policies about when a patient's records are deleted, such as five years after the patient's last visit to the practice. In most instances, it is more appropriate to close a case than to delete it. Cases are closed by clicking the Case Closed box in the Personal tab of the Case dialog box.

Cases are deleted in the Patient List dialog box. With the Case radio button clicked, the specific case to be deleted is selected by clicking the line that displays the case number and description. The case is then deleted by clicking the Delete Case button at the bottom of the dialog box. The system will ask, "Are you sure you want to delete this case?" Clicking the Yes button deletes the case from the system.

Copy Case   The Copy Case button copies all the information from an existing case into a new case. This feature is useful when creating a new case for a patient who already has a case in the system. Copy Case makes it unnecessary to reenter the information in all eleven tabs; instead, the information in the existing case is copied into a new case. Then the information that needs to be changed can be edited to reflect the new case. Sometimes the new case requires few changes; other times data must be changed in all the tabs of the Case folder. For this reason, when copying a case it is important to check each tab to make sure the copied information is accurate for the new case. The information that remains the same from the previous case can be left as is.

Print Grid   The Print Grid button is used to select or deselect columns of information for printing purposes.

Quick Entry   The Quick Entry button is used in practices that customize the way patient data are entered.

Close   The Close button closes the Patient List dialog box.

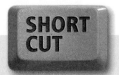

SHORT CUT

USING COPY CASE
When creating a new case for an established patient, it is faster to use the Copy Case button than to create a new case using the New Case button.

THE CASE DIALOG BOX

Clicking the New Case button brings up the Case dialog box (see Figure 5-2). Information about a patient is entered in eleven different tabs in the Case dialog box:

1. Personal
2. Account
3. Diagnosis
4. Policy 1
5. Policy 2

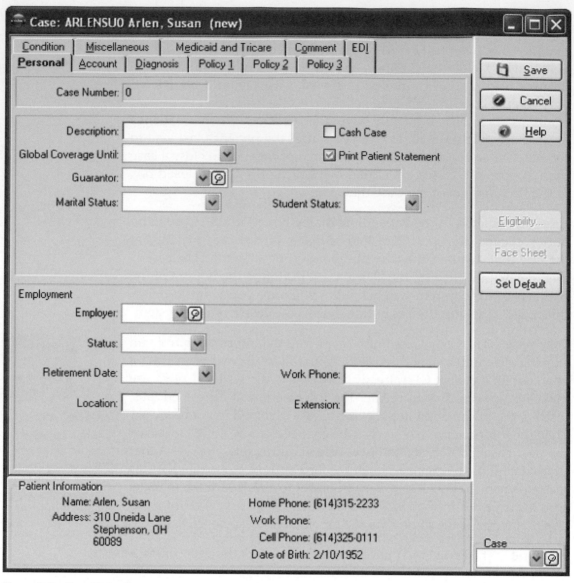

Figure 5-2 Case Dialog Box

6. Policy 3

7. Condition

8. Miscellaneous

9. Medicaid and Tricare

10. Comment

11. EDI

chart a folder that contains all records pertaining to a patient

The information required to complete the eleven tabs comes from documents found in a patient's chart. The **chart** is a folder that contains all records pertaining to a patient. The new patient information form supplies basic information, such as name and address, as well as information about insurance coverage, allergies, whether the condition is related to an accident, and the referral source. The **record of treatment and progress** contains the physician's notes about a patient's condition and diagnosis. The encounter form is a list of services performed and the charges for them.

record of treatment and progress a physician's notes about a patient's condition and diagnosis

Several buttons are located on the right side of the Case folder. These buttons are

Save   Saves the information entered in the dialog box.

Cancel   Closes the dialog box and discards any information entered.

Help   Displays the Medisoft help window for the Case folder.

Eligibility   Displays an option to verify eligibility for the patient and case.

Face Sheet   Prints a sheet of information about the patient and case.

Set Default   Sets the information in the case as the default for new cases for this patient. To remove the default, hold down the CTRL key, and this button changes to a Remove Default button.

Case   Displays a list of the patient's cases.

5.3 ENTERING PATIENT AND ACCOUNT INFORMATION

The Personal tab and the Account tab contain basic information about the patient, such as name, address, date of birth, marital status, and employment status. Much of the information is filled in by the program, using the information already entered in the Patient/Guarantor dialog box. The Account tab lists the patient's assigned provider, referral source, authorized number of visits, and more.

PERSONAL TAB

The Personal tab contains basic information about a patient and his or her employment (see Figure 5-3).

Case Number   The case number is a sequential number assigned by Medisoft. To avoid confusion, case numbers are unique; no two patients ever have the same case number.

Case Closed   A case is marked as closed by placing a check mark in the Case Closed box. At times it is appropriate to close a case. Closing a case indicates that no more data will be entered into the case. When is it appropriate to close a case? Policies vary from practice to practice, but generally cases are closed when a patient changes insurance carriers, has recovered completely from a condition (such as the flu), or is no longer a patient at the practice. *Note:* The Case Closed box does not appear until a case is created and saved.

Description   Information entered in the Description box indicates a patient's complaint, or reason for seeing a physician. For example, if a

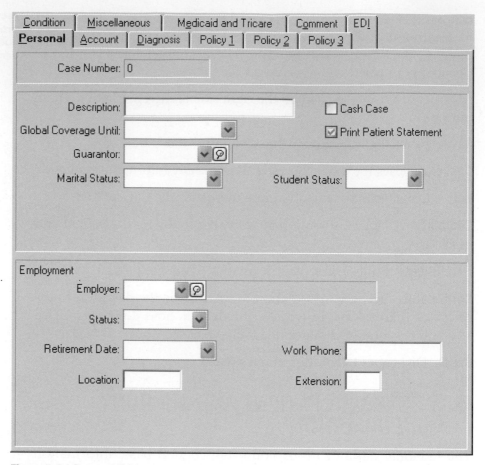

Figure 5-3 Personal Tab

patient comes to see a physician for an annual physical examination, the Description box would read "annual physical." Other examples of entries are sore throat, stomach pains, dog bite, and accident at work. A patient's complaint can be found in his or her chart.

Cash Case   If the Cash Case box is checked, the patient is paying cash and has no insurance coverage.

Global Coverage Until   Certain services are paid for under what are known as "global fees." These fees include reimbursement for services performed at different times by the same provider (or group) when performed in conjunction with one medical procedure or episode of care. For example, preoperative, intraoperative, and post-operative services are included in the single payment for a global surgical procedure. The entry in this field indicates the date on which charges are no longer considered part of the global fee.

Print Patient Statement   If this box is checked, a statement for the patient is automatically printed when statements for the practice are printed.

Guarantor   The Guarantor box lists the name of the person responsible for paying the bill. The drop-down list contains the chart numbers and names of all potential guarantors in the database.

Marital Status   The drop-down list provides the following choices to indicate a patient's marital status: Divorced, Legally separated, Married, Single, Unknown, or Widowed.

Student Status   The Student Status drop-down list is used to indicate whether a patient is a full-time student, a part-time student, or a non-student. If a patient's status is not known, the box should be left blank.

Employer   The Employer box contains the default employer information that has been entered in the Patient/Guarantor dialog box. If it is necessary to change the employer, the default can be overridden by clicking another employer code on the drop-down list.

Status   The Status box lists a patient's employment status as recorded in the Patient/Guarantor dialog box. To change the selection that appears in the Status box, another selection is clicked on the drop-down list. The options are Full-time, Not employed, Part-time, Retired, and Unknown.

Retirement Date   The Retirement Date box should be filled in only when a patient is already retired. There are two ways of entering the retirement date. It can be entered in the Retirement Date box, or it can be selected from the pop-up calendar that appears when the triangle button to the right of the box is clicked.

Work Phone   The Work Phone box contains a patient's work phone number.

Location   If a patient has supplied a specific work location, such as "Fifth Avenue Branch," it is entered in the Location box.

Extension   The Extension box lists a patient's work phone extension.

ENTERING DATA IN THE PERSONAL TAB	EXERCISE 5-1

Create a new case for patient Hiro Tanaka, and enter information in the Personal tab. The information needed to complete this exercise is found on Source Document 1.

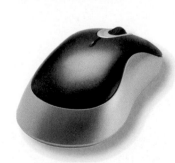

Date: October 3, 2016

1. Start Medisoft and restore the data from your last work session.

2. Change the Medisoft Program Date to the date listed above, October 3, 2016.

3. On the Lists menu, click Patients/Guarantors and Cases. The Patient List dialog box is displayed.

4. Search for Hiro Tanaka by keying *T* in the Search for box. The arrow should point to the entry line for Hiro Tanaka.

5. Click the Case radio button to activate the case portion of the Patient List dialog box.

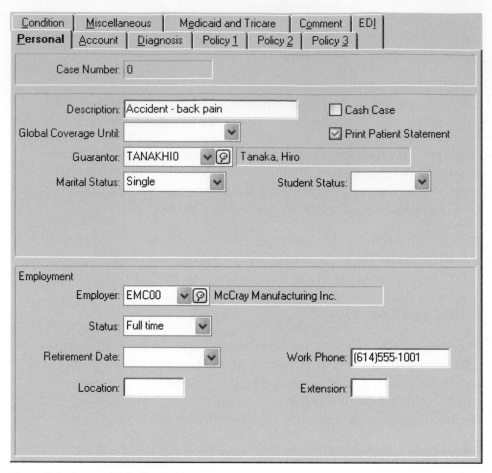

Figure 5-4   Personal Tab, Hiro Tanaka

6. Click the New Case button. The dialog box labeled Case: TANAKHIØ Tanaka, Hiro (new) is displayed. The Personal tab is the current active tab. Notice that some information is already filled in.

7. Enter Tanaka's reason for seeing the doctor in the Description box.

8. Choose the correct entry for Tanaka's marital status from the drop-down list in the Marital Status box. The Student Status box can be left blank.

9. Notice that the information on Tanaka's employment is already filled in. The system copies the information entered in the Patient/Guarantor dialog box to the case file for you.

10. Use the completed Personal tab in Figure 5-4 to check your entries for accuracy.

11. Click the Save button to save the case information you just entered. The Patient List dialog box redisplays. Notice that the case you just created is listed in the right side of the dialog box in the area labeled List of cases for: Tanaka, Hiro.

12. Do not close the Patient List dialog box.

 You have completed Exercise 5-1.

Condition	Miscellaneous		Medicaid and Tricare	Comment	EDI
Personal	**Account**	Diagnosis	Policy 1	Policy 2	Policy 3

Assigned Provider: 1 ⌄ 🔍 Katherine Yan MD

Referring Provider: ⌄ 🔍

Supervising Provider: ⌄ 🔍

Referral Source: ⌄ 🔍

Attorney: ⌄ 🔍

Facility: ⌄ 🔍

Case Billing Code: A ⌄ 🔍 Default Billing Code

Price Code: A   Other Arrangements:

Treatment Authorized Through: ⌄

Visit Series
Authorization Number: Last Visit Date: ⌄

Authorized Number of Visits: 0   ID: Last Visit Number: 0

Figure 5-5   Account Tab

ACCOUNT TAB

The Account tab includes information on a patient's assigned provider, referring provider, and referral source, as well as other information that may be used in some medical practices but not others (see Figure 5-5).

Assigned Provider   The Assigned Provider box is automatically filled in with the code number and name of the assigned provider listed in the Patient/Guarantor dialog box. The drop-down list includes a complete list of providers in the practice. If necessary, the Assigned Provider selection can be changed by clicking another provider on the list.

Referring Provider   A **referring provider** is a physician who recommends that a patient see a specific other physician. The Referring Provider box contains the name of the physician who referred the patient to the practice. The referring provider's name and code are selected from the drop-down list. If the referring provider is not listed on the drop-down list, he or she will need to be added to the Referring Provider list, which is found on the Lists menu. It is not necessary to close the Case dialog box to add a referring provider to the database. To add a new referring provider, click in the Referring Provider box and press the F8 key, or click Referring Providers on

referring provider a physician who recommends that a patient see a specific other physician

the Lists menu. The Referring Provider List dialog box opens in front of the other dialog boxes displayed on the screen, and a new provider can be entered.

Supervising Provider   When the provider rendering services is being supervised by a physician, the supervising physician's information is included on the claim.

Referral Source   If known, the source of a patient's referral is selected from the drop-down list of choices.

Attorney   The Attorney box is used for accident cases. If a patient has an attorney, the name of the attorney should be selected from the drop-down list. If the attorney is not listed, he or she will need to be added to the system by clicking Addresses on the Lists menu and entering information about the attorney.

Facility   The Facility box lists the place where a patient is receiving treatment. A facility is selected from the drop-down list. When necessary, facilities can be added to the database by clicking Facilities on the Lists menu and entering the necessary information.

Case Billing Code   The Case Billing Code box is a one- or two-character box used by some practices to classify and sort patients by insurance carrier, diagnosis, billing cycle, or other kinds of information.

Price Code   The Price Code box determines which set of fees is used when entering transactions for this case. The Price Code fees are entered and stored in the Amounts tab of the Procedure/Payment/Adjustment List dialog box, accessed through the Lists menu.

Other Arrangements   If a special arrangement is made for billing, it is indicated in the Other Arrangements box.

Treatment Authorized Through   A date can be entered in this box if the insurance carrier has authorized treatment only through a certain date.

Visit Series   Information in the Visit Series section of the Account tab is used primarily by psychotherapy practices and chiropractors.

EXERCISE 5-2	ENTERING DATA IN THE ACCOUNT TAB

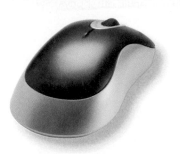

Complete the Account tab for Hiro Tanaka. The information needed to complete this exercise is found on Source Document 1.

Date: October 3, 2016

1. Confirm that Hiro Tanaka is still listed in the Patient List dialog box and that the Case radio button is selected.

2. Click the Edit Case button to add information to Tanaka's case file. The Case dialog box is displayed, with the Personal tab active.

3. Make the Account tab active. The word *Account* should now be displayed in boldface type, and the boxes on the Account tab should be visible.

4. Notice that the Assigned Provider box is already filled in with the name of Tanaka's assigned provider, Katherine Yan. The system copies this information from data stored in the Patient/Guarantor dialog box.

5. Click the name of Tanaka's referring provider on the Referring Provider drop-down list. Press Tab.

6. Accept the default entry of "A" in the Price Code box.

7. Check your work for accuracy.

8. Save the changes. The Patient List dialog box is redisplayed.

9. Do not close the Patient List dialog box. **CiMC**

 You have completed Exercise 5-2.

5.4 ENTERING INSURANCE INFORMATION

The **primary insurance carrier** is the first carrier to whom claims are submitted. There may also be a secondary carrier (Policy 2 tab) or a tertiary carrier (Policy 3 tab). The Medicaid and Tricare tab is used to enter specific information for Medicaid and TRICARE claims.

primary insurance carrier the first carrier to whom claims are submitted

POLICY 1 TAB

The Policy 1 tab is where information about a patient's primary insurance carrier and coverage is recorded (see Figure 5-6).

Insurance 1   The Insurance 1 box lists the code number and name of the insurance carrier. The drop-down list shows the carriers already in the system. If the carrier is not listed, it must be added to the database. It is not necessary to close the Case dialog box to add an insurance carrier to the database. When Insurance is clicked on the Lists menu, and Carriers is clicked on the submenu, the Insurance Carrier List dialog box is displayed in front of the other dialog boxes on the screen.

Policy Holder 1   The Policy Holder box lists the person who is the insured under a particular policy. For example, if the patient is a child covered under his or her parent's insurance plan, the parent's chart number would be entered in this box. The insured's chart number is selected from the choices on the drop-down list. (If the insured is not a patient of the practice, he or she must be entered as a guarantor in Medisoft, and a chart number must be established.)

Relationship to Insured   This box describes a patient's relationship to the individual listed in the Policy Holder 1 box.

Policy Number   A patient's policy number is entered in the Policy Number box.

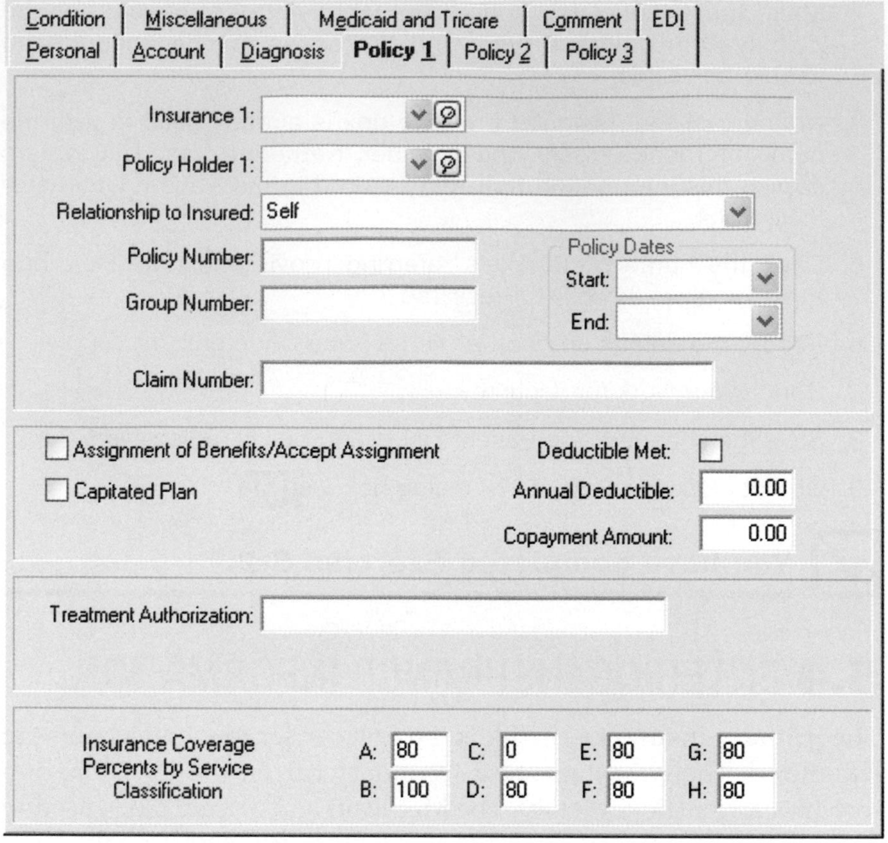

Figure 5-6 Policy 1 Tab

Group Number The group number for a patient's policy is entered in the Group Number box.

Policy Dates—Start/End The date a patient's insurance policy went into effect is entered in the Policy Dates—Start box. If the date is not known, the date the patient first came to the practice for treatment can be entered. If the policy has ended, for example, because the carrier changed or the coverage expired, the date on which coverage terminated is entered in the Policy Dates—End box.

Claim Number This field is used on property, casualty, and auto claims. The number is assigned by the property and casualty payer, usually during eligibility determinations.

Assignment of Benefits/Accept Assignment For physicians who are participating in an insurance plan, a check mark in the Accept Assignment box indicates that the provider accepts payment directly from the insurance carrier. For the exercises in this book, this information is located on the bottom of the patient information form.

Capitated Plan In a **capitated plan,** prepayments are made to the physician from a managed care company to cover the physician's services to a plan member for a specified period of time, whether members seek medical care or not. A check mark in this box indicates that this insurance plan is capitated.

capitated plan an insurance plan in which prepayments made to a physician cover the physician's services to a plan member for a specified period of time

Copayment Amount   The dollar amount of a patient's copayment per visit is entered in the Copayment Amount box.

Annual Deductible   The dollar amount of the insured's insurance plan deductible is entered in this box.

Deductible Met   This box is checked if the patient has met the deductible for the current year.

Treatment Authorization   This field is used to record the treatment authorization code from an insurance company for UB-04 claims. The UB-04 is the standard uniform bill (UB) that is used for institutional health care providers such as hospitals. The UB-04 replaced the UB-92 in 2007.

Insurance Coverage Percents by Service Classification   The percentage of fees that an insurance carrier covers is entered in the Insurance Coverage Percents by Service Classification box. Some insurance plans pay different percentages of charges based on the type of service provided. For example, a plan may pay 80 percent of necessary medical procedures, 100 percent of lab work, and 50 percent of outpatient mental health charges.

ENTERING DATA IN THE POLICY 1 TAB	EXERCISE 5-3

Complete the Policy 1 tab for Hiro Tanaka. The information needed to complete this exercise is found on Source Document 1.

Date: October 3, 2016

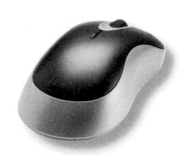

1. Edit the case for Hiro Tanaka.

2. Make the Policy 1 tab active.

3. Select Tanaka's primary insurance carrier from the drop-down list in the Insurance 1 box. Press Tab.

4. The program completes the Policy Holder 1 field with the name of the patient. Since Tanaka is the policyholder, accept this entry.

5. Notice that the Relationship to Insured box already has "Self" entered. Since this is correct, do not make any changes.

6. Enter Tanaka's insurance policy number in the Policy Number box. Press Tab.

7. Enter Tanaka's group number in the Group Number box. Press Tab.

8. In the Policy Dates—Start box, key **01012016** (January 1, 2016) as the start date of the policy. Press Tab. The program displays a Confirm message stating that the date entered is in the future and asking whether you want to change it. Click No.

9. Dr. Yan accepts assignment for this carrier, so click the Assignment of Benefits/Accept Assignment box.

10. The insurance plan is capitated, so check the Capitated Plan box.

11. Key **20** in the Copayment Amount box if it does not already appear. Press Tab.

12. Key *100* in each of the Insurance Coverage Percents by Service Classification boxes.

13. Check your work for accuracy.

14. Save the changes.

15. Do not close the Patient List dialog box.

✓ **You have completed Exercise 5-3.**

POLICY 2 TAB

Claims are usually not submitted to a secondary carrier until the primary carrier has paid. The secondary carrier must have access to the remittance advice of the primary carrier to see what has already been paid on the claim. Delayed secondary billing may be set up so a claim is not created for the secondary carrier until a response has been received from the primary carrier.

The boxes in the Policy 2 tab are the same as those in the Policy 1 tab, with a few exceptions. The Copayment Amount, Capitated Plan, Annual Deductible, and Deductible Met boxes are only in the Policy 1 tab. Only the Policy 2 tab has a Crossover Claim box (see Figure 5-7).

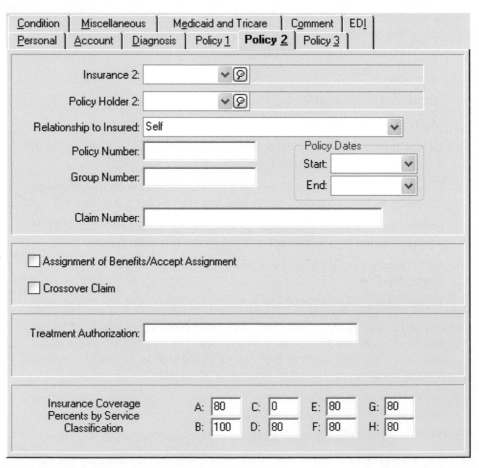

Figure 5-7 Policy 2 Tab

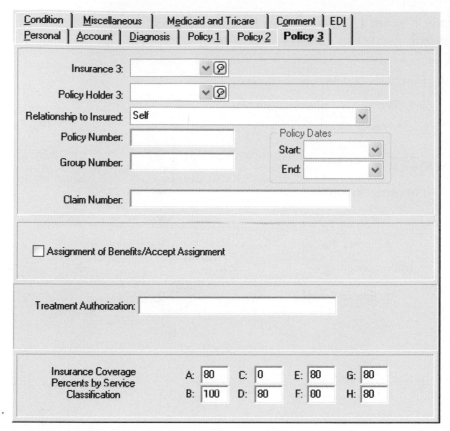

Figure 5-8   Policy 3 Tab

Crossover Claim   The Crossover Claim box is used when a patient has Medicare as the primary carrier and Medicaid as the secondary carrier. Because Medicare is the primary carrier, it pays first on a claim and then submits the claim directly to the Medicaid carrier.

POLICY 3 TAB

The Policy 3 tab does not contain the Copayment Amount, Capitated Plan, Annual Deductible, Deductible Met, or Crossover Claim boxes. Otherwise, the boxes are the same as those in the Policy 1 and Policy 2 tabs (see Figure 5-8).

MEDICAID AND TRICARE TAB

For patients covered by Medicaid or TRICARE, the Medicaid and Tricare tab is used to enter additional information about the government programs (see Figure 5-9).

Medicaid
EPSDT   *EPSDT* stands for Early and Periodic Screening, Diagnosis, and Treatment. This is a Medicaid program for patients under the age of twenty-one who need screening and diagnostic services to determine physical or mental problems as well as treatment for conditions discovered. It also includes well-baby checkup examinations. A check mark in the EPSDT box indicates that a patient's visit is part of the EPSDT program.

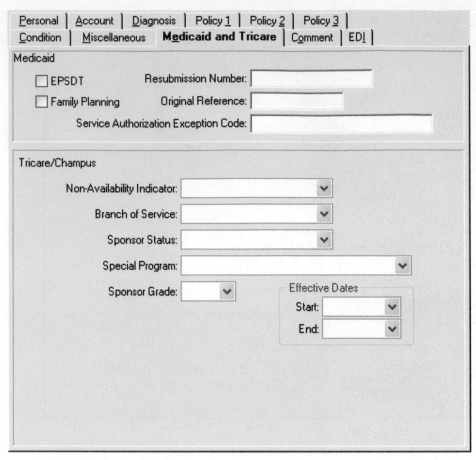

Figure 5-9 Medicaid and Tricare Tab

Family Planning A check mark in the Family Planning box specifies that a patient's condition is related to Medicaid family planning services.

Resubmission Number For claims being resubmitted to Medicaid, the resubmission number is entered in this box.

Original Reference For claims being resubmitted to Medicaid, the original reference number is recorded in the Original Reference box.

Service Authorization Exception Code This code is required on some Medicaid claims. If a service authorization code was not obtained before seeing the patient, enter one of the following codes:

1 Immediate/Urgent Care

2 Services Rendered in a Retroactive Period

3 Emergency Care

4 Client as Temporary Medicaid

5 Request from County for Second Opinion to Recipient Can Work

6 Request for Override Pending

7 Special Handling

TRICARE/CHAMPUS

TRICARE is the government insurance program that serves spouses and children of active-duty service members, military retirees and their families, some former spouses, and survivors of deceased military members (Army, Navy, Air Force, Marine Corps, Coast Guard, Public Health Service, and NOAA, the National Oceanic and Atmospheric Administration). TRICARE was previously known as CHAMPUS.

Non-Availability Indicator   The Non-Availability Indicator box specifies whether a nonavailability (NA) statement is required. The choices on the drop-down list are NA statement not needed, NA statement obtained, and Other carrier paid at least 75%.

Branch of Service   The Branch of Service box indicates the particular branch of service: Army, Air Force, Marines, Navy, Coast Guard, Public Health Service, NOAA, and ChampVA.

Sponsor Status   The **sponsor** is the active-duty service member. The sponsor's family members are covered by the TRICARE insurance plan. The drop-down list in the Sponsor Status box provides choices to indicate the sponsor's status in the service, such as Active, Civilian, and National Guard.

sponsor in TRICARE, the active-duty service member

Special Program   The Special Program drop-down list contains codes for special TRICARE programs.

Sponsor Grade   The two-character sponsor grade is entered in the Sponsor Grade box.

Effective Dates   The start date of the TRICARE policy is entered in the Effective Dates—Start box. If there is an end date, it is entered in the Effective Dates—End box. Specific dates can be entered, or a selection can be made from the pop-up calendar.

5.5 ENTERING HEALTH INFORMATION

Information about a patient's health is recorded in the Diagnosis and Condition tabs in Medisoft.

DIAGNOSIS TAB

The Diagnosis tab contains a patient's diagnosis, information about allergies, and electronic media claim (EDI) notes (see Figure 5-10).

Principal Diagnosis and Default Diagnosis 2, 3, and 4   A patient's diagnosis is selected from the drop-down list of diagnoses. If a patient has more than one diagnosis for the same condition, the primary diagnosis is entered in the Principal Diagnosis field. Additional diagnoses are entered in the Default Diagnosis 2, 3, and 4 fields. The program options can be changed to display up to eight diagnoses if required.

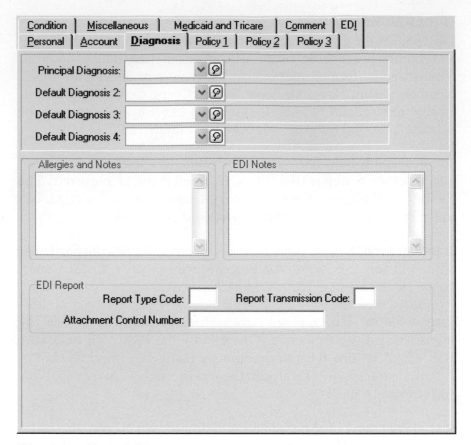

Figure 5-10   Diagnosis Tab

Allergies and Notes   If a patient has allergies or other special conditions that need to be recorded, they are entered in the Allergies and Notes box.

EDI Notes   If a patient's claims require special handling when submitted electronically, notes about the procedure, such as an explanation about the charges for supplies, are listed in this box.

EDI Report   The Report Type Code is a two-character code that indicates the title or contents of a document, report, or supporting item sent with electronic claims. The Report Transmission Code is a two-character code that defines the timing, transmission method, or format by which reports are sent with electronic claims. The value entered in the Attachment Control Number field is a unique reference number up to seven digits long.

EXERCISE 5-4   ENTERING DATA IN THE DIAGNOSIS TAB

Complete the Diagnosis tab for Hiro Tanaka. The information needed to complete this exercise is found on Source Documents 1 and 3.

Date: October 3, 2016

1. Edit the case for Hiro Tanaka.

2. Make the Diagnosis tab active.

3. From the list of choices in the drop-down list, select Tanaka's diagnosis.

4. In the Allergies and Notes box, enter information on Tanaka's allergies.

5. Check your work for accuracy.

6. Save the changes. The Patient List dialog box is redisplayed.

7. Do not close the Patient List dialog box.

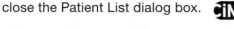 **You have completed Exercise 5-4.**

CONDITION TAB

The Condition tab stores data about a patient's illness, accident, disability, and hospitalization (see Figure 5-11). This information is used by insurance carriers to process claims.

Injury/Illness/LMP Date   The date of a patient's injury, illness, or last menstrual period (LMP) is entered in the Injury/Illness/LMP Date box. (For an illness, the date when the symptoms first appeared is entered.)

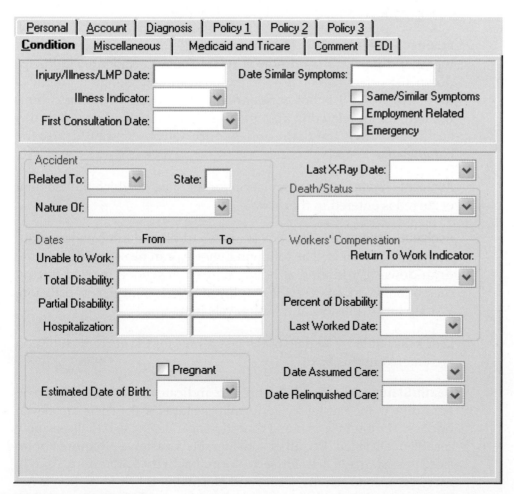

Figure 5-11   Condition Tab

Illness Indicator   The Illness Indicator box specifies whether a patient's condition is an illness, a last menstrual period in the case of a pregnancy, or an injury.

First Consultation Date   The date of a patient's first visit for a particular condition is entered in the First Consultation Date box. The actual date can be entered, or the pop-up calendar can be activated and dates selected.

Date Similar Symptoms   If a patient has had similar symptoms in the past, enter the date of those symptoms in the Date Similar Symptoms box.

Same/Similar Symptoms   A check mark in the Same/Similar Symptoms box indicates that a patient has had the same or similar symptoms in the past.

Employment Related   If the Employment Related box is checked, it means that the illness or accident is in some way related to a patient's employment.

Emergency   If a patient sees the provider on an emergency visit, a check mark is entered in the Emergency box.

Accident—Related To   The Accident—Related To box indicates whether a patient's condition is related to an accident. The drop-down list offers three choices: Auto, if an automobile accident is involved; No, if it is not accident-related; and Yes, if it is accident-related but not related to an auto accident. If a patient's condition is accident-related, the State and Nature Of boxes should also be completed.

Accident—State   The abbreviation for the state in which the accident occurred is entered in this box.

Accident—Nature Of   This box provides additional information about the type of accident. The following choices can be selected from the drop-down list: Injured at home, Injured at school, Injured during recreation, Work injury/Self employed, Work injury/Non-collision, Work injury/Collision, and Motorcycle injury.

Last X-Ray Date   The date of the last X-rays for the current condition are entered in this box.

Death/Status   The Death/Status box indicates a patient's condition according to the Karnofsky Performance Status Scale. There are eleven options: Moribund (a terminal condition near death), Very sick, Severely disabled, Disabled, Requires considerable assistance, Requires occasional assistance, Cares for self, Normal activity with effort, Able to carry on normal activity, Dead, and Normal. If this information is not provided by the physician, the box should be left blank.

Dates—Unable to Work   If a patient is unable to work, the dates of the absence from work are listed in these boxes.

Dates—Total Disability   If a patient is totally disabled, the dates of the total disability are entered in these boxes.

Dates—Partial Disability   If a patient is partially disabled, the dates of the partial disability are listed in these boxes.

Dates—Hospitalization   If a patient is hospitalized, the dates of the hospitalization are entered in these boxes.

Workers' Compensation—Return to Work Indicator   If a patient has been out of work on workers' compensation, the patient's return to work status is selected from the drop-down list of choices: Limited, Normal, or Conditional. If the status is Conditional or Limited, the Percent of Disability box should also be completed.

Workers' Compensation—Percent of Disability   This box indicates a patient's percentage of disability upon returning to work.

Last Worked Date   The last day the patient worked is listed in this box.

Pregnant   This box is checked if a woman is pregnant.

Estimated Date of Birth   If the patient is pregnant, enter the date the baby is due.

Date Assumed Care   This field is used when providers share post-operative care. Enter the date the provider assumed care for this patient.

Date Relinquished Care   This field is used when providers share postoperative care. Enter the date the provider relinquished care of the patient.

ENTERING DATA IN THE CONDITION TAB	EXERCISE 5-5

Complete the Condition tab for Hiro Tanaka. The information needed to complete this exercise is found on Source Documents 1, 3, and 4.

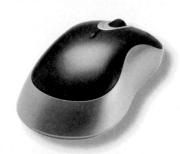

Date: October 3, 2016

1. Edit the case for Hiro Tanaka.

2. Make the Condition tab active.

3. Enter the date of the injury in the Injury/Illness/LMP Date box.

4. Select Injury in the Illness Indicator box.

5. In the First Consultation Date box, enter the date Tanaka first saw Dr. Yan for this condition, which is 10/3/2016. Press Tab. The program displays a Confirm message stating that the date entered is in the future, and asking whether you want to change it. Click No.

6. Since this visit resulted from a non-work-related accident, leave the Date Similar Symptoms box, the Same/Similar Symptoms box, and the Employment Related box blank.

7. Since this was an emergency visit, place a check mark in the Emergency box by clicking it.

8. Choose Auto in the Accident—Related To box.

9. In the Accident—State box, enter the two-letter abbreviation for the state in which the accident occurred.

10. Tanaka was injured while driving home from a softball game. Complete the Accident—Nature Of box regarding the type of accident with Injured during recreation.

11. Enter the dates Tanaka was unable to work in the Dates—Unable to Work boxes.

12. Enter the dates Tanaka was totally disabled in the Dates—Total Disability boxes.

13. Enter the dates Tanaka was partially disabled in the Dates—Partial Disability boxes.

14. Enter the dates Tanaka was hospitalized in the Dates—Hospitalization boxes.

15. Leave the remaining fields blank.

16. Check your work for accuracy.

17. Save the changes.

18. Do not close the Patient List dialog box.

☑ **You have completed Exercise 5-5.**

5.6 ENTERING OTHER INFORMATION
MISCELLANEOUS TAB

The Miscellaneous tab records a variety of miscellaneous information about the patient and his or her treatment (see Figure 5-12).

Outside Lab Work   If the Outside Lab Work box is checked, the lab work was performed by a lab other than the physician's office. If the lab bills the provider rather than the patient, then the provider bills the patient for the lab work even though it was performed by an outside lab.

Lab Charges   The charges for lab work, whether performed inside or outside the practice, are entered in the Lab Charges box.

Local Use A and B   These boxes may be used by some medical practices to record information specific to the local office.

Indicator   If an indicator code is used to categorize patients or services, it is entered in the Indicator box. For example, patients

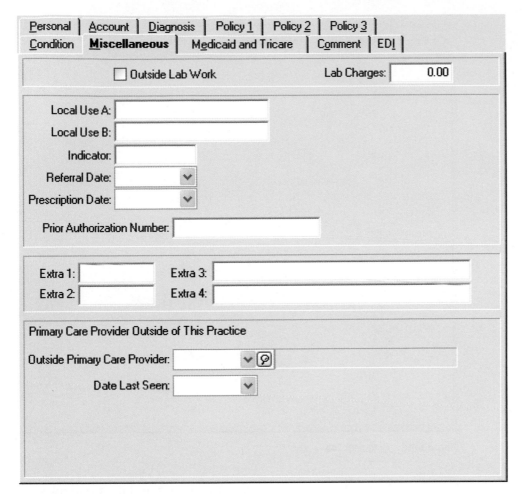

Personal | Account | Diagnosis | Policy 1 | Policy 2 | Policy 3 |
Condition | **Miscellaneous** | Medicaid and Tricare | Comment | EDI |

Outside Lab Work   Lab Charges: 0.00

Local Use A:
Local Use B:
Indicator:
Referral Date:
Prescription Date:

Prior Authorization Number:

Extra 1:   Extra 3:
Extra 2:   Extra 4:

Primary Care Provider Outside of This Practice

Outside Primary Care Provider:
Date Last Seen:

Figure 5-12   Miscellaneous Tab

might be categorized according to the primary diagnosis. Services might be divided into such categories as lab work, consultations, and hospital visits.

Referral Date   If the patient was referred to the provider, enter the date of the referral.

Prescription Date   This field is required for hearing and vision claims.

Prior Authorization Number   Before some services are performed, prior authorization must be obtained from the appropriate insurance carrier. If an insurance carrier has issued an authorization number for treatment that has not yet occurred, the number is entered in the Prior Authorization Number box.

Extra 1, 2, 3, and 4   The Extra 1, 2, 3, and 4 boxes are used for different purposes depending on the medical practice.

Outside Primary Care Provider   If a patient is covered by a managed care plan and the patient's primary care provider is outside the medical practice, the name of the provider is selected from the drop-down list in this box.

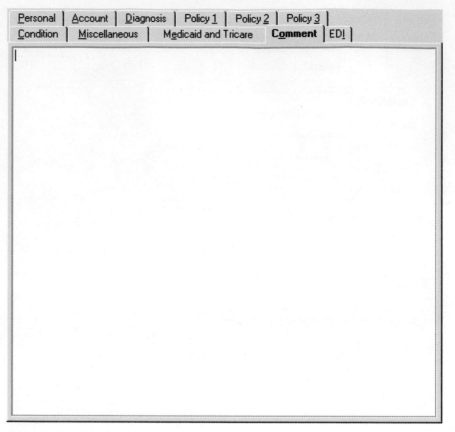

Figure 5-13 Comment Tab

Date Last Seen   The Date Last Seen box lists the date a patient was last seen by the outside primary care provider.

COMMENT TAB

The Comment tab is used to enter case notes (see Figure 5-13). Notes entered in this box will print on statements if statements are formatted to include case comments.

EDI TAB

The EDI tab is used to enter information for electronic claims specific to this case (see Figure 5-14). Only fields that are relevant for the particular case need to be completed.

Care Plan Oversight #   If a physician is billing for home health and hospice care plan oversight (CPO), enter the care plan oversight number.

Assignment Indicator   The entry in this field is the assignment indicator for this case. Valid codes are

   A   Assigned

   B   Assignment accepted on clinical lab services only

   C   Not assigned

   P   Patient refuses to assign benefits

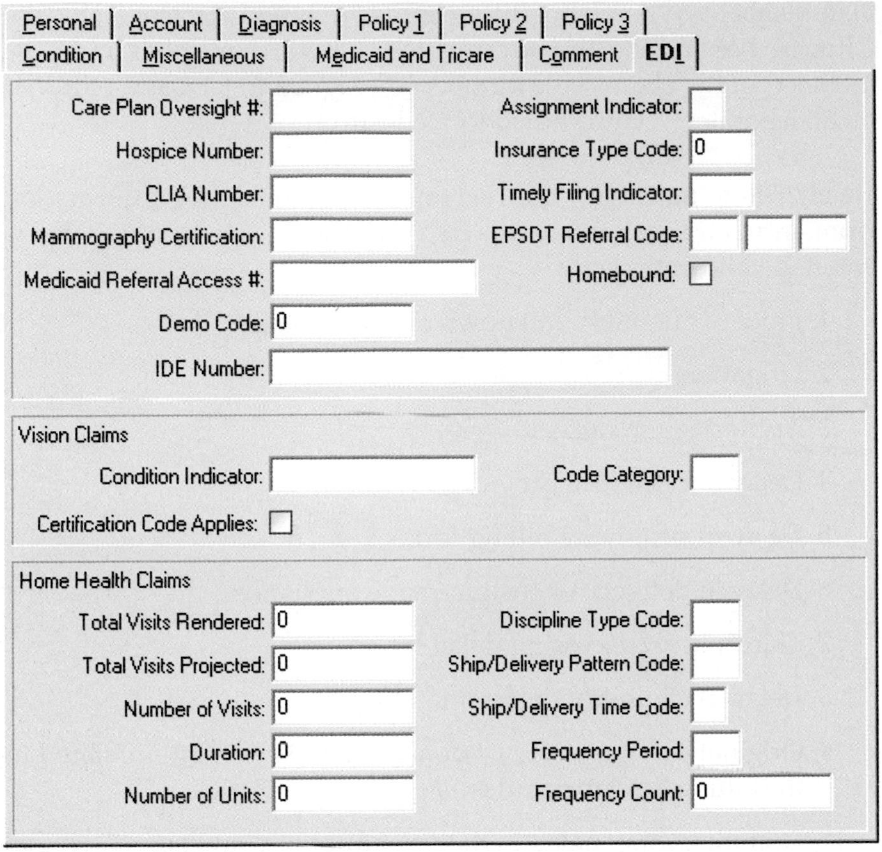

Figure 5-14 EDI Tab

Hospice Number If a physician is billing for hospice care, enter the hospice number.

Insurance Type Code The type of insurance that the patient has is selected in the Insurance Type Code field. This is required when sending Medicare secondary claims. Valid codes are

12 Medicare secondary working-aged beneficiary or spouse with employer group health plan

13 Medicare secondary end-stage renal disease beneficiary in the twelve-month coordination period with an employer's group health plan

14 Medicare secondary, no-fault insurance including auto is primary

15 Medicare secondary workers' compensation

16 Medicare secondary public health service (PHS) or other federal agency

41 Medicare secondary black lung

42 Medicare secondary Veterans Administration

43 Medicare secondary disabled beneficiary under age sixty-five with large-group health plan (LGHP)

47 Medicare secondary, other liability insurance is primary

CLIA Number   When laboratory claims are billed electronically, the Clinical Laboratory Improvement Act (CLIA) number must be included in the claim. This number is assigned to labs and required on all laboratory claims billed to Medicare.

Timely Filing Indicator   If a response to a request for information from an insurance carrier was delayed, the reason for the delay is entered. Valid entries are

1 Proof of eligibility unknown or unavailable

2 Litigation

3 Authorization delays

4 Delay in certifying provider

5 Delay in supplying billing forms

6 Delay in delivery of custom-made appliances

7 Third-party processing delay

8 Delay in eligibility determination

9 Original claim rejected or denied due to a reason unrelated to the billing limitation rules

10 Administration delay in the prior approval process

11 Other

Mammography Certification   This box lists the provider's or facility's mammography certification number.

EPSDT Referral Code   The patient's referral code for the EPSDT program is entered in this field.

Medicaid Referral Access #   The referring physician's Medicaid referral access number for the patient is entered in this field.

Homebound   If the patient is under homebound care, this box should be checked.

Demo Code   This field is used when filing claims for this patient under demonstration projects.

IDE Number   The IDE number is required when there is an investigational device exemption on the claim. This is usually for vision claims but can also be assigned for other types of claims.

Vision Claims
If a provider submits vision claims, entries are made in these fields.

Condition Indicator   The code indicator is entered in this field.

Code Category   The code category for the vision device is entered in this field.

Certification Code Applies   This box is checked if a certification code is applicable.

Home Health Claims

If a provider submits home health claims, these fields are filled in.

Total Visits Rendered   This field indicates the total number of visits.

Discipline Type Code   The provider's discipline type code is entered.

Total Visits Projected   This field lists the total number of visits projected.

Ship/Delivery Pattern Code   Enter the pattern code for the home visits.

Number of Visits   The total number of visits is entered in this field.

Ship/Delivery Time Code   This field records the time code for the home visits.

Duration   The duration of the home health visits is recorded in this field.

Frequency Period   The frequency period for the home visits is listed.

Number of Units   This field contains the number of units for the home visits.

Frequency Count   The frequency count for the home visits is entered.

5.7 EDITING CASE INFORMATION

Information in an existing case is modified by selecting the case to be edited and clicking the Edit Case button at the bottom of the Patient List dialog box. (The Case radio button must be clicked for the Edit Case button to be displayed.) Alternatively, a case can be opened for editing by double clicking directly on the case line in the right half of the dialog box.

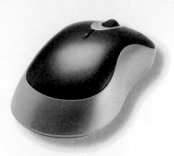

John Fitzwilliams, an established patient, has just divorced. Edit the information in his Case dialog box to reflect this change.

Date: October 3, 2016

1. Click in the Search for field and press the backspace key to delete the *T* that was entered to search for Hiro Tanaka. The Patient List once again displays the complete list of patients.

2. Enter *F* in the Search for field. All patients who have last names beginning with the letter *F* are displayed. Click anywhere in the listing for John Fitzwilliams to select his entry.

3. Click the Case radio button. Verify that Acute Gastric Ulcer is listed in the Case area of the dialog box.

4. Click the Edit Case button.

5. In the Personal tab, change the entry in the Marital Status box from Married to Divorced.

6. Check your work for accuracy.

7. Save the changes.

8. Close the Patient List dialog box.

 You have completed Exercise 5-6.

APPLYING YOUR SKILLS
2: CREATING A CASE FOR A NEW PATIENT

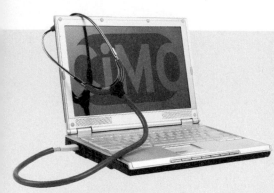

October 3, 2016

Lisa Wright is a new patient who has just arrived for her office visit with Dr. Jessica Rudner. Dr. Rudner accepts assignment from Blue Cross/Blue Shield. Using Source Document 2, complete the Personal, Account, and Policy 1 tabs in the Case dialog box. In the Policy 1 tab, enter 100 in all the Insurance Coverage by Service Classification boxes. (*Note:* Not all tabs and text boxes will have entries.)

Remember to create a backup of your work before exiting Medisoft! To help you keep track of your work, name the backup file after the chapter you are working on, for example, StudentID-c5.mbk.

ELECTRONIC HEALTH RECORD EXCHANGE

Creating Cases for Imported Transactions

Transactions received from an electronic health record will not always be related to an existing case in Medisoft. As illustrated below, the Unprocessed Transactions Edit dialog box contains a blank Case field and a message, "Case number does not exist. [Error]".

To process the transaction, a new case must be created. This can be done from the Unprocessed Transactions Edit dialog box, simply by pressing the F8 shortcut key, which opens a new Case dialog box in Medisoft.

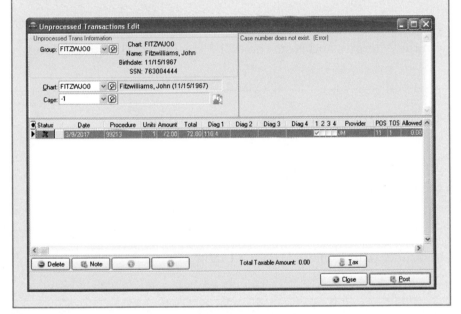

Name: _____ Date: _____

After completing all the exercises in the chapter, answer the following questions in the spaces provided.

1. *[LO 5.3]* What is the entry in the Referring Provider box for Hiro Tanaka (Account tab)?

_____

2. *[LO 5.5]* What is the entry in the Allergies and Notes box for Hiro Tanaka (Diagnosis tab)?

_____

3. *[LO 5.3]* What is the code for John Fitzwilliams's employer (Personal tab)?

_____

4. *[LO 5.5]* What is listed in the Principal Diagnosis field for Hiro Tanaka (Diagnosis tab)?

_____

5. *[LO 5.4]* Is Hiro Tanaka's insurance plan capitated (Policy 1 tab)?

_____

6. *[LO 5.4]* What is the entry in the Copayment Amount box for Hiro Tanaka (Policy 1 tab)?

_____

7. *[LO 5.4]* What code is entered in the Insurance 1 box for Hiro Tanaka (Policy 1 tab)?

_____

8. *[LO 5.3]* What is entered in the Description box for Lisa Wright (Personal tab)?

_____

9. *[LO 5.3]* What is the entry in the Price Code box for Lisa Wright (Account tab)?

_____

10. *[LO 5.4]* Has Lisa Wright met her deductible for the year (Policy 1 tab)?

_____

5.1 Describe when it is necessary to create a new case in Medisoft. Pages 136–137

Cases are organized around a common element. Most often this element is the patient's medical condition. A new case must be created when the patient is treated for a different medical condition. A new case must also be created when the patient changes insurance plans, or when treatment is covered by another policy, such as in the case of workers' compensation injuries.

5.2 List the eleven tabs in the Case dialog box. Pages 138–141

1. Personal
2. Account
3. Diagnosis
4. Policy 1
5. Policy 2
6. Policy 3
7. Condition
8. Miscellaneous
9. Medicaid and Tricare
10. Comment
11. EDI

5.3 Review the information contained in the Personal tab and the Account tab. Pages 141–147

The Personal tab contains basic information about a patient, including

- A description of the case
- Name of guarantor
- Marital and student status
- Employment information

The Account tab tracks basic information about the patient's account, including: providers, referral source, attorney, and facility. It also includes accounting codes and visit authorization information.

5.4 Discuss the information recorded in the Policy 1, 2, 3, and Medicaid and Tricare tabs in Medisoft. Pages 147–153	The Policy 1, 2, and 3 tabs contain information about the patient's insurance coverage, including - Insurance carrier - Policy holder - Relationship to insured - Policy and group number - Policy start and end dates There is also information about the assignment of benefits, deductible, and copayment, as well as other insurance-related information. The Medicaid and Tricare tab is used to enter information specific to those claims.
5.5 Describe the information contained in the Diagnosis tab and the Condition tab in Medisoft. Pages 153–158	- The Diagnosis tab contains the patient's principal diagnosis and three additional diagnoses. There are also fields for entering allergies and information specific to electronic claims. - The Condition tab contains information about the general status or condition of the patient. There are many fields for recording data about the dates of an illness or injury. It also includes workers' compensation information.
5.6 Review the purpose of the Miscellaneous, Comment, and EDI tabs in Medisoft. Pages 158–163	The Miscellaneous tab is used to enter information that may be required to submit a claim, including outside lab work and lab charges, a prior authorization number, or the name of an outside primary care provider. The Comment tab is used to enter notes that can be printed on patient statements. The EDI tab contains numerous fields in which carrier-specific information for electronic claims is entered.
5.7 Describe how to edit information in a case. Pages 163–164	Information in an existing case is edited in the same way it is entered; changes are made directly in the field that contains the information that requires editing.

USING TERMINOLOGY

Match the terms on the left with the definitions on the right.

_____ **1.** *[LO 5.4]* capitated plan

_____ **2.** *[LO 5.1]* case

_____ **3.** *[LO 5.2]* chart

_____ **4.** *[LO 5.4]* primary insurance carrier

_____ **5.** *[LO 5.2]* record of treatment and progress

_____ **6.** *[LO 5.3]* referring provider

_____ **7.** *[LO 5.4]* sponsor

a. A folder that contains a patient's medical records.

b. Physician's notes about a patient's condition and diagnosis.

c. A physician who recommends that a patient make an appointment with a particular doctor.

d. An insurance plan in which payments are made to primary care providers whether patients visit the office or not.

e. The insurance company that receives claims before they are submitted to any other payer.

f. A grouping of transactions organized around a common element.

g. The active-duty service member on the TRICARE government insurance program.

CHECKING YOUR UNDERSTANDING

Answer the questions below in the space provided.

1. *[LO 5.4]* Sarina Bell has no insurance of her own but is covered by her father's insurance policy. How would this be indicated in the Policy 1 tab for Sarina Bell?

_____

_____

2. *[LO 5.5]* Where in the Case dialog box can you find information about a patient's allergies?

_____

_____

3. *[LO 5.1]* Is it necessary to set up a new case when a patient changes insurance carriers? Why?

_____

_____

4. *[LO 5.5]* In the Case dialog box, where would you enter information about a work-related accident?

_____

_____

5. *[LO 5.5]* Where is information needed to complete the Diagnosis tab usually found?

_____

_____

6. *[LO 5.1]* A patient has been seeing the doctor regularly for treatment of diabetes. She was hospitalized yesterday, and the doctor saw her in the hospital for treatment of her diabetes. Do you need to set up a new case for the hospitalization?

_____

_____

APPLYING YOUR KNOWLEDGE

Answer the questions below in the space provided.

5.1. *[LO 5.3]* While you are entering case information for a new patient, you realize that the patient's referring provider is not one of the choices in the Referring Provider box in the Account tab. What should you do?

_____

_____

5.2. *[LO 5.4]* An established patient has changed insurance carriers from Blue Cross and Blue Shield to OhioCare HMO. What specific boxes need to be changed in the Case dialog box?

_____

_____

THINKING ABOUT IT

Answer the question below in the space provided.

5.1. *[LO 5.1]* Why are patient transactions grouped into cases? What could happen if transactions were not organized by case?

_____

_____

AT THE COMPUTER

Answer the following questions at the computer.

5.1. *[LO 5.4]* Using the information contained in the Case dialog box, list Randall Klein's primary and secondary insurance carriers.

_____

_____

5.2. *[LO 5.3]* Who is the guarantor for Janine Bell's account?

_____

_____

chapter
6

Entering Charge Transactions and Patient Payments

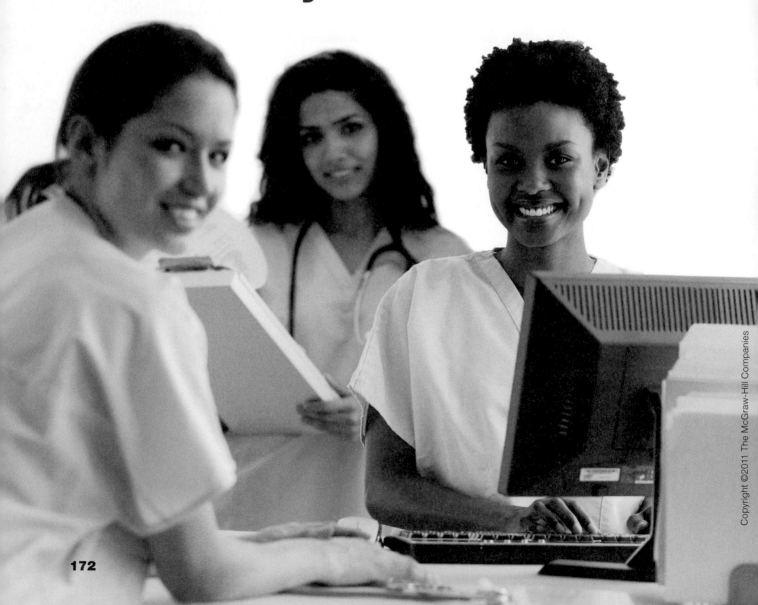

key terms

adjustments
charges
MultiLink codes
NSF check
payments

learning outcomes

When you finish this chapter, you will be able to:

6.1 Describe the three types of transactions recorded in Medisoft.

6.2 Discuss how to select a patient and case in Transaction Entry.

6.3 Demonstrate how to enter charge transactions in Medisoft.

6.4 Demonstrate how to enter payments made at the time of an office visit.

6.5 Demonstrate how to print a walkout receipt.

6.6 Demonstrate how to process a refund for a patient.

6.7 Demonstrate how to post a nonsufficient funds (NSF) check.

what you need to know

To use this chapter, you need to know how to:

- Start Medisoft, use menus, and enter and edit text.
- Enter patient information in Medisoft.
- Work with chart and case numbers.

6.1 UNDERSTANDING CHARGES, PAYMENTS, AND ADJUSTMENTS

charges amounts a provider bills for the services performed

payments monies received from patients and insurance carriers

adjustments changes to patients' accounts that alter the amounts charged or paid

Three types of transactions are recorded in Medisoft®: charges, payments, and adjustments. **Charges** are the amounts a provider bills for the services performed. **Payments** are monies received from patients and insurance carriers. **Adjustments** are changes to patients' accounts. Examples of adjustments include returned checks, refunding of overpayments, and differences between the amount billed and the amount allowed per contract. This chapter covers charge transactions and patient payments and adjustments. Chapter 8 covers insurance payment and adjustment transactions.

The primary document needed to enter charge transactions in Medisoft is a patient's encounter form. Typically, the physician indicates the appropriate procedure and diagnosis codes on the encounter form during or just after the patient visit. Charges and payments listed on an encounter form are later entered in the Transaction Entry dialog box in Medisoft by an insurance billing specialist. If the office uses an electronic health record program that exchanges data with Medisoft, the charges may not require manual posting. After charge transactions are entered, they are checked for accuracy. If all the information is correct, the transaction data are saved, and a walkout receipt is printed for the patient. If it is incorrect, the data are edited and then saved.

In Medisoft, transactions are entered in the Transaction Entry dialog box, which is accessed by selecting Enter Transactions on the Activities menu. The Transaction Entry dialog box consists of three main sections, each consuming about a third of the window (see Figure 6-1):

1. Patient/Account Information: The top third contains information about the patient, the insurance coverage, and the patient's account.

2. Charge Transactions: The middle section is where charge transactions are entered.

3. Payment/Adjustment Transactions: The bottom third is where patient payments and different types of adjustments are entered and applied. The topic of entering payments from insurance carriers is discussed in Chapter 8.

6.2 SELECTING A PATIENT AND CASE

The Patient/Account Information section of the Transaction Entry dialog box consists of the top third of the Transaction Entry dialog box (see Figure 6-2). It contains two critical pieces of information: chart number and case number. Boxes for entering these numbers are found at the top left of the dialog box.

CHART

The Chart drop-down list includes all patients in the practice. In large practices, the list of chart numbers could be very long, so it is

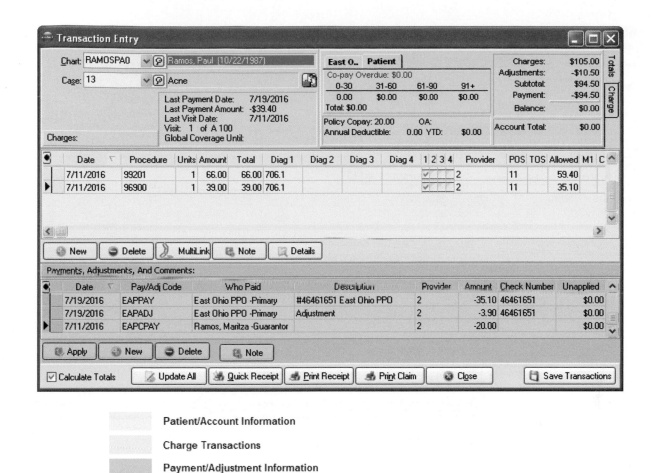

Figure 6-1 Transaction Entry Dialog Box with Three Sections Highlighted

Patient/Account Information

Charge Transactions

Payment/Adjustment Information

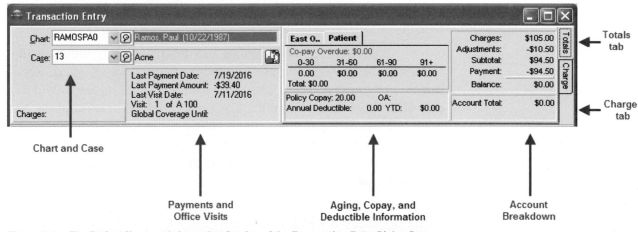

Figure 6-2 The Patient/Account Information Section of the Transaction Entry Dialog Box

important to know how to search for a chart number. One way to locate a chart number is to key the first several letters of a patient's last name. As the letters are keyed, the first chart number in the list that matches is highlighted. In the example in Figure 6-3, the letters *RAMOSP* were keyed. The program highlights the first patient with a chart number beginning with those letters—in this case, Paul Ramos.

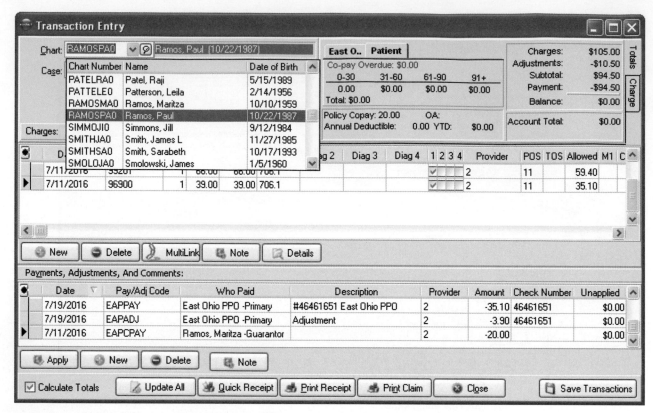

Figure 6-3   Chart Drop-down List After *RAMOSP* Is Keyed

If this is the correct patient, pressing Tab selects the patient and closes the drop-down list. If a different patient is desired, the up and down arrow keys are used to move up or down in the list.

CASE

Once the patient's chart number has been located, the case that relates to the current charges or payments must be selected. Recall from what you learned in Chapter 5 that transactions are linked to a case. The drop-down list in the Case box displays case numbers and descriptions for the patient (see Figure 6-4). By default, the transactions for the most recent case are displayed. Transactions for other cases can be displayed by changing the selection in the Case box. Only one case can be opened at a time.

ADDITIONAL INFORMATION

The remaining areas in the Patient/Account Information section of the Transaction Entry dialog box contain information that is entered automatically by the program and cannot be edited. The dates and figures are automatically updated after a new transaction is entered and saved.

The Aging, Copay, and Deductible section (see Figure 6-2) displays account aging information for the patient and the insurance carrier(s).

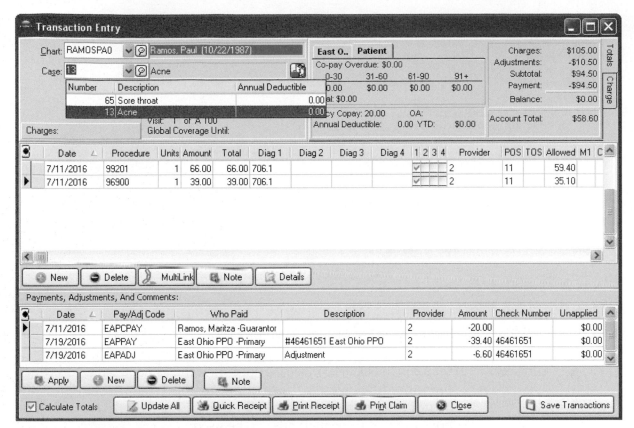

Figure 6-4 Case Drop-down List for the Patient Listed in the Chart Box

By default, the Patient tab is displayed. The Patient tab contains the following information:

- Whether a copayment is overdue
- The outstanding balance for 0–30, 31–60, 61–90, and 91+ days, and the total amount outstanding
- The amount of the copayment per the patient's health plan
- The amount of the annual deductible and the amount paid toward the deductible year-to-date

The Insurance tab, which is not visible until you click on the tab title (the name of the patient's insurance carrier), contains similar information, except it displays aging information for the carrier.

6.3 ENTERING CHARGE TRANSACTIONS

Charges for procedures performed by a provider are entered in the Charges section in the middle of the Transaction Entry dialog box (see Figure 6-5). The process of entering a charge transaction in Medisoft begins with clicking the New button, located just below the list of individual charges.

Date　When the New button is clicked, the program automatically enters the current date (the date that the Medisoft Program Date is

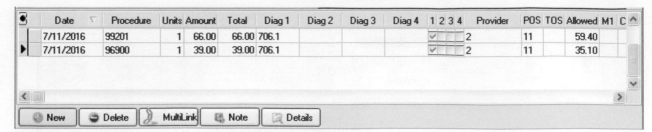

Date	Procedure	Units	Amount	Total	Diag 1	Diag 2	Diag 3	Diag 4	1 2 3 4	Provider	POS	TOS	Allowed	M1	C
7/11/2016	99201	1	66.00	66.00	706.1				✓	2	11		59.40		
7/11/2016	96900	1	39.00	39.00	706.1				✓	2	11		35.10		

New   Delete   MultiLink   Note   Details

Figure 6-5   Charges Area in the Transaction Entry Dialog Box, with the New Button Highlighted

Date	Procedure	Units	Amount	Total	Diag 1	Diag 2	Diag 3	Diag 4	1 2 3 4	Provider	POS	TOS	Allowed	M1	C
7/11/2016	99201	1	66.00	66.00	706.1				✓	2	11		59.40		
7/11/2016	96900	1	39.00	39.00	706.1				✓	2	11		35.10		
7/19/2016		1	0.00	0.00	706.1				✓	2			0.00		

New   Delete   MultiLink   Note   Details

Figure 6-6   Date Displayed in the Date Column After the New Button Is Clicked (New Entry Highlighted in Yellow)

set to) in the Date box (see Figure 6-6). If this is not the date on which the procedures were performed, it must be changed to reflect the actual date of the procedures. To change the default date for these boxes, any of these methods can be used:

- The Set Program Date command on the File menu can be clicked.

- The Date button in the lower-right corner of the screen can be clicked. (This must be done before the New button is clicked in the Transaction Entry dialog box.)

- The information that is already in the Date box can be keyed over with the desired date.

Procedure   After the date is entered, the next information required is the code for the procedure performed by the provider. The procedure code is selected from a drop-down list of CPT codes already in the database. Again, it is more efficient to locate a code by entering the full code number or the first several digits than to scroll through the entire list of codes. In the example in Figure 6-7, the numbers *8, 0,* and *0* were entered, and the first CPT code that matches is highlighted. To select the code, press Tab. If a different code is desired, use the up and down arrow keys on the keyboard to move up or down in the list.

Only one procedure code can be selected for each transaction. If multiple procedures were performed for a patient, each must be entered as a separate transaction (unless a MultiLink code, which is discussed later in the chapter, is used).

If a CPT code for a procedure is not listed, it can be added to the database by pressing the F8 key or by clicking Procedure/Payment/Adjustment Codes on the Lists menu. This may be done without exiting the Transaction Entry dialog box.

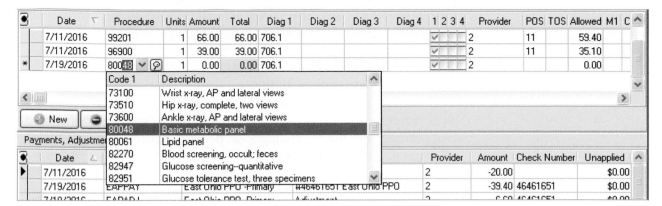

	Date ▽	Procedure	Units	Amount	Total	Diag 1	Diag 2	Diag 3	Diag 4	1 2 3 4	Provider	POS	TOS	Allowed	M1	C
	7/11/2016	99201	1	66.00	66.00	706.1				✓	2	11		59.40		
	7/11/2016	96900	1	39.00	39.00	706.1				✓	2	11		35.10		
*	7/19/2016	80048 ▼ ⊘	1	0.00	0.00	706.1				✓	2			0.00		

Code 1	Description
73100	Wrist x-ray, AP and lateral views
73510	Hip x-ray, complete, two views
73600	Ankle x-ray, AP and lateral views
80048	Basic metabolic panel
80061	Lipid panel
82270	Blood screening, occult; feces
82947	Glucose screening--quantitative
82951	Glucose tolerance test, three specimens

New ⊖

Payments, Adjustme

	Date △			Provider	Amount	Check Number	Unapplied
▶	7/11/2016	East Ohio PPO -Primary	#46461651 East Ohio PPO	2	-20.00		$0.00
	7/19/2016	EAPPAY East Ohio PPO -Primary	#46461651 East Ohio PPO	2	-39.40	46461651	$0.00
	7/19/2016	EAPADJ East Ohio PPO -Primary	Adjustment	2	-6.60	46461651	$0.00

Figure 6-7 Procedure Drop-down List After the Numbers *8, 0,* and *0* Are Entered

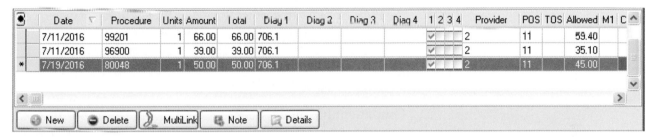

	Date ▽	Procedure	Units	Amount	Total	Diag 1	Diag 2	Diag 3	Diag 4	1 2 3 4	Provider	POS	TOS	Allowed	M1	C
	7/11/2016	99201	1	66.00	66.00	706.1				✓	2	11		59.40		
	7/11/2016	96900	1	39.00	39.00	706.1				✓	2	11		35.10		
*	7/19/2016	80048	1	50.00	50.00	706.1				✓	2	11		45.00		

New ⊖ Delete MultiLink Note Details

Figure 6-8 Charges Section of the Transaction Entry Dialog Box After a Procedure Code Is Selected

After the code is selected and the Tab key is pressed, the program automatically enters data in the other columns (see Figure 6-8). These entries are described in the paragraphs that follow. If additional information must be added, use the Tab key to move to the box in the appropriate column.

Units The Units box indicates the quantity of the procedure. Normally, the number of units is one. In some cases, however, it may be more than one.

Amount The Amount box lists the charge amount for a procedure. The amount is entered automatically by the system based on the CPT code and insurance carrier. Each CPT code stored in the system has a charge amount associated with it. The charge amount can be edited if necessary. These amounts are determined by the fee schedule(s) for a particular office.

Total To the right of the Amount box is the Total box. This field displays the total charges for the procedures performed. The amount is calculated by the system; the number in the Units box is multiplied by the number in the Amount box. For example, suppose a patient had three X-rays done at a charge of $45.00 per X-ray. The Units box would read "3," and the Amount box would read "$45.00." The Total box would read "$135.00," which is 3 × $45.00.

Diagnosis The Diag 1, 2, 3, and 4 boxes correspond to the information in the Diagnosis tab of the Case folder. If a patient has several different diagnoses, the diagnosis that is most relevant to the procedure is used.

1, 2, 3, 4   The 1, 2, 3, and 4 boxes to the right of the Diag 1, 2, 3, and 4 boxes indicate which diagnoses should be used for this charge. A check mark appears in each Diagnosis box for which a diagnosis was entered in the Diag 1, 2, 3, 4 boxes. Some insurance carriers do not permit more than one diagnosis per procedure. Diagnoses can be checked or unchecked as needed.

Provider   The Provider box lists the code number of a patient's assigned provider. If a patient sees a different provider for a visit, the Provider box can be changed to list that provider instead.

POS   The POS, or place of service, box indicates where services were performed. The standard numerical codes used are

- 11   Provider's office
- 21   Inpatient hospital
- 22   Outpatient hospital
- 23   Hospital emergency room

When Medisoft is set up for use in a practice, an option is provided to set a default POS code. In addition, POS codes can be assigned to specific procedure codes when they are set up in the Procedure/Payment/Adjustment Codes List. For purposes of this book, the default code has been set to 11 for provider's office.

TOS   *TOS* stands for "type of service." Medical offices may set up a list of codes to indicate the type of service performed. For example, 1 may indicate an examination, 2 a lab test, and so on. The TOS code is specified in the Procedure/Payment/Adjustment entry for each CPT code.

Allowed   This is the amount allowed by the payer for this procedure. This value comes from the Allowed Amounts tab of the Procedure/Payment/Adjustment dialog box.

M1   The M1 box is for a CPT code modifier. The grid in the Transaction Entry dialog box can be changed to allow entry of up to four modifiers per line.

Co-Pay   A check mark in this box indicates that the code entered in the Procedure column requires a copayment.

BUTTONS IN THE CHARGES AREA OF THE TRANSACTION ENTRY DIALOG BOX

Five buttons are provided at the bottom of the Charges area: New, Delete, MultiLink, Note, and Details. The New button, used to create a new charge entry, has already been discussed.

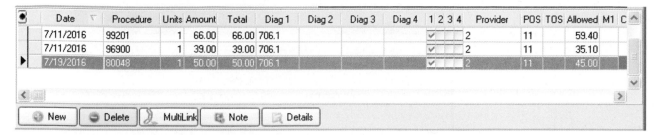

	Date	Procedure	Units	Amount	Total	Diag 1	Diag 2	Diag 3	Diag 4	1 2 3 4	Provider	POS	TOS	Allowed	M1	C
	7/11/2016	99201	1	66.00	66.00	706.1				✓	2	11		59.40		
	7/11/2016	96900	1	39.00	39.00	706.1				✓	2	11		35.10		
▶	7/19/2016	80048	1	50.00	50.00	706.1				✓	2	11		45.00		

New   Delete   MultiLink   Note   Details

Figure 6-9   Transaction Selected for Deletion Indicated by Line Pointer at Left

Delete Button To delete a charge transaction, it is necessary to select the particular charge that is to be deleted. This is accomplished by clicking in any of the boxes associated with that transaction (Date, Procedure, Units, Amount, and so on). Clicking in a box selects the transaction, indicated by the black triangle pointer at the far left box on the line (see Figure 6-9).

Once the desired transaction is selected, it is ready for deletion. Clicking the Delete button causes a confirmation message to be displayed (see Figure 6-10). To continue with the deletion, click the Yes button. To cancel the deletion, click the No button.

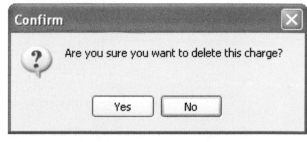

Figure 6-10   Confirm Dialog Box Displayed After Clicking the Delete Button

 All transactions can be deleted from within the Transaction Entry dialog box. Caution should be exercised when using the Delete feature. Deleted data cannot be recovered!

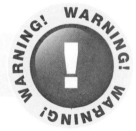

MultiLink Button Medisoft provides a feature that saves time when entering multiple CPT codes that are related to the same activity. **MultiLink codes** are groups of procedure code entries that relate to a single activity. For example, a MultiLink code could be created for the procedures related to diagnosing a strep throat: 99211 OF—Established patient, minimal; 87430 Strep test; and 85025 Complete CBC w/auto diff. WBC.

MultiLink codes groups of procedure code entries that relate to a single activity

When the MultiLink button is clicked, the code STREPM is selected from a drop-down list of MultiLink codes already in the database (see Figures 6-11 and 6-12). All three procedure codes associated with diagnosing a strep throat are entered automatically by the system, eliminating the need to enter each CPT code separately. The MultiLink feature saves time by reducing the number of procedure code entries, and it also reduces omission errors. When procedure codes are entered as a MultiLink, it is impossible to forget to enter a procedure, since all the codes that are in the MultiLink group are entered automatically.

Figure 6-11
MultiLink Button

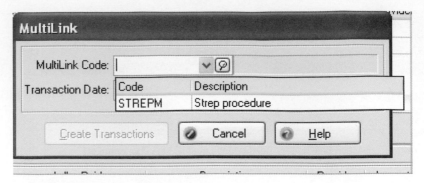

Figure 6-12   MultiLink Code Drop-down List

Clicking the MultiLink button (see Figure 6-11) in the Transaction Entry dialog box displays the MultiLink dialog box (see Figure 6-12). After a MultiLink code is selected from the MultiLink drop-down list, the Create Transactions button is clicked.

The codes and charges for each procedure are automatically added to the list of transactions at the bottom of the Transaction Entry dialog box (see Figure 6-13).

Note Button   The Note button is used to enter additional information about a particular procedure. When the Note button is clicked, the Transaction Documentation dialog box is displayed (see Figure 6-14).

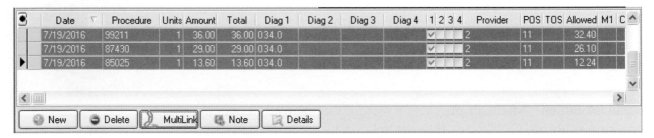

Figure 6-13   Charge Transactions Created with STREPM MultiLink Code

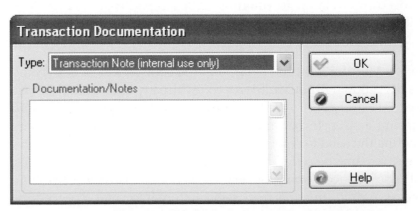

Figure 6-14   Transaction Documentation Dialog Box, Where Notes About a Transaction Are Entered

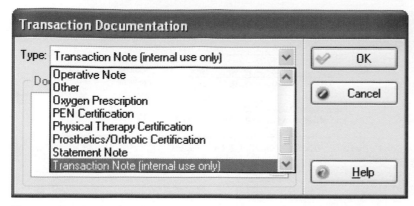

Figure 6-15 Some of the Many Types of Transaction Documentation Available in Medisoft

In the Type field, Medisoft provides a list of types of documentation in the drop-down list (see Figure 6-15). Some of the information entered here is transmitted with an insurance claim when claims are transmitted electronically.

Details Button When clicked, the Details button displays a dialog box that is used to enter drug/prescription information for a charge.

COLOR CODING IN TRANSACTION ENTRY

Transactions in Medisoft are color-coded, making it easy to determine the status of a charge or payment. No color can be assigned to more than one transaction type at the same time. Color codes are set up using the Program Options selection on the File menu.

In the medical practice used in this text/workbook, the codes have already been determined. Three color codes are applied to the status of a charge:

1. No payment (gray)

2. Partially paid charge (aqua)

3. Overpaid charge (yellow)

Charges that have been paid in full are not colored and appear white.

To display a list of color codes used in the Transaction Entry dialog box, click the right mouse button in the white area below the list of transactions, and a shortcut menu is displayed (see Figure 6-16).

When the Show Color Legend option is selected, the Color Coding Legend box appears on the screen (see Figure 6-17). The box lists the meaning of the color codes used in Transaction Entry—three for charges, and three for payments. The color codes used to indicate the status of a payment are discussed later in the chapter.

In Figure 6-16, there is one charge entry on 7/19/2016 for procedure 99211. The line is shaded light blue, to indicate that it has been partially paid. The other two charges are gray, indicating that no payment has been made for these charges.

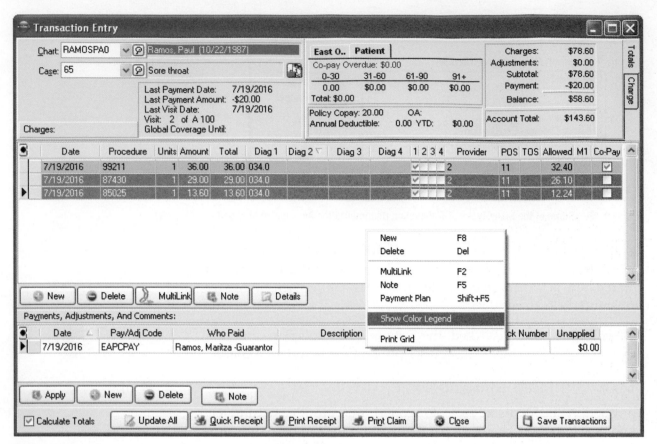

Figure 6-16 Shortcut Menu with Show Color Legend Option Highlighted

SAVING CHARGES

When all the charge information has been entered and checked for accuracy, the transactions must be saved. Transactions are saved by clicking the Save Transactions button, which is located at the bottom of the Transaction Entry dialog box (see Figure 6-18).

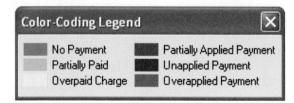

Figure 6-17 Color-Coding Legend Box

Transactions can also be saved by clicking the Update All button located in the same row of buttons. When Update All is clicked, the transactions are saved, and the program checks all fields for missing or invalid information and displays various messages, such as a warning that the date entered is in the future.

The other buttons located in this row, Quick Receipt and Print Receipt, are used to print a walkout receipt for a patient (covered later in this chapter). The Print Claim button is discussed in Chapter 7. The Close button simply closes the Transaction Entry dialog box.

EDITING TRANSACTIONS

The most efficient way to edit a transaction is to click in the field that needs to be changed and enter the correct information. For example, to change the procedure code, click in the Procedure box, and either key a new code or select a new code from the drop-down list. After

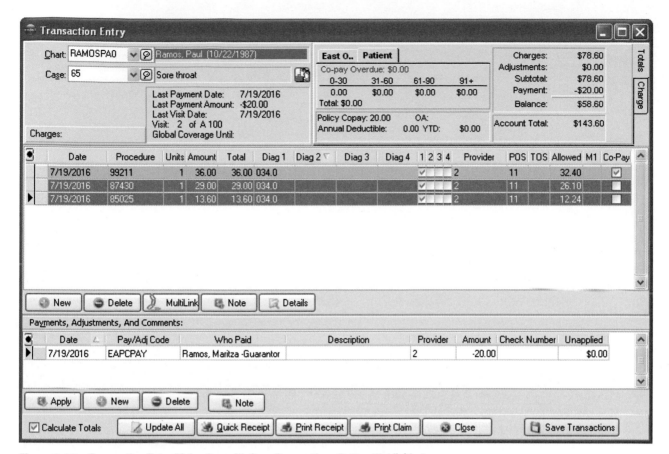

Figure 6-18 Transaction Entry Dialog Box with Save Transactions Button Highlighted

changes are made, the data must be saved. To view the updated amounts in the Patient/Account Information area, click the Update All button near the bottom of the Transaction Entry dialog box.

Depending on the type of edit, the program may display several message boxes. For example, if an attempt is made to change the Payment Type or Who Paid fields, a message is displayed to confirm the change. If someone tries to change a diagnosis code that is already included in a claim, the program asks whether to remove the transaction from the existing claim and create a new claim, or to replace the original diagnosis code in the transaction.

ENTERING A CHARGE FOR HIRO TANAKA	EXERCISE 6-1

Using Source Document 3, enter a charge transaction for Hiro Tanaka's accident case.

Date: October 3, 2016

1. Start Medisoft and restore the data from your last work session.

2. Change the Medisoft Program Date to October 3, 2016, if it is not already set to that date.

3. On the Activities menu, click Enter Transactions. The Transaction Entry dialog box is displayed.

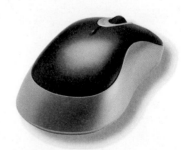

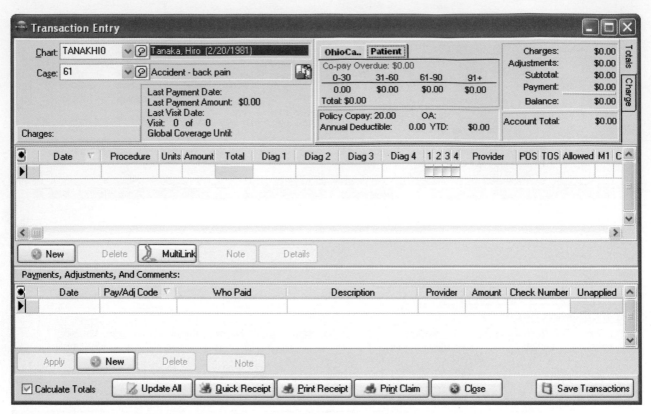

Figure 6-19 Transaction Entry Dialog Box with Hiro Tanaka Selected

4. Key *T* in the Chart box, and then press Tab to select Hiro Tanaka. An Information dialog box is displayed with a message about Tanaka's allergies. Click the OK button to close the box.

5. Verify that the Accident—back pain case is the active case in the Case box. Compare your screen to Figure 6-19.

6. In the Charges section of the dialog box, click the New button.

7. Verify that the entry in the Date box is 10/3/2016.

8. Click in the Procedure box, and enter **99202** to select the procedure code for the service checked off on the encounter form. Press Tab. Notice that the Diag 1 box and the Units box have been automatically completed. The Amount box is also automatically completed ($88.00). If necessary, these entries can be edited by clicking in the box and entering new data.

9. Review the entries in the Provider (1) and POS (11) boxes. Since there are no modifiers to the procedure code, the M1 box is left blank.

10. Check your entries against Figure 6-20 for accuracy.

11. Click the Save Transactions button. A Date of Service Validation message appears. Click Yes to save the transaction.

12. A message appears that a $20.00 copayment is due. This will be entered later in the chapter, in the section on copayments. Click the OK button.

13. At the top of the Transaction Entry dialog box, notice that the Co-pay Overdue field in red now lists $20.00 and the Account Total field displays $88.00.

14. Check your work against Figure 6-21.

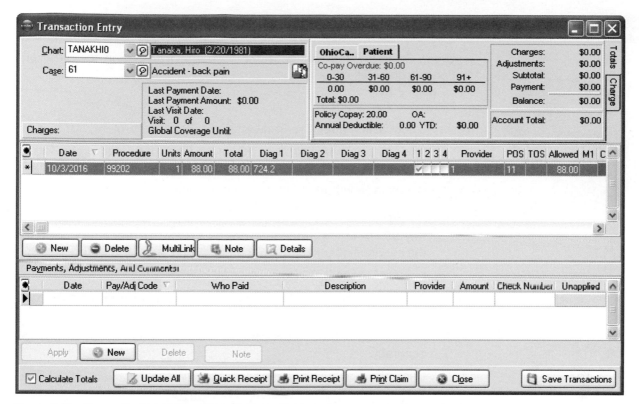

Figure 6-20 Transaction Entry Dialog Box with Charge Entered

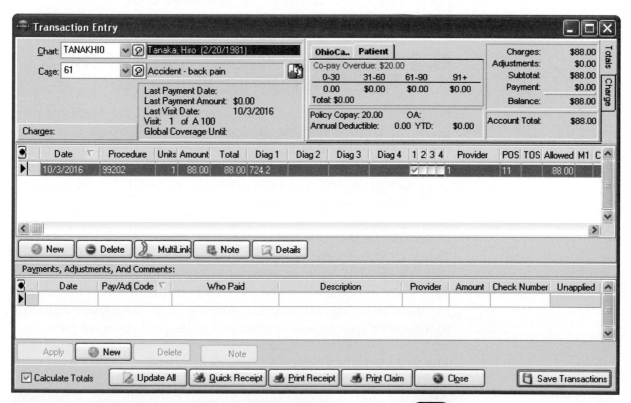

Figure 6-21 Transaction Entry Dialog Box with Transaction Saved

 You have completed Exercise 6-1.

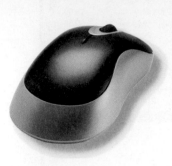

Using Source Document 5, enter a charge transaction for Elizabeth Jones's diabetes case.

Date: October 3, 2016

1. If necessary, open the Transaction Entry dialog box.

2. Click in the Chart field; key **JO** in the Chart box; and press Tab to select Elizabeth Jones. Verify that the Diabetes case is selected.

3. Click the New button in the Charges section of the window.

4. Accept the default in the Date box (10/3/2016).

5. Key **99213** in the Procedure box to select the procedure code for the services checked off on the encounter form. Press Tab.

6. Keep "1" in the Units box.

7. Accept the charge for the procedure that is displayed in the Amount box ($72.00).

8. Review the entries in the other boxes, and check your entries for accuracy.

9. Click the Save Transactions button. When the Date of Service Validation box appears, click Yes.

☑ **You have completed Exercise 6-2.**

6.4 ENTERING PAYMENTS MADE AT THE TIME OF AN OFFICE VISIT

Payments are entered in two different areas of the Medisoft program: the Transaction Entry dialog box, and the Deposit List dialog box, which will be discussed in Chapter 8. Practices have different preferences for how payments are entered, depending on their billing procedures. In this text/workbook, you will be introduced to both methods of payment entry.

Patient payments made at the time of an office visit are entered in the Transaction Entry dialog box. Payments that are received electronically or by mail, such as insurance payments and mailed patient payments, are entered in the Deposit List dialog box. The Deposit List feature is very efficient for entering large insurance payments that must be split up and applied to a number of different patients.

The first step when entering a patient payment is to select a patient's chart number and case number in the Transaction Entry dialog box. After the chart and case numbers have been selected, a payment transaction can be entered. Payments are entered in the Payments, Adjustments, and Comments section of the Transaction Entry dialog box (see Figure 6-22).

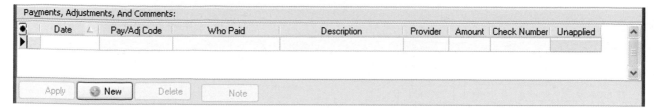

Figure 6-22   Payments, Adjustments, and Comments Area of the Transaction Entry Dialog Box

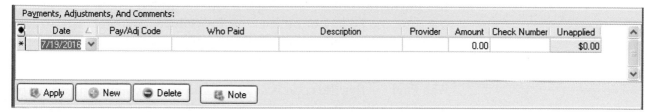

Figure 6-23   Payments, Adjustments, and Comments Area After Clicking the New Button

The process of creating a payment transaction begins with clicking the New button. When the New button is clicked, the program automatically enters the current date (the date that the Medisoft program date is set to) in the Date box (see Figure 6-23).

If this is not the date on which the payment was received, the date must be changed to reflect this date. To change the default date for these boxes, any of these methods can be used:

- The Set Program Date command on the File menu can be clicked.

- The Date button in the lower-right corner of the screen can be clicked. (This must be done before the New button is clicked in the Transaction Entry dialog box.)

- The date that is already in the Date box can be keyed over.

Pay/Adj Code   Once the correct date is entered, pressing the Tab key moves the cursor to the Payment/Adjustment Code box. The code for a payment is selected from the drop-down list of payment codes already entered in the system (see Figure 6-24).

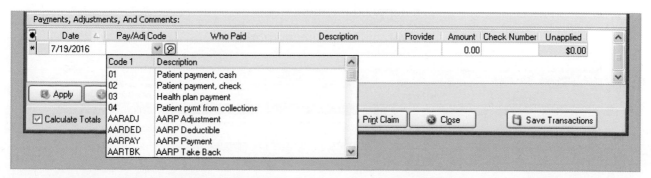

Figure 6-24   Payment/Adjustment Code Drop-down List

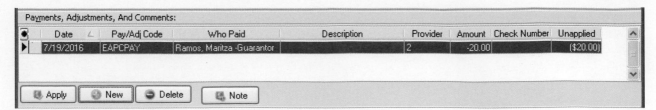

Figure 6-25 Payments, Adjustments, and Comments Area After Payment/Adjustment Code Is Entered

If a payment code is not listed, it can be added to the database by pressing the F8 key or by clicking Procedure/Payment/Adjustment Codes on the Lists menu. This may be done without exiting the Transaction Entry dialog box.

Who Paid   After the code is selected and the Tab key is pressed, the program automatically completes the Who Paid box based on information stored in the database (see Figure 6-25). The Who Paid field displays a drop-down list of guarantors and carriers that are assigned in the patient case folder.

Description   The Description field can be used to enter other information about the payment, if desired.

Provider   The Provider column lists the code number of the provider.

Amount   The Amount field contains the amount of payment received. If the payment is a copayment from a patient, this box is completed automatically when a payment/adjustment code is selected. Again, the program uses information stored in the database.

Check Number   The Check Number field is used to record the number of the check used for payment.

Unapplied   The dollar value in the Unapplied box is the amount that has not yet been applied to a charge transaction.

APPLYING PAYMENTS TO CHARGES

Payments are color-coded to indicate payment status (see Figure 6-26). Three color codes are applied to the status of a payment:

1. Partially applied payment (blue)

2. Unapplied payment (red)

3. Overapplied payment (pink)

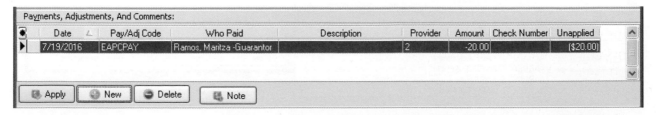

Figure 6-26 Payments, Adjustments, and Comments Area with a Color-Coded Unapplied Payment and Apply Button Highlighted

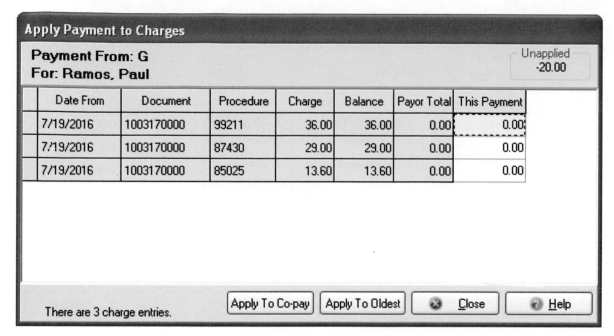

Apply Payment to Charges

Payment From: G
For: Ramos, Paul

Unapplied
-20.00

Date From	Document	Procedure	Charge	Balance	Payor Total	This Payment
7/19/2016	1003170000	99211	36.00	36.00	0.00	0.00
7/19/2016	1003170000	87430	29.00	29.00	0.00	0.00
7/19/2016	1003170000	85025	13.60	13.60	0.00	0.00

There are 3 charge entries.

Apply To Co-pay   Apply To Oldest   Close   Help

Figure 6-27   Apply Payment to Charges Dialog Box with This Payment Box Highlighted

Payments that have been fully applied are not colored and appear white.

Once all the necessary information is entered, it is time to apply the payment to specific charges. This is accomplished by clicking the Apply button, which causes the Apply Payment to Charges dialog box to be displayed. The Apply Payment to Charges dialog box lists information about all unpaid charges for a patient, including the date of the procedure, the document number, the procedure code, the charge, the balance, and the total amount paid (see Figure 6-27).

In the upper-right corner of the dialog box, the amount of payment that has not yet been applied to charges is listed in the Unapplied box.

The first step in applying a payment is to determine the charge(s) to which the payment should be applied. Payments may be applied to charges that require a copayment, charges that are the oldest, or any other charges.

If the payment is a copayment, then the Apply to Co-pay button is clicked. When the Apply to Co-pay button is clicked, the program automatically applies the payment to the charge on that date that requires a copayment. Information about whether a procedure code requires a copayment is located in the General tab of the Procedure/Payment/Adjustment dialog box for that code. In the exercises in this text/workbook, copayments are required for Evaluation and Management Codes—procedure codes that cover physicians' services performed to determine the optimum course for patient care.

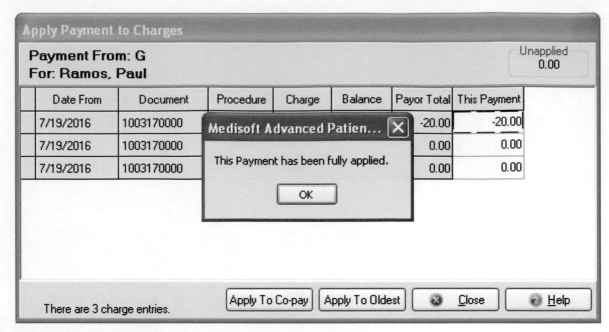

Figure 6-28 Apply Payment to Charges Dialog Box with Payment Entered

If the payment should be applied to the oldest charge, then the Apply to Oldest button is clicked. When the Apply to Oldest button is used, the program automatically applies the payment to the oldest charge.

Payments may also be manually applied by clicking in the box in the This Payment column on the line that contains the charge. To select a box, click in it; a dotted rectangle appears around the outside of the box. Enter the amount of the payment (without a decimal point), and press the Enter key. The payment is applied, and the Unapplied Amount entry is lowered by the amount of the payment.

Notice in Figure 6-28 that the payment amount has been entered in the appropriate This Payment box.

Payments can be applied to more than one charge. For example, suppose that the payment is $200.00 and three charges have not been paid. The $200.00 payment can be applied to one, two, or all three of the charges.

Once the box is closed, the payment appears in the Payments, Adjustments, and Comments area of the Transaction Entry dialog box (see Figure 6-29).

SAVING PAYMENT INFORMATION

When all the information on a payment has been entered and checked for accuracy, it must be saved. Payment transactions are saved in the manner described earlier for charge transactions, by clicking the Save Transactions button.

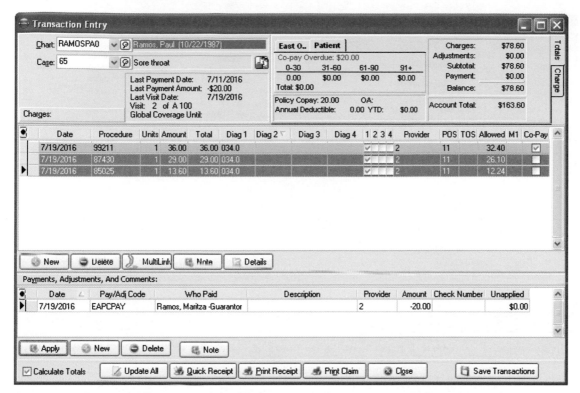

Figure 6-29 Payments, Adjustments, and Comments Area with Payment Listed and Charges Color-Coded as Partially Paid (Aqua) and No Payment (Gray)

| ENTERING A COPAYMENT | EXERCISE 6-3 |

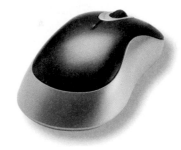

Using Source Documents 1 and 3, enter the copayment made by Hiro Tanaka for her October 3, 2016, office visit.

Date: October 3, 2016

1. Open the Transaction Entry dialog box if it is not already open.

2. In the Chart box, key **T,** and press Tab to select Hiro Tanaka. An Information box is displayed with information about Tanaka's allergies. Click the OK button.

3. Verify that Accident—back pain is the active case in the Case box.

4. Click the New button in the Payments, Adjustments, and Comments section of the dialog box.

5. Accept the default entry of 10/3/2016 in the Date box.

6. Click in the Pay/Adj Code box. From the drop-down list, select OHCCPAY (the code for OhioCare HMO copayment), and press Tab. *Note:* You can also select OHCCPAY by entering the letters in the box. Once you press Tab, the entire line will be highlighted in red. Notice that some of the boxes have been completed by the program.

7. Verify that Tanaka, Hiro—Guarantor is listed in the Who Paid box.

8. Notice that −20.00 has already been entered in the Amount box. Confirm that this is the correct amount of the copay by looking at Source Document 1.

9. The Unapplied Amount box should read ($20.00).

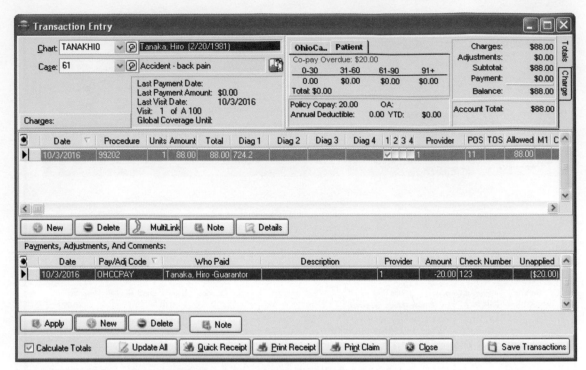

Figure 6-30   Transaction Entry Dialog Box with Copayment Entered

10. Click in the Check Number box; enter **123;** and press Tab. Your screen should look like the dialog box in Figure 6-30.

11. Click the Apply button. The Apply Payment to Charges dialog box is displayed.

12. Notice that the amount of this payment (−20.00) is listed in the Unapplied box at the upper-right of the dialog box (see Figure 6-31).

13. Click the Apply to Co-pay button. When the box appears that states "This payment has been fully applied," click OK. The program automatically enters −20.00 in the box in the This Payment column for the 99202 procedure charge. The Unapplied box is now zero. (*Note:* If zero is not displayed yet, click once in the empty space below the This Payment box, and the program will update the Unapplied box.) See Figure 6-32.

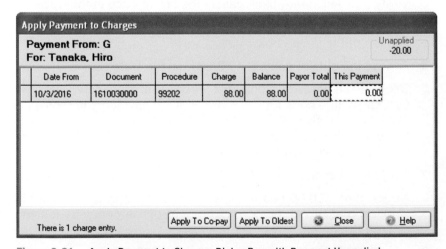

Figure 6-31   Apply Payment to Charges Dialog Box with Payment Unapplied

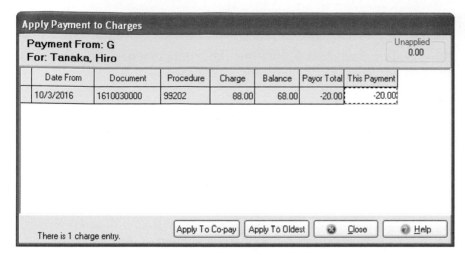

Figure 6-32   Apply Payment to Charges Dialog Box with Payment Applied

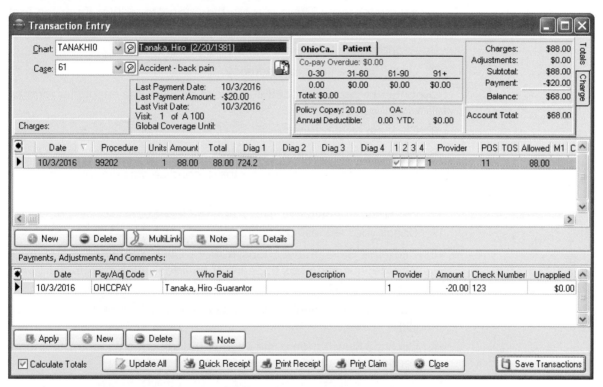

Figure 6-33   Transaction Entry Dialog Box with Copayment Entry Applied and Saved

14. Click the Close button.

15. Click the Save Transactions button. When the date warning box appears, click Yes. If an Information box appears with a reminder about the copay, click OK.

16. Notice that the line listing the procedure charge has changed from gray (not paid) to aqua (partially paid), indicating that a portion of the charge has been paid (see Figure 6-33). **CiMC**

 You have completed Exercise 6-3.

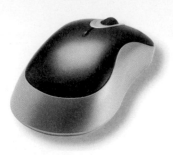

Using Source Document 6, enter the procedure charges and copayment for John Fitzwilliams's acute gastric ulcer case.

Date: October 3, 2016

1. Open the Transaction Entry dialog box, if it is not already open. Click in the Chart box, and key **F.** Notice that the chart number for John Fitzwilliams is highlighted on the drop-down list. Press the Tab key. Verify that Acute gastric ulcer is the active case in the Case box.

2. Notice that there are already charges and payments listed for this case, since this is an existing medical condition for which the patient has been treated in the past.

3. Click the New button in the Charges section of the dialog box.

4. Accept the default in the Date box (10/3/2016).

5. Select the procedure code for the services checked off on the encounter form. There is more than one procedure. Enter the first procedure code (99212). Press Tab.

6. Accept the default entries in the other boxes.

7. Check your entries for accuracy.

Now enter the second procedure code marked on the encounter form by following these steps.

8. Click the New button.

9. Accept the default in the Date box.

10. Select the procedure code for the second service checked off on the encounter form (82270). Press Tab.

11. Accept the default entries in the other boxes.

12. Check your entries for accuracy.

13. Click the Save Transactions button. Click Yes when the Date of Service Validation box appears. If an Information box appears with a reminder about the copay, click OK.

Now enter the copayment listed on the encounter form by completing the remaining steps.

14. Click the New button in the Payments, Adjustments, and Comments section of the dialog box.

15. Accept the default entry of 10/3/2016 in the Date box.

16. On the Pay/Adj Code drop-down list, click CHVCPAY (CHAMPVA Copayment), and press Tab. Notice that all the remaining boxes except Check Number and Description are once again filled in. Verify that the entries are correct.

17. Enter **456** in the Check Number box, and press Tab.

18. Click the Apply button. The Apply Payment to Charges dialog box is displayed.

19. Notice that the amount of this payment (–15.00) is listed in the Unapplied box at the upper-right of the dialog box.

20. Click the Apply to Co-pay button. When the box appears that states "This payment has been fully applied," click OK.

21. Click the Close button.

22. Click the Save Transactions button. When the date warning box appears, click the Yes button. If an Information box appears with a reminder about the copay, click OK.

23. Notice that the amount listed in the Unapplied Amount column is now zero. Also notice that the line listing the 99212 charge on 10/3/2016 is now aqua rather than gray, indicating that the charge has been partially paid.

24. Notice also that the program moves the most recent transaction in the Payments, Adjustments, and Comments section (the transaction dated 10/3/2016) up to the first row after it is applied. Clicking once on a Date column heading in the Transaction Entry dialog box reorders the transaction dates chronologically from newest to oldest. Clicking again reorders them in the reverse way, from oldest to newest. The order of the dates can be toggled back and forth, depending on your preference.

 You have completed Exercise 6-4. **CiMO**

6.5 PRINTING WALKOUT RECEIPTS

After a patient payment has been entered in the Transaction Entry dialog box, a walkout receipt is printed and given to the patient before he or she leaves the office. A walkout receipt, also known as a walkout statement, includes information on the procedures, diagnosis, charges, and payments for a visit. If there is a balance due, the receipt serves as a reminder to the patient of the amount owed.

In the Transaction Entry dialog box, walkout receipts are created via the Print Receipt or Quick Receipt button (see Figure 6-34). The Quick Receipt option remembers the user's preferred report format and eliminates several steps in the creation of a receipt. (*Note:* A Print Claim button also appears in the Transaction Entry dialog box; claim management is discussed in detail in Chapter 7.)

When the Print Receipt button is clicked, the Open Report window appears with the first report highlighted, Walkout Receipt (All Transactions), as shown in Figure 6-35.

After clicking the OK button in the Open Report window, the Print Report Where? dialog box is displayed, and three options are provided (see Figure 6-36):

1. Preview the report on the screen

2. Print the report on the printer

3. Export the report to a file

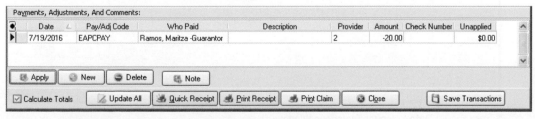

Figure 6-34 Quick Receipt and Print Receipt Buttons Highlighted in Yellow

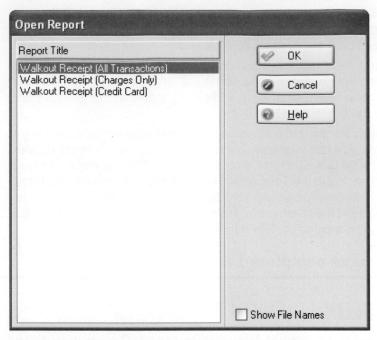

Figure 6-35   Open Report Window with Walkout Receipt (All Transactions) Selected

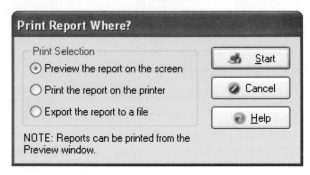

Figure 6-36   Print Report Where? Dialog Box

Once a printing choice is made, clicking the Start button causes the Data Selection Questions window to open (see Figure 6-37). This is where the data for the receipt are selected.

Finally, when the OK button is clicked, the report is sent to its destination (on screen, to the printer, to a file; see Figure 6-38).

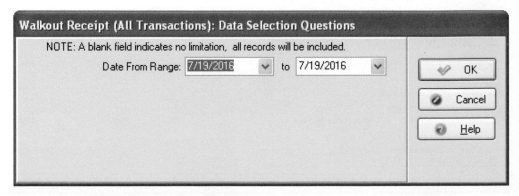

Figure 6-37   Data Selection Questions Window

Family Care Center
285 Stephenson Boulevard
Stephenson, OH 60089
(614)555-0000

Page: 1

7/19/2016

Patient:	Paul Ramos	Instructions:

Patient: Paul Ramos
39 Locust Avenue
Stephenson, OH 60089

Chart #: RAMOSPA0
Case #: 65

Instructions:
Complete the patient information portion of your insurance claim form. Attach this bill, signed and dated, and all other bills pertaining to the claim. If you have a deductible policy, hold your claim forms until you have met your deductible. Mail directly to your insurance carrier.

Date	Description	Procedure	Modify	Dx 1	Dx 2	Dx 3	Dx 4	Units	Charge
7/19/2016	OF--established patient, minimal	99211		034.0				1	36.00
7/19/2016	Strep test	87430		034.0				1	29.00
7/19/2016	Complete CBC w/auto diff WDC	85025		034.0				1	13.60
7/19/2016	East Ohio PPO Copayment	EAPCPAY						1	-20.00

Provider Information

Provider Name:	John Rudner MD
License:	84701
Insurance PIN:	
SSN or EIN:	339-67-5000

Total Charges:	$ 78.60
Total Payments:	-$ 20.00
Total Adjustments:	$ 0.00
Total Due This Visit:	**$ 58.60**
Total Account Balance:	$ 143.60

Assign and Release: I hereby authorize payment of medical benefits to this physician for the services described above. I also authorize the release of any information necessary to process this claim.

Patient Signature: _____   Date: _____

Figure 6-38   Sample Walkout Receipt

CREATING A WALKOUT RECEIPT

Create a walkout receipt for John Fitzwilliams.

Date: October 3, 2016

1. With the Transaction Entry dialog box open to John Fitzwilliams's acute gastric ulcer case, click the Quick Receipt button. The Print Report Where? dialog box is displayed.

2. In the Print Report Where? dialog box, accept the default selection to preview the report on the screen. Click the Start button. The Preview Report window opens, displaying the walkout receipt.

3. Review the charge and payment entries listed in the top half of the receipt.

4. Scroll down and review the total charges, payments, and adjustments listed in the lower-right area of the receipt.

5. Click the Close button to exit the Preview Report window.

✔ **You have completed Exercise 6-5.**

6.6 PROCESSING A PATIENT REFUND

Sometimes it is necessary to make an adjustment to a patient account. This can happen for a number of reasons. Some practices ask patients to make an estimated payment at the time of the office visit. This amount is an estimate of the amount the patient will owe after the expected payment is received from the insurance company. When the actual payment is received from the insurance carrier, it may be greater or less than the estimated amount. If it is greater than estimated, the practice must issue the patient a refund of the overpayment.

Adjustments to patient accounts are entered in the same manner as payments are recorded, in the lower third of the Transaction Entry dialog box. Clicking the New button begins the process of entering an adjustment. When the New button is clicked, the program automatically enters the current date (the date that the Medisoft program date is set to) in the Date box. The other fields include the following:

Payment/Adjustment Code This code indicates the type of adjustment transaction, such as PTREFUND (patient refund).

Who Paid In the case of a refund, the chart number of the patient who is receiving the refund is entered.

Description The reason for the refund, such as "patient payment more than expected," is entered.

Provider The provider column lists the code number of the provider.

Amount The amount of the refund is shown.

Check Number The number of the check used for the refund is entered.

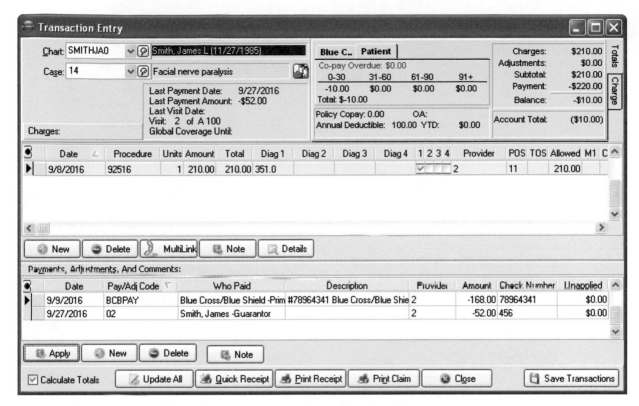

Figure 6-39 Transaction Entry Dialog Box with the Overpaid Charge Highlighted in Yellow

Unapplied The dollar value in the Unapplied box is the amount that has not yet been applied to a transaction.

If the patient's account has a positive balance because the patient overpaid, the patient's charge in the Transaction Entry dialog box is color-coded yellow (see Figure 6-39). This indicates the patient is due a refund for that procedure, and an adjustment needs to be made.

| PROCESSING A REFUND | EXERCISE 6-6 |

Process a refund for a patient who has overpaid on his account.

Date: October 3, 2016

1. Open the Transaction Entry dialog box, if it is not already open.

2. In the Chart box, key **SM,** and press Tab to select James L. Smith.

3. Verify that Facial nerve paralysis is displayed in the Case box.

4. Notice that the entry in the Charges section of the window is highlighted in yellow, indicating that this is an overpaid charge. According to the patient's insurance plan, the plan pays 80 percent of charges and the patient pays 20 percent. In this case, 20 percent of the charges ($210.00) would be $42.00. However, the patient paid $52, and is therefore due a refund of $10.00.

5. Click the New button in the Payments, Adjustments, and Comments section of the dialog box.

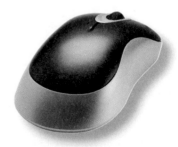

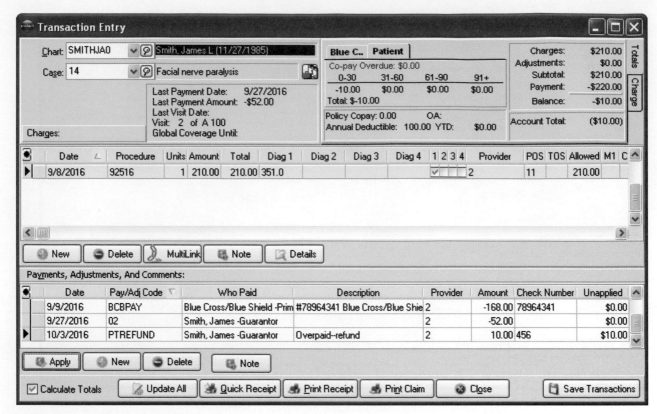

Figure 6-40 Transaction Entry Dialog Box with Unapplied Patient Refund Adjustment

6. Accept the default entry of 10/3/2016 in the Date box.

7. Click in the Pay/Adj Code box. Select PTREFUND (the code for a patient refund) from the drop-down list, and press Tab.

8. Select Smith, James—Guarantor in the Who Paid box.

9. Enter **Overpaid—refund** in the Description box, and press Tab twice to get to the Amount box.

10. Enter **10** in the Amount box, and press Tab. Notice that the amount is listed as a positive amount.

11. The Unapplied Amount box should read $10.00.

12. Enter **456** in the Check Number box, and press Tab. Check your work against Figure 6-40.

13. Click the Apply button. The Apply Adjustment to Charges dialog box is displayed.

14. Notice that the amount of this refund ($10.00) is listed in the Unapplied box at the upper-right of the dialog box.

15. Click in the white box in the This Adjust. column. Enter **10,** and press Enter. Your screen should look like Figure 6-41.

16. Click the Close button.

17. Click the Save Transactions button. When a box appears indicating that the statement has been marked done, click OK.

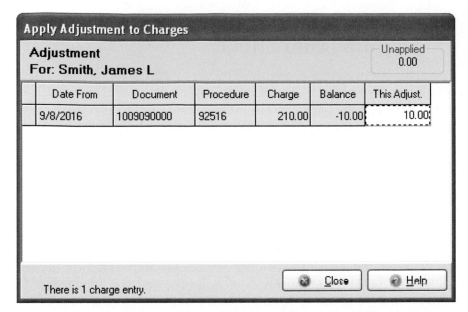

Figure 6-41   Apply Adjustment to Charges Dialog Box with $10.00 Refund Adjustment Applied

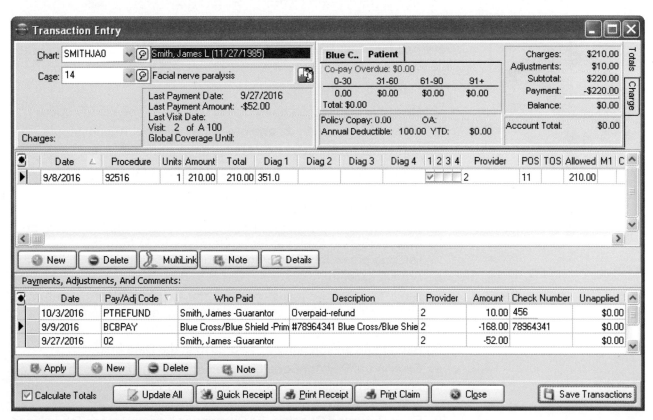

Figure 6-42   Transaction Entry Dialog Box No Longer Showing Overpayment

18. Notice that the line listing the procedure charge has changed from yellow (overpaid) to white (fully paid), indicating that the expected amount has been paid (see Figure 6-42).   **ciMO**

 You have completed Exercise 6-6.

6.7 PROCESSING A NONSUFFICIENT FUNDS (NSF) CHECK

NSF check a check that is not honored by a bank because the account it was written on does not have sufficient funds to cover it

When a patient makes a payment by check and does not have adequate funds in his or her checking account to cover the check, it is not honored by the bank. These checks are referred to as **NSF checks**, for "nonsufficient funds." They are also commonly called "bounced" and "returned" checks. A bank may also not honor a check if the account has been closed. When a practice receives an NSF notice from a bank, an adjustment is made in the patient's account, since the patient now owes the practice the amount of the returned check. In addition, most practices charge a fee for a returned check. The maximum amount of the fee is governed by state laws.

In Medisoft, the fee for the returned check is entered in the Charges section of the Transaction Entry dialog box, and the adjustment is entered in the Payments, Adjustments, and Comments section.

EXERCISE 6-7	PROCESSING AN NSF CHECK

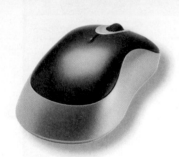

Kristin Zapata's check number 1033, in the amount of $247.50, was returned for insufficient funds. Process an NSF fee and adjustment for the returned check.

Date: October 3, 2016

1. Open the Transaction Entry dialog box, if it is not already open.
2. In the Chart box, key **Z,** and press Tab to select Kristin Zapata.
3. Verify that Preventive Exam is displayed in the Case box.
4. Click the New button in the Charges section of the Transaction Entry dialog box.
5. Accept the date entry of 10/3/2016.
6. To enter the fee for the returned check, click in the Procedure box. Select NSFFEE (NSF fee for a returned check) from the drop-down list, and press Tab. The program automatically enters $35.00 in the Amount column.
7. Next, to enter the adjustment for the full amount of the returned check, click the New button in the Payments, Adjustments, and Comments section of the dialog box.
8. Accept the default entry of 10/3/2016 in the Date box.
9. Click in the Pay/Adj Code box. Select NSF (the code for a returned check) from the drop-down list, and press Tab twice (no information is entered in the Who Paid box).
10. Enter **Returned Check** in the Description box, and press Tab twice to go to the Amount box.
11. Enter **$247.50** in the Amount box, and press Tab. Notice that the amount is listed as a positive amount.
12. Press Tab and enter the check number in the Check Number field.
13. Click the Apply button. The Apply Adjustment to Charges dialog box is displayed.
14. Notice that the amount of the adjustment ($247.50) is listed in the Unapplied box at the upper-right of the dialog box.

15. Click in the white box in the This Adjust. column for the $247.50 charge on 8/29/2016. Enter **247.50**, and press Enter.

16. Click the Close button.

17. In the Charges section of the dialog box, notice that the line for the charge that was white (fully paid) is now gray (no payment received). The line for the $35.00 fee (NSFFEE) is also gray, since it has not been paid.

18. Click the Save Transactions button. When the date warning box appears, click Yes.

19. *Note:* To see the NSF adjustment you just entered, you may need to scroll down in the Payments, Adjustments, and Comments section of the dialog box.

✓ **You have completed Exercise 6-7.**

APPLYING YOUR SKILLS

3: ADD A DIAGNOSIS AND ENTER PROCEDURE CHARGES

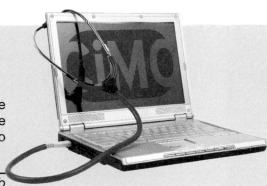

October 3, 2016
Lisa Wright has just been seen by Dr. Jessica Rudner. Using Source Document 7, enter the diagnosis in the Case folder, and then enter the procedure charges in the Transaction Entry dialog box. Be sure to enter the charge in the second column of the encounter form.

Remember to create a backup of your work before exiting Medisoft! To help you keep track of your work, name the backup file after the chapter you are working on, for example, StudentID-c6.mbk.

ELECTRONIC HEALTH RECORD EXCHANGE

Importing Transactions

Transactions imported from an electronic health record (EHR) are held as unprocessed transactions until they are reviewed and posted by a member of the billing staff. In Medisoft, the Unprocessed Charges window displays transactions transmitted from the EHR program that have yet to be posted in Medisoft. The dialog box provides editing capability should changes need to be made before posting.

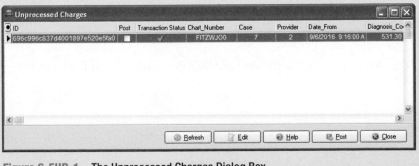

Figure 6-EHR-1   The Unprocessed Charges Dialog Box

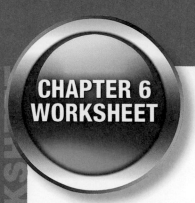

Name: _____   Date: _____

After completing all the exercises in the chapter, answer the following questions in the spaces provided.

1. *[LO 6.5]* What are the total charges listed on John Fitzwilliams's walkout receipt?

   _____

2. *[LO 6.4]* What is entered in the Pay/Adj Code box for Hiro Tanaka's copayment on 10/3/2016 (Transaction Entry dialog box)?

   _____

3. *[LO 6.4]* What is listed as the annual deductible for John Fitzwilliams (Transaction Entry dialog box)?

   _____

4. *[LO 6.3]* What is listed in the Allowed Amount box for procedure 99212 on 10/3/2016 for John Fitzwilliams (Transaction Entry dialog box)?

   _____

5. *[LO 6.3]* What is entered in the Total box for procedure 99213 on 10/3/2016 for Elizabeth Jones (Transaction Entry dialog box)?

   _____

6. *[LO 6.3]* What is entered in the Diag 1 box for procedure 99202 on 10/3/2016 for Hiro Tanaka (Transaction Entry dialog box)?

   _____

7. *[LO 6.3]* What is entered in the Provider box for procedure 99202 on 10/3/2016 for Hiro Tanaka (Transaction Entry dialog box)?

   _____

8. *[LO 6.7]* What is the amount of the returned check fee for Kristin Zapata on 10/3/2016 (Transaction Entry dialog box)?

   _____

9. *[LO 6.3]* What is entered in the Amount box for procedure 99203 on 10/3/2016 for Lisa Wright (Transaction Entry dialog box)?

   _____

10. *[LO 6.3]* What two procedure codes are listed for Lisa Wright on 10/3/2016 (Transaction Entry dialog box)?

   _____

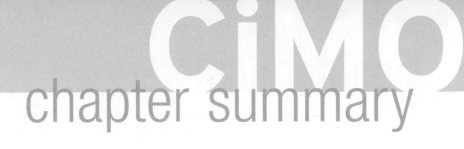
6.1 Describe the three types of transactions recorded in Medisoft. Page 174	1. Charges are the amounts a provider bills for the services performed. 2. Payments are monies received from patients and insurance carriers. 3. Adjustments are changes to patients' accounts.
6.2 Discuss how to select a patient and case in Transaction Entry. Pages 174–177	To select a patient, click the Chart drop-down list. Enter the first few letters of the patient's last name, and when you find the patient's entry, click to select it. To select a case for the patient, click the Case drop-down list and click on the desired case.
6.3 Demonstrate how to enter charge transactions in Medisoft. Pages 177–188	1. Select the patient and case in the Transaction Entry dialog box. 2. In the Charges section of the dialog box, click the New button. 3. Accept or change the date listed. 4. Click the Procedure drop-down list, and find the correct code. Click the code to enter it. You may also key in the code manually. Press the Tab key to get to the end of the line. 5. Review the information you entered. 6. Click the Save Transactions button. (If a Date of Service Validation box opens because the date is in the future, click Yes to continue saving.)
6.4 Demonstrate how to enter payments made at the time of an office visit. Pages 188–197	1. Select the patient and case in the Transaction Entry dialog box. 2. In the Payments, Adjustments, and Comments section of the dialog box, click the New button. 3. Accept or change the date listed. 4. Click the Pay/Adj Code drop-down list, and find the correct code. Click the code to enter it. Press the Tab key. 5. Click in the Who Paid column, and select the appropriate entry. Press the Tab key. 6. Entering information in the Description field is optional. 7. To record a check number, press Tab to get to the Check Number field. 8. Review the information you entered.

9. Click the Apply button. The Apply Payment to Charges window appears.

   - If the payment is a copayment, click the Apply to Co-pay button. Click OK in response to the message that the payment has been fully applied. Then click the Close button.

   - If the payment is not a copayment, click in the box in the This Payment column next to the appropriate charge. Enter the amount of the payment and press Enter. Then click the Close button.

10. Click the Save Transactions button. (If a Date of Service Validation box opens because the date is in the future, click Yes to continue saving.)

6.5 Demonstrate how to print a walkout receipt. Pages 197–200

1. Select the patient and case in the Transaction Entry dialog box.

2. Click the Print Receipt or Quick Receipt button in the Transaction Entry dialog box.

3. In the Open Report window, confirm that the Walkout Receipt (All Transactions) option is selected, then click OK.

4. In the Print Report Where? dialog box, select an option to preview the report, print the report, or save the report as a file, and then click Start.

5. In the Walkout Receipt (All Transactions) box, confirm that the correct dates are selected in both Date From Range boxes and click OK.

6. The receipt is created and appears on the screen (if a preview), is sent to a printer, or is saved to a file.

6.6 Demonstrate how to process a refund for a patient. Pages 200–203

1. Select the patient and the appropriate case in the Transaction Entry dialog box.

2. In the Payments, Adjustments, and Comments section of the dialog box, click the New button.

3. Accept or change the date listed.

4. Click the Pay/Adj Code drop-down list, and select the PTREFUND code. Press the Tab key.

5. Click in the Who Paid column and select the patient. Press the Tab key.

6. Enter *Overpaid—refund* in the Description field. Press Tab twice.

7. Enter the amount of the refund, and press Tab.

8. Review the information you entered.

	9. Click the Apply button. The Apply Adjustment to Charges dialog box appears.
	10. Click in the white box in the This Adjust. column next to the overpaid charge. Enter the amount of the refund, and press Enter. Then click the Close button.
	11. Click the Save Transactions button. (If a Date of Service Validation box opens because the date is in the future, click Yes to continue saving.)
6.7 Demonstrate how to post a nonsufficient funds (NSF) check. Pages 204–205	Begin by entering the NSF fee for the returned check.
	1. Select the patient and case in the Transaction Entry dialog box.
	2. In the Charges section of the dialog box, click the New button.
	3. Accept or change the date listed.
	4. Click the Procedure drop-down list, and select the NSFFEE code. Click the code to enter it. Press the Tab key. Confirm that the correct amount is listed in the Amount field.
	5. Review the information you entered.
	Now enter the returned check as an adjustment to the account.
	6. In the Payments, Adjustments, and Comments section of the dialog box, click the New button.
	7. Accept or change the date listed.
	8. Click the Pay/Adj Code drop-down list, and select the NSF code. Leave the Who Paid field blank. Press the Tab key.
	9. Enter *Returned Check* in the Description box. Press Tab twice.
	10. Enter the amount of the returned check in the Amount field, and press Tab.
	11. Review the information you entered.
	12. Click the Apply button. The Apply Adjustment to Charges window appears.
	13. Click in the white box in the This Adjust. column next to the entry for the check. Enter the amount of the returned check, and press Enter. Then click the Close button.
	14. Click the Save Transactions button. (If a Date of Service Validation box opens because the date is in the future, click Yes to continue saving.)

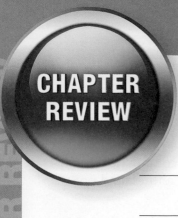

USING TERMINOLOGY

Match the terms on the left with the definitions on the right.

_____ **1.** *[LO 6.1]* adjustments

_____ **2.** *[LO 6.1]* charges

_____ **3.** *[LO 6.3]* MultiLink codes

_____ **4.** *[LO 6.7]* NSF check

_____ **5.** *[LO 6.1]* payments

a. Changes to patients' accounts.

b. The amounts billed by a provider for particular services.

c. A payment not honored by a bank because the account it was written on does not have sufficient funds to cover the check.

d. Monies paid to a medical practice by patients and insurance carriers.

e. Groups of procedure code entries that are related to a single activity.

CHECKING YOUR UNDERSTANDING

Answer the questions below in the space provided.

1. *[LO 6.3]* What are the two key pieces of information you must have before entering a procedure charge?

_____

_____

2. *[LO 6.3]* List two advantages of using MultiLink codes.

_____

_____

3. *[LO 6.5]* When is it appropriate to print a walkout receipt?

_____

_____

4. *[LO 6.3]* What color code indicates that no payment has been made on a charge transaction?

_____

_____

5. *[LO 6.4]* What is the color code for an unapplied payment?

_____

_____

APPLYING YOUR KNOWLEDGE

Answer the questions below in the space provided.

6.1. *[LO 6.3]* After you have entered a charge for procedure code 99393, you realize it should have been 99394. What should you do?

_____

_____

6.2. *[LO 6.3]* The receptionist working at the front desk phones to tell you that Maritza Ramos has just seen the physician and would like to know—before she leaves the office—what the charges were for her September 8, 2016, office visit. You are in the middle of entering charges from an encounter form for another patient. What should you do first? What is your reasoning?

_____

_____

6.3. *[LO 6.4]* After you have entered a patient copayment for $20.00, you realize it should have been $30.00. What should you do?

_____

_____

THINKING ABOUT IT

Answer the questions below in the space provided.

6.1. *[LO 6.1]* What is the purpose of entering charges in Medisoft? What would happen to a medical practice that did not record charges?

_____

_____

6.2. *[LO 6.4]* Why is it necessary to enter patient payments in Medisoft? Would it be sufficient to give the patient a receipt instead of entering the payment in Medisoft?

_____

_____

6.3 *[LO 6.6]* Describe a situation in which an office would need to issue a refund to a patient.

_____

_____

AT THE COMPUTER

Answer the following questions at the computer.

6.1. *[LO 6.3, 6.4]* What are the procedure codes and charges for Randall Klein for September 6, 2016?

_____

_____

6.2. *[LO 6.3]* What is the amount of the procedure charge entered on September 9, 2016, for patient Jo Wong?

_____

_____

6.3. *[LO 6.3]* What is the total amount that John Fitzwilliams paid in copayments in September 2016? (*Hint:* Include his daughter Sarah in the calculation.)

_____

_____

chapter

7

Creating Claims

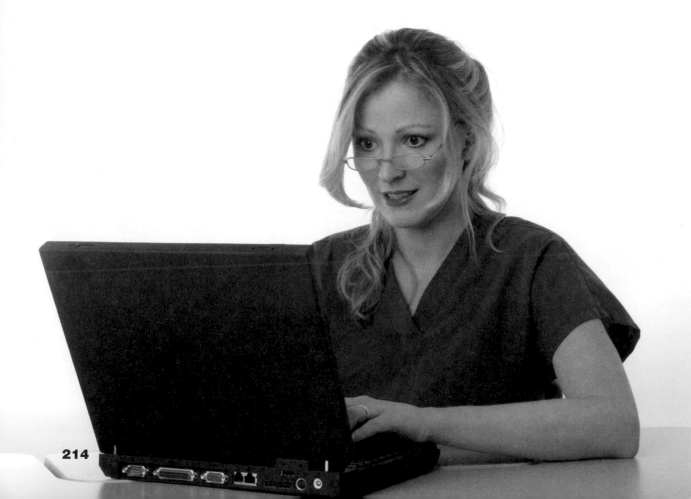

key terms

clean claims
filter
navigator buttons

learning outcomes

When you finish this chapter, you will be able to:

7.1 Describe the role of claims in the billing cycle.

7.2 Discuss the information contained in the Claim Management dialog box.

7.3 Demonstrate how to create claims in Medisoft.

7.4 Describe how to locate a claim that has already been submitted.

7.5 Discuss how claims are edited in Medisoft.

7.6 Explain how to change the status of a claim.

7.7 List the steps required to submit electronic claims in Medisoft.

7.8 Describe how to add attachments to electronic claims.

what you need to know

To use this chapter, you need to know how to:

- Start Medisoft, use menus, and enter and edit text.
- Work with chart numbers and codes.

7.1 THE ROLE OF CLAIMS IN THE BILLING CYCLE

Once the services a patient has received from a provider have been entered into the practice management program, the next step is to create insurance claims. The insurance claim is the most important document for correct reimbursement. Claims communicate information about a patient's diagnosis, procedures, and charges to a payer.

A physician practice depends on the billing specialist to submit **clean claims**—claims with all the correct information necessary for payer processing. An error on a claim may cause the claim to be delayed or denied. Rejected claims can cost the practice twice as much as clean claims and can result in reduced cash flow. Claims that are not paid in full also have a negative effect on the practice's bottom line.

Today, almost all claims are sent electronically. The HIPAA standard transaction for electronic claims is the HIPAA X12 837 Health Care Claim or Equivalent Encounter Information (837P). The paper format is known as the CMS-1500 claim form. Both types of insurance claims are prepared in the practice management program.

The National Uniform Claim Committee (NUCC), led by the American Medical Association, determines the content of both the 837P and the CMS-1500. The CMS-1500 claim has 33 numbered boxes representing about 150 discrete data elements, while the 837P has a maximum of 244 segments representing about 1,054 elements. However, many of these data elements are conditional and apply to particular specialties only. The CMS-1500 is pictured in Figure 7-1.

A listing of the data elements on the CMS-1500 and the corresponding location of those data in Medisoft® is provided in Table 7-1.

7.2 CLAIM MANAGEMENT IN MEDISOFT

Within the Claim Management area of Medisoft, insurance claims are created, edited, and submitted for payment. Claims are created from transactions previously entered in Medisoft. After claims are created, they can either be printed and mailed or transmitted electronically.

The Claim Management dialog box is displayed by clicking Claim Management on the Activities menu or by clicking the Claim

1500

HEALTH INSURANCE CLAIM FORM

APPROVED BY NATIONAL UNIFORM CLAIM COMMITTEE 08/05

☐☐ PICA

PICA ☐☐

CARRIER

1. MEDICARE ☐ (Medicare #) MEDICAID ☐ (Medicaid #) TRICARE CHAMPUS ☐ (Sponsor's SSN) CHAMPVA ☐ (Member ID#) GROUP HEALTH PLAN ☐ (SSN or ID) FECA BLK LUNG ☐ (SSN) OTHER ☐ (ID)

1a. INSURED'S I.D. NUMBER   (For Program in Item 1)

2. PATIENT'S NAME (Last Name, First Name, Middle Initial)

3. PATIENT'S BIRTH DATE MM ☐ DD ☐ YY   SEX M ☐ F ☐

4. INSURED'S NAME (Last Name, First Name, Middle Initial)

5. PATIENT'S ADDRESS (No., Street)

6. PATIENT RELATIONSHIP TO INSURED
Self ☐ Spouse ☐ Child ☐ Other ☐

7. INSURED'S ADDRESS (No., Street)

CITY   STATE

8. PATIENT STATUS
Single ☐ Married ☐ Other ☐
Employed ☐ Full-Time Student ☐ Part-Time Student ☐

CITY   STATE

ZIP CODE   TELEPHONE (Include Area Code)
(   )

ZIP CODE   TELEPHONE (Include Area Code)
(   )

PATIENT AND INSURED INFORMATION

9. OTHER INSURED'S NAME (Last Name, First Name, Middle Initial)

10. IS PATIENT'S CONDITION RELATED TO:

11. INSURED'S POLICY GROUP OR FECA NUMBER

a. OTHER INSURED'S POLICY OR GROUP NUMBER

a. EMPLOYMENT? (Current or Previous)
☐ YES ☐ NO

a. INSURED'S DATE OF BIRTH MM ☐ DD ☐ YY   SEX M ☐ F ☐

b. OTHER INSURED'S DATE OF BIRTH MM ☐ DD ☐ YY   SEX M ☐ F ☐

b. AUTO ACCIDENT?   PLACE (State)
☐ YES ☐ NO

b. EMPLOYER'S NAME OR SCHOOL NAME

c. EMPLOYER'S NAME OR SCHOOL NAME

c. OTHER ACCIDENT?
☐ YES ☐ NO

c. INSURANCE PLAN NAME OR PROGRAM NAME

d. INSURANCE PLAN NAME OR PROGRAM NAME

10d. RESERVED FOR LOCAL USE

d. IS THERE ANOTHER HEALTH BENEFIT PLAN?
☐ YES ☐ NO If yes, return to and complete item 9 a-d.

READ BACK OF FORM BEFORE COMPLETING & SIGNING THIS FORM.
12. PATIENT'S OR AUTHORIZED PERSON'S SIGNATURE I authorize the release of any medical or other information necessary to process this claim. I also request payment of government benefits either to myself or to the party who accepts assignment below.

SIGNED _____ DATE _____

13. INSURED'S OR AUTHORIZED PERSON'S SIGNATURE I authorize payment of medical benefits to the undersigned physician or supplier for services described below.

SIGNED _____

14. DATE OF CURRENT: MM ☐ DD ☐ YY ◄ ILLNESS (First symptom) OR INJURY (Accident) OR PREGNANCY(LMP)

15. IF PATIENT HAS HAD SAME OR SIMILAR ILLNESS. GIVE FIRST DATE MM ☐ DD ☐ YY

16. DATES PATIENT UNABLE TO WORK IN CURRENT OCCUPATION MM ☐ DD ☐ YY TO MM ☐ DD ☐ YY
FROM

17. NAME OF REFERRING PROVIDER OR OTHER SOURCE

17a.
17b. NPI

18. HOSPITALIZATION DATES RELATED TO CURRENT SERVICES MM ☐ DD ☐ YY TO MM ☐ DD ☐ YY
FROM

19. RESERVED FOR LOCAL USE

20. OUTSIDE LAB? $ CHARGES
☐ YES ☐ NO

21. DIAGNOSIS OR NATURE OF ILLNESS OR INJURY (Relate Items 1, 2, 3 or 4 to Item 24E by Line)

1. ⌊___ . ___⌋   3. ⌊___ . ___⌋

2. ⌊___ . ___⌋   4. ⌊___ . ___⌋

22. MEDICAID RESUBMISSION CODE   ORIGINAL REF. NO.

23. PRIOR AUTHORIZATION NUMBER

24. A. DATE(S) OF SERVICE						B. PLACE OF SERVICE	C. EMG	D. PROCEDURES, SERVICES, OR SUPPLIES (Explain Unusual Circumstances)		E. DIAGNOSIS POINTER	F. $ CHARGES	G. DAYS OR UNITS	H. EPSDT Family Plan	I. ID. QUAL.	J. RENDERING PROVIDER ID. #
From			To					CPT/HCPCS	MODIFIER						
MM	DD	YY	MM	DD	YY										
1														NPI	
2														NPI	
3														NPI	
4														NPI	
5														NPI	
6														NPI	

25. FEDERAL TAX I.D. NUMBER   SSN ☐ EIN ☐

26. PATIENT'S ACCOUNT NO.

27. ACCEPT ASSIGNMENT? (For govt. claims, see back)
☐ YES ☐ NO

28. TOTAL CHARGE
$

29. AMOUNT PAID
$

30. BALANCE DUE
$

31. SIGNATURE OF PHYSICIAN OR SUPPLIER INCLUDING DEGREES OR CREDENTIALS (I certify that the statements on the reverse apply to this bill and are made a part thereof.)

SIGNED _____ DATE _____

32. SERVICE FACILITY LOCATION INFORMATION

a. NPI   b.

33. BILLING PROVIDER INFO & PH # (   )

a. NPI   b.

PHYSICIAN OR SUPPLIER INFORMATION

NUCC Instruction Manual available at: www.nucc.org

APPROVED OMB-0938-0999 FORM CMS-1500 (08/05)

Figure 7-1   The CMS-1500 Claim Form

Box	CMS-1500 Field Name	Data Source in Medisoft	Dialog Box/Tab/Field Name in Medisoft
Top 1	Insurance Name/Address	Insurance	*Insurance Carrier,* Address, *Name, etc.*
Top 2	Primary, Secondary, Tertiary	Insurance	Determined by claim form selected
1	Insurance Type	Insurance	*Insurance Carrier,* EDI/Eligibility, *Type*
1a	Insured's ID No.	Case	*Case,* Policy 1, 2, 3, *Policy No.*
2	Patient's Name	Patient	*Patient/Guarantor,* Name, Address, *Last Name, First Name, Middle Initial*
3	Patient Birth Date, Sex	Patient	*Patient/Guarantor,* Name, Address, *Birth Date, Sex*
4	Insured's Name	Case	*Case,* Policy 1, 2, 3, *Policy Holder 1, 2, 3*
5	Patient's Address	Patient	*Patient/Guarantor,* Name, Address, *Street, City, State, Zip*
6	Patient Relation to Insured	Case	*Case,* Policy 1, 2, 3, *Relationship to Insured*
7	Insured's Address	Patient	*Patient/Guarantor,* Name, Address, *Street, City, State, Zip*
8	Patient Status	Case	*Case,* Personal, *Marital Status, Student Status, Employment Status*
9	Other Insured's Name	Case	*Case,* Policy 1, 2, 3, *Policy Holder 1, 2, 3*
9a	Other Insured's Policy/Group No.	Case	*Case,* Policy 1, 2, 3, *Policy Number, Group Number*
9b	Other Insured's Date of Birth, Sex	Patient	*Patient/Guarantor,* Name, Address, *Birth Date, Sex*
9c	Employer/School	Patient	*Patient/Guarantor,* Other Information, *Employer*
9d	Insurance Plan Name, Program	Insurance	*Insurance Carrier,* Address, *Plan Name;* if empty, prints carrier name
10a	Condition Related to Employment	Case	*Case,* Condition, *Employment Related* check box
10b	Condition Related to Auto Accident	Case	*Case,* Condition, *Accident, Related To*
10c	Condition Related to Other Accident	Case	*Case,* Condition, *Accident, Related To*
10d	Local Use	Case	*Case,* Miscellaneous, *Local Use A*
11	Insured's Policy Group/FECA#	Case	*Case,* Policy 1, *Policy Number, Group Number*
11a	Insured's Date of Birth, Sex	Patient	*Patient/Guarantor,* Name, Address, *Birth Date, Sex*
11b	Employer/School	Patient	*Patient/Guarantor,* Other Information, *Employer*
11c	Insurance Plan Name/Program	Insurance	*Insurance Carrier,* Address, *Plan Name;* if empty, prints carrier name
11d	Another Health Benefit Plan?	Case	*Case,* Policy 2, 3
12	Patient Signature or Authorized Signature	Patient	*Patient/Guarantor,* Other Information, *Signature on File; Insurance Carrier,* Options and Codes, *Patient Signature on File*
13	Insured's Signature or Authorized Signature	Patient	*Patient/Guarantor,* Other Information, *Signature on File; Insurance Carrier,* Options and Codes, *Insured Signature on File*

TABLE 7-1 *(continued)*

Box	CMS-1500 Field Name	Data Source in Medisoft	Dialog Box/Tab/Field Name in Medisoft
14	Date Current Ill/Inj/LMP	Case	**Case,** Condition, *Injury/Illness/LMP Date*
15	Same/Similar Date	Case	**Case,** Condition, *Date Similar Symptoms*
16	Dates Unable to Work	Case	**Case,** Condition, *Dates—Unable to Work*
17	Referring Provider	Case	**Case,** Account, *Referring Provider*
17a	Referring Provider, Other Identifier, Qualifier	Referring Provider	**Referring Provider,** Referring Provider IDs, *NPI*
17b	Referring Provider NPI	Referring Provider	**Referring Provider,** Referring Provider IDs, *NPI*
18	Hospitalization Dates	Case	**Case,** Condition, *Dates—Hospitalization*
19	Local Use	Case	**Case,** Miscellaneous, *Local Use B*
20	Outside Lab? $ Charges	Case	**Case,** Miscellaneous, *Outside Lab Work*
21	Diagnosis	Case	**Case,** Diagnosis, Principal Diagnosis, *Default Diagnosis 2, 3, 4*
22	Medicaid Resubmission	Case	**Case,** Medicaid and Tricare, *Resubmission No., Original Reference*
23	Prior Authorization #	Case	**Case,** Miscellaneous, *Prior Authorization Number*
24A	Dates of Service	Transaction	**Transaction Entry,** *Date From, Date To*
24B	Place of Service	Transaction	**Transaction Entry,** *Place of Service*
24C	EMG		**Payer Specific Code**
24D	Procedures, Services, or Supplies	Transaction	**Transaction Entry,** *Procedure, M1, M2, M3, M4*
24E	Diagnosis Pointer	Transaction	**Transaction Entry,** *Diag 1, Diag 2, Diag 3, Diag 4*
24F	$ Charges	Transaction	**Transaction Entry,** *Amount*
24G	Days or Units	Transaction	**Transaction Entry,** *Units*
24H	EPSDT	Case	**Case,** Medicaid and Tricare, *EPSDT*
24I	Rendering Provider, Other ID, Qualifier	Provider	**Provider,** Provider IDs
24J	Rendering Provider ID#	Provider	**Provider,** Provider IDs
25	Federal Tax ID	Practice	**Provider,** Provider IDs, *Tax ID/SSN*
26	Patient's Account No.	Patient	**Patient/Guarantor,** Name, Address, *Chart No.*
27	Accept Assignment?	Case	**Case,** Policy 1, 2, 3, *Assignment of Benefits/Accept Assignment*
28	Total Charge	Transaction	Calculated field
29	Amount Paid	Transaction	**Transaction Entry,** *Payment*
30	Balance Due	Transaction	Calculated field
31	Physician's Signature	Provider	**Provider,** Address, *Signature on File;* **Insurance Carrier,** Address, *Signature on File*
32	Facility Address	Practice	**Facility,** Address
32A	Facility NPI	Address	**Facility,** Facility IDs, *NPI*
33	Billing Provider Information	Provider	**Provider,** Address, *First Name, Middle Initial, Last Name, Street, City, State, Zip*
33A	Billing Provider NPI	Provider	**Provider:** Provider IDs, *NPI*

Figure 7-2
Claim Management
Shortcut Button

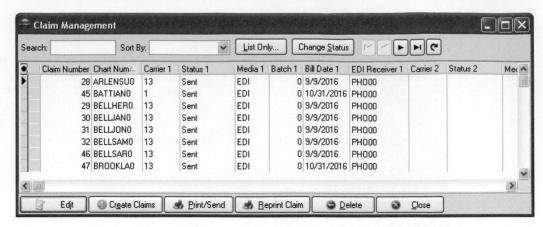

Figure 7-3   Claim Management Dialog Box

Management shortcut button on the toolbar (see Figure 7-2). The dialog box (see Figure 7-3) lists all claims that have already been created. In this dialog box, several actions can be performed: existing claims can be reviewed and edited, new claims can be created, the status of existing claims can be changed, and claims can be printed or submitted electronically.

navigator buttons buttons that simplify the task of moving from one entry to another

The upper-right corner of the Claim Management dialog box contains five **navigator buttons** that simplify the task of moving from one entry to another (see Figure 7-4). The First Claim button selects the first claim in the list and makes it active. The Previous Claim button reactivates the claim that was most recently active. The Next Claim button makes the next claim in the list active. The Last Claim button makes the last claim in the list active. The Refresh Data button is used to restore data when necessary.

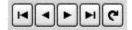

Figure 7-4   Navigator Buttons

The bottom of the Claim Management dialog box contains a number of buttons that are used for various functions (see Figure 7-3).

Edit   Opens a claim for editing.

Create Claims   Opens the Create Claims dialog box.

Print/Send   Begins the process of sending electronic claims or printing paper claims.

Reprint Claim   Reprints a claim that has already been printed.

Delete   Deletes the selected claim and releases the transactions bound to the claim.

Close   Closes the Claim Management dialog box.

7.3 CREATING CLAIMS

Claims are created in the Create Claims dialog box. The Create Claims dialog box (see Figure 7-5) is accessed by clicking the Create Claims button in the Claim Management dialog box. This dialog box provides several filters to customize the creation of claims. A **filter** is a condition that data must meet to be selected. For example, claims can be created for services performed between the first and the fifteenth of the month. In this case, the filter is the condition that services must have been performed between the first and fifteenth of the month. Transactions that meet this criterion are included in the selection; transactions that do not fall within the date range are not included. Filters can be used to create claims for a specific patient, for a specific insurance carrier, and for transactions that exceed a certain dollar amount, among others. The following filters can be applied within the Create Claims dialog box.

filter a condition that data must meet to be selected

Transaction Dates The Transaction Dates boxes are used to specify the starting and ending dates for which claims will be created. If the boxes are left blank, transactions for all dates will be included.

Chart Numbers In the Chart Numbers boxes, the starting and ending chart numbers for which claims will be created are entered. If the boxes are left blank, all chart numbers will be included.

Primary Insurance The carrier code for the insurance company is entered in the Primary Insurance box. If claims are being sent to a clearinghouse, more than one insurance carrier code can be entered.

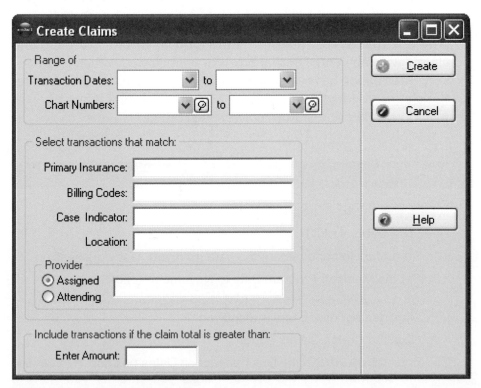

Figure 7-5 Create Claims Dialog Box

When more than one code is entered, commas must be placed between the codes. If claims are being sent directly to the carrier, only that carrier's code is entered.

Billing Codes The billing code is entered in the Billing Codes box. If more than one code is entered, commas must be placed between the codes.

Case Indicator If case indicators are used to classify patients (such as by type of illness for workers' compensation cases), the case indicator can be listed in the Case Indicator box. If more than one indicator is entered, commas must be placed between them.

Location Sometimes a sort is needed by location, such as all procedures done at a hospital. The location code is entered in the Location box. If more than one code is entered, commas must be placed between the codes.

Assigned The radio buttons in the Provider box indicate whether the provider is the assigned or attending provider. The assigned provider is the patient's regular physician. In the box to the right of the radio button, the provider code is entered. If more than one code is entered, commas must be placed between the codes.

Attending The attending provider is someone other than the patient's regular physician who provides treatment to the patient. In the box to the right of the radio button, the provider code is entered.

Enter Amount The dollar amount entered in this box is the minimum total amount required for a case before a claim can be created.

Any box that is not filled in will default to include all data, and claims with any entry in that box will be included. When all necessary information has been entered, clicking the Create button creates the claims. Medisoft will create a file of matching claims but will include only those that have not yet been billed.

EXERCISE 7-1   CREATING CLAIMS

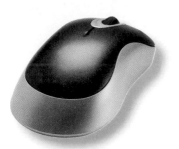

Create insurance claims for patients.

Date: November 4, 2016

1. Start Medisoft and restore the data from your last work session.
2. Set the Medisoft Program Date to November 4, 2016.
3. On the Activities menu, click Claim Management. The Claim Management dialog box is displayed.
4. Click the Create Claims button.
5. Enter **09/01/2016** in the first Transaction Dates box and **11/4/2016** in the second. When the program asks you whether you want to change the date (because it is in the future), click the No button.

Copyright ©2011 The McGraw-Hill Companies

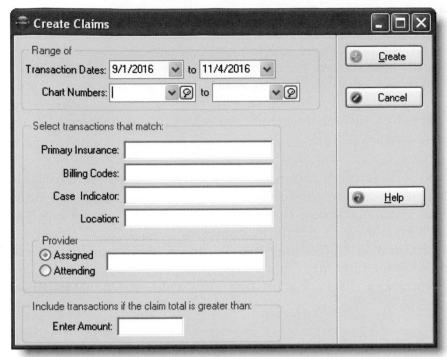

Figure 7-6 Create Claims Dialog Box with Dates Entered

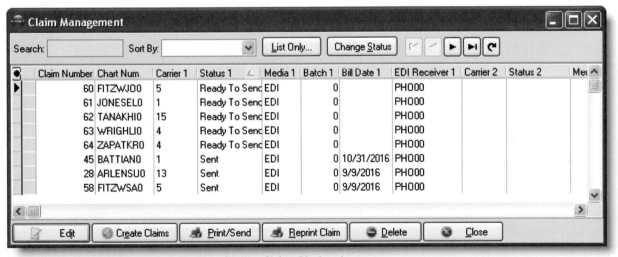

Figure 7-7 Claim Management Dialog Box with New Claims Displayed

6. Leave the remaining boxes in the Create Claims dialog box blank to create claims for all patients. Your screen should look like Figure 7-6.

7. Click the Create button.

8. Use the scroll bars to view the claims just created. Confirm that you have created the claims with a Ready to Send status that are visible in Figure 7-7.

9. Before you close the dialog box, write your answers to questions 1 and 2 in the space provided on the Chapter 7 Worksheet on page 240.

10. Click the Close button. **CiMC**

☑ **You have completed Exercise 7-1.**

7.4 LOCATING CLAIMS

At times it is necessary to select and view specific claims that have already been created. For example, any claims prepared for submission to an insurance carrier must be selected and then reviewed for completeness and accuracy. In addition, all claims that have been rejected by insurance carriers are selected and reviewed before resubmission.

Medisoft's List Only feature is used when it is necessary to list claims that match certain criteria. Filters are applied in the List Only Claims That Match dialog box. They can be used to view claims selectively, such as claims for a specific insurance carrier and claims created on a certain date. Unlike the filters in the Create Claims dialog box, those in the List Only Claims That Match dialog box do not create claims; they simply list existing claims that meet the specified criteria.

Once the filters have been applied, only those claims that match the criteria are listed at the bottom of the main Claim Management dialog box. Claims can be sorted by chart number, date the claim was created, insurance carrier, electronic claim (EDI) receiver, billing method, billing date, batch number, and claim status. Not all the boxes need to be filled in, only the ones that will be used to select the desired claims.

The List Only feature is activated by clicking the List Only . . . button in the Claim Management dialog box (see Figure 7-8). Clicking the button causes the List Only Claims That Match dialog box to be displayed (see Figure 7-9).

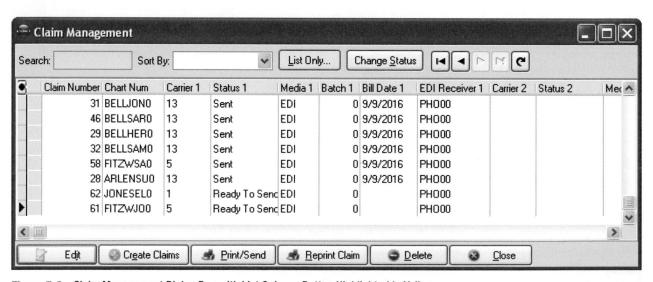

Figure 7-8 Claim Management Dialog Box with List Only . . . Button Highlighted In Yellow

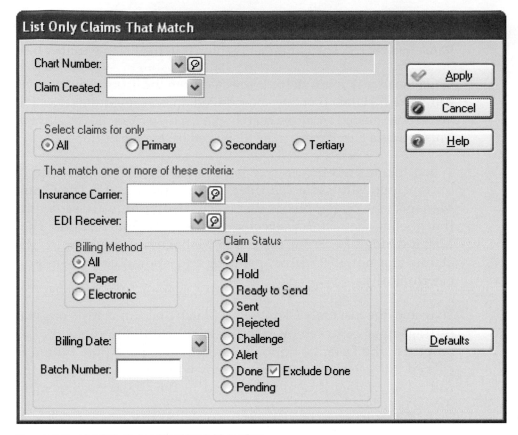

Figure 7-9 List Only Claims That Match Dialog Box

The following filters are available in the List Only Claims That Match dialog box.

Chart Number   A patient's chart number is selected from the drop-down list of patients' chart numbers.

Claim Created   The date that a claim was created is entered in MMDDCCYY format.

Select Claims for Only   A radio button is clicked for either all insurance carriers, primary insurance carrier only, secondary insurance carrier only, or tertiary insurance carrier only. When a patient has insurance coverage with more than one carrier, the primary carrier is billed first, and then, if appropriate, the second and third (tertiary) carriers are billed.

Insurance Carrier   An insurance carrier is selected from the drop-down list of choices.

EDI Receiver   An EDI receiver is selected from the choices on the drop-down list.

Billing Method   In the Billing Method box, the radio button for All, Paper, or Electronic is clicked.

Billing Date   The date of billing is entered in the Billing Date box.

Batch Number   A batch number is entered in the Batch Number box.

Claim Status   A claim status is selected from the list of radio buttons provided. If claims that have been billed and accepted (not rejected) are to be excluded from the search, the Exclude Done box is clicked. This causes a check mark to be displayed beside the option.

When the desired boxes have been filled in, clicking the Apply button applies the selected filters to the claims data. The Claim Management dialog box is displayed, listing only those claims that match the criteria selected in the List Only Claims That Match dialog box. From the Claim Management dialog box, the claims can now be edited, printed, and mailed or transmitted electronically.

To restore the List Only Claims That Match dialog box to its original settings (that is, to remove the filters selected), the dialog box is reopened; the Defaults button is clicked; and the Apply button is clicked. All the boxes in the dialog box will become blank, and the full list of claims is again displayed in the Claim Management dialog box.

EXERCISE 7-2	USING THE LIST ONLY FEATURE

Find all insurance claims for Medicare that have a status of Sent.

Date: November 4, 2016

1. If necessary, open the Claim Management dialog box by selecting it on the Activities menu. The Claim Management dialog box is displayed.

2. Click the List Only . . . button. The List Only Claims That Match dialog box is displayed.

3. Leave the Chart Number and Claim Created fields blank.

4. In the Select Claims for Only section, make sure All is selected.

5. Select 1-Medicare from the drop-down list in the Insurance Carrier field.

6. Leave the EDI Receiver field blank.

7. Select Electronic as the Billing Method.

8. Leave the Billing Date and Batch Number fields blank.

9. Select Sent as the Claim Status.

10. Click the Apply button.

11. Your screen should look like the window in Figure 7-10.

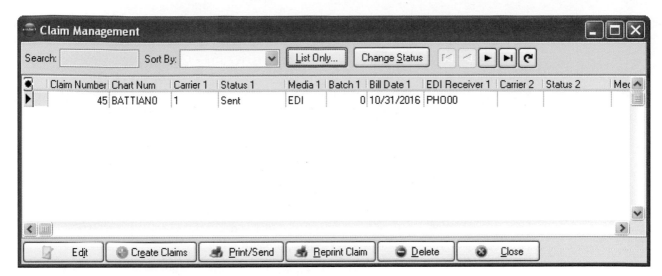

Figure 7-10 Claim Management Dialog Box with Selected Claim Displayed

12. To restore the full list of claims in the Claim Management box, click the List Only . . . button, and then click the Defaults button.

13. Click the Apply button.

☑ **You have completed Exercise 7-2.**

7.5 EDITING CLAIMS

Medisoft's Claim Edit feature allows claims to be reviewed and edited before they are submitted to insurance carriers for payment. The more problems that can be spotted and solved before claims are sent to insurance carriers, the sooner the practice will receive payment.

When a claim is active in the Claim Management dialog box, it can be edited by clicking the Edit button or by double clicking the claim itself. The Claim dialog box is displayed (see Figure 7-11). The top section of the Claim dialog box lists the claim number, the date the claim was created, the chart number, the patient's name, and the case number. This information cannot be edited, although the information in the five tabs can be edited.

CARRIER 1 TAB

The Carrier 1 tab displays information about claims being submitted to a patient's primary insurance carrier. The following boxes are listed in the Carrier 1 tab:

Claim Status The Claim Status box indicates the status of a particular claim: Hold, Ready to Send, Sent, Rejected, Challenge, Alert, Done, and Pending. The radio button that reflects a claim's status should be clicked.

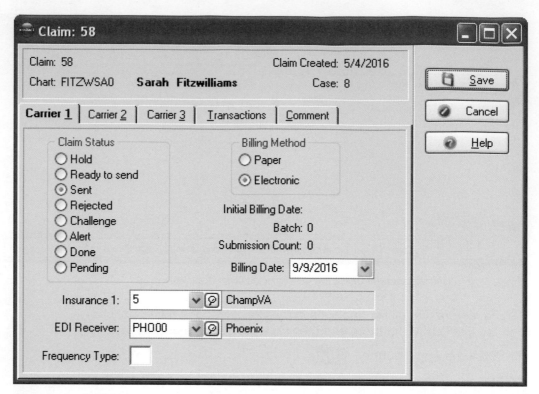

Figure 7-11 Claim Dialog Box

Billing Method   The Billing Method box displays two choices: Paper and Electronic. The radio button that describes the billing method should be clicked.

Initial Billing Date   If the claim was sent more than once, this box automatically displays the initial billing date.

Batch   If the claim has been assigned to a batch, the batch number is displayed.

Submission Count   The Submission Count area lists the number of claims submitted.

Billing Date   The Billing Date box lists the most recent date the bill was sent (if the claim was submitted more than once).

Insurance 1   The Insurance 1 box lists a patient's primary insurance carrier.

EDI Receiver   The EDI receiver is selected from the drop-down list.

Frequency Type   This field is used with some insurance carriers when sending claims electronically. Allowed entries in this field are

    1-Original (admission through discharge claim)

    6-Corrected (adjustment of prior claim)

    7-Replacement (replacement of prior claim)

    8-Void (voiding/cancellation of prior claim)

CARRIER 2 AND CARRIER 3 TABS

The Carrier 2 and Carrier 3 tabs display information about claims being submitted to a patient's secondary (Carrier 2) and tertiary (Carrier 3) insurance carriers. The boxes in these tabs are the same as the boxes in the Carrier 1 tab, with the exception of the Claim Status box and the Frequency Type box. In the Carrier 2 and Carrier 3 tabs, there is no Pending radio button in the Claim Status box, and there is no Frequency Type box. Otherwise the three tabs are the same.

TRANSACTIONS TAB

The Transactions tab lists information about the transactions included in a claim. The scroll bars can be used to view all the information in the Transactions tab (see Figure 7-12).

Diagnosis   The diagnosis for the listed transactions is displayed.

Date From   The Date From box lists the date on which service was provided.

Document   The Document box lists the document number of a transaction.

Procedure   The Procedure box displays the procedure code for a performed procedure.

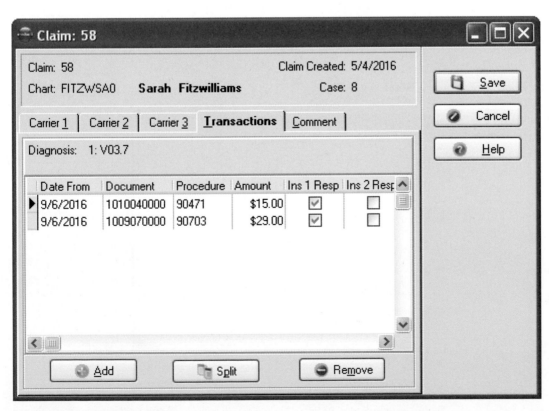

Figure 7-12   Transactions Tab

Amount   In the Amount box, the dollar cost of a service is displayed.

Ins 1 Resp   If this box is checked, the primary insurance carrier is responsible for the claim.

Ins 2 Resp   If this box is checked, the secondary insurance carrier is responsible for the claim.

Ins 3 Resp   If this box is checked, the tertiary insurance carrier is responsible for the claim.

The Transactions tab also contains three buttons at the bottom of the dialog box:

Add   The Add button is used to add a transaction to an existing claim.

Split   The Split button removes a single transaction from an existing claim and places it on a new claim.

Remove   The Remove button deletes a transaction from the claim database.

COMMENT TAB

The Comment tab provides a place to include any specific notes or comments about the claim (see Figure 7-13). The comments are for internal use and are not transmitted or printed.

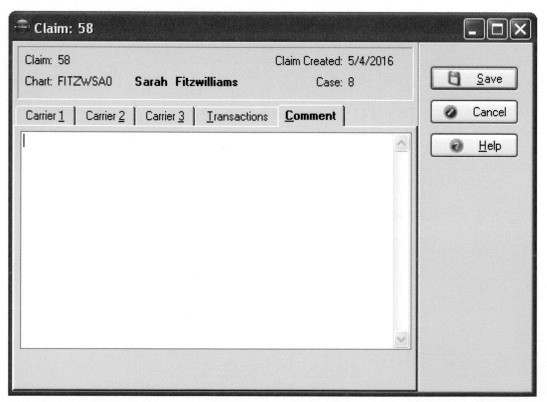

Figure 7-13   Comment Tab

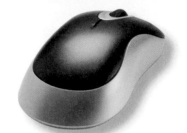

Review insurance claims for patients with East Ohio PPO as their insurance carrier.

Date: November 4, 2016

1. Open the Claim Management dialog box, if it is not already open.

2. Click the List Only . . . button.

3. Click 13 East Ohio PPO on the drop-down list in the Insurance Carrier box.

4. Click the Apply button. You are returned to the Claim Management dialog box. Notice that only claims for patients who have East Ohio PPO as their insurance carrier are listed.

5. Click the claim for Lawana Brooks (chart number BROOKLAØ).

6. Click the Edit button to review the claim. The Claim dialog box is displayed.

7. Review the information in the Carrier 1 tab.

8. Review the information in the Transactions tab.

9. Click the Cancel button to exit the Claim dialog box without saving any changes. (The Cancel button does not cancel the claim; it just cancels any changes that may have been made.)

10. To restore the full list of claims in the Claim Management box, click the List Only . . . button, and then click the Defaults button.

11. Click the Apply button. **ciMO**

✓ **You have completed Exercise 7-3.**

7.6 CHANGING THE STATUS OF A CLAIM

If claims were transmitted electronically, the Claim Status for each claim would automatically change from Ready to Send to Sent once the claims were sent. Since it is not possible to actually send electronic claims during these exercises, for the purposes of this text/workbook, you will be asked to change the claim status manually from Ready to Send to Sent for claims you create. In the next exercise, you change the claim status for the claims created earlier in the chapter.

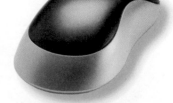

Change the Claim Status for the claims created on November 4, 2016, from Ready to Send to Sent.

Date: November 4, 2016

1. In the Claim Management dialog box, click the Change Status button. The Change Claim Status/Billing Method dialog box appears.

2. Click Batch, and accept the default entry of 0.

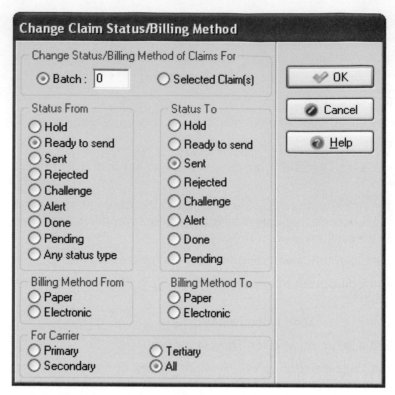

Figure 7-14   Selections in Change Claim Status/Billing Method Dialog Box

3. Select Ready to Send in the Status From column.

4. Select Sent in the Status To column. Check your screen against Figure 7-14.

5. Click the OK button. The dialog box closes, and the Claim Management dialog box reappears with the Claim Status column displaying Sent for the two new claims at the bottom of the list.

6. Before you close the dialog box, write your answer to question 4 in the space provided on the Chapter 7 Worksheet on page 240.

7. Close the Claim Management dialog box.

☑ **You have completed Exercise 7-4.**

7.7 SUBMITTING ELECTRONIC CLAIMS

Before the implementation of the HIPAA Electronic Health Care Transactions and Code Sets standards in 2003, physician practices used many different electronic data interchange (EDI) systems to submit electronic claims. The HIPAA standards describe a particular electronic format that providers and payers must use to send and receive health care transactions. They also establish standard medical code sets, such as ICD and CPT, for use in health care transactions. Most of the setup and data entry requirements for electronic claims are handled by the medical office's systems manager.

STEPS IN TRANSMITTING ELECTRONIC CLAIMS

1. Select Revenue Management > Revenue Management . . . on the Activities menu (see Figure 7-15).

2. The Revenue Management main window opens (see Figure 7-16).

3. Select Claims on the Process menu (see Figure 7-17).

4. Select an EDI receiver. A list of claims ready to be sent is displayed (see Figure 7-18).

5. To perform an edit check on the claims, click Check Claims and the EDI receiver. The claims are checked against a number of edits, including MCD (Medicare Coverage Database), CCI (Correct Coding Initiative), and Common Edits.

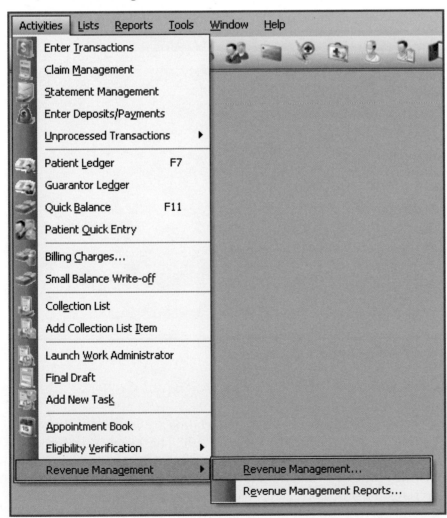

Figure 7-15   Revenue Management Selected on the Activities Menu

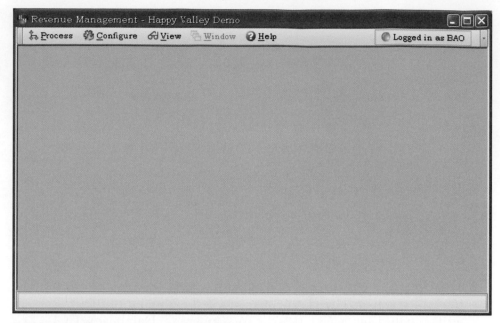

Figure 7-16 The Revenue Management Window

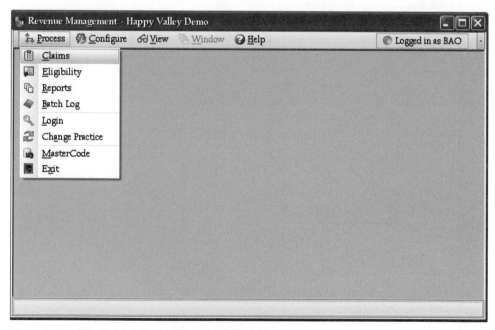

Figure 7-17 The Process Menu with Claims Selected

6. When the edit check is finished, claims are marked with a green flag or a red flag (see Figure 7-19). The green flag indicates that the claim passed the edits and is ready to send, and a red flag indicates that the claim did not pass. Claims with red flags must be corrected before they can be sent. You can view and correct the errors now or print an error report and fix the claims at a later time.

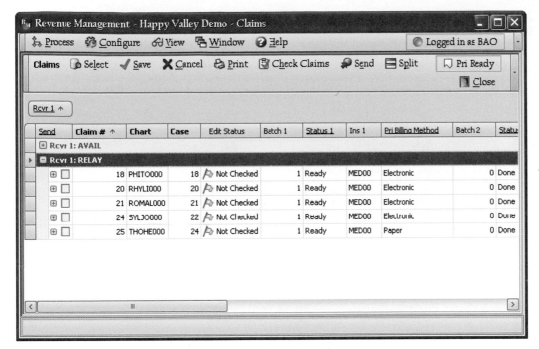

Figure 7-18 List of Claims Ready to be Sent, by EDI Receiver

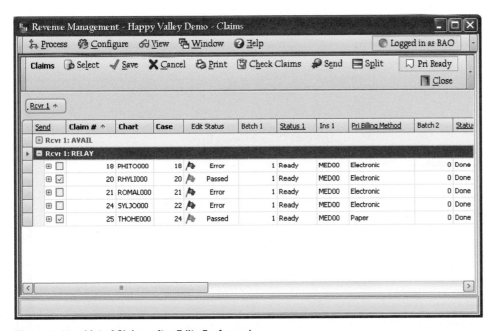

Figure 7-19 List of Claims after Edits Performed

7. To continue with the ready-to-send claims, select Send, select Claims, and select the EDI receiver. Medisoft creates a claims file and displays a preview report (see Figure 7-20).

8. The preview report checks the claims for ANSI (American National Standards Institute) errors. If any errors are found, the claims must be edited before they can be transmitted. Clicking the Remove Claims button removes the selected claim from the claims file.

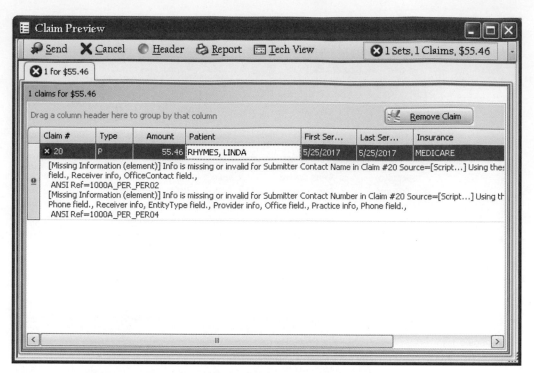

Figure 7-20   Claim Preview Window with Remove Claim Button Highlighted

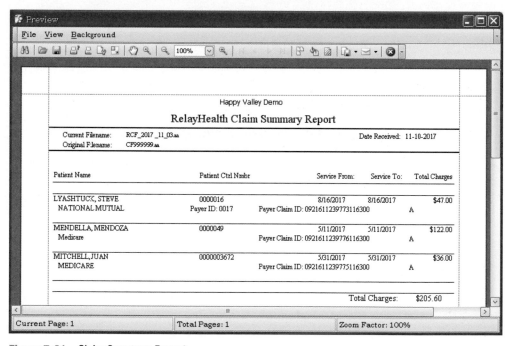

Figure 7-21   Claim Summary Report

9. Click the Send button to send the claims files. The file is transmitted to the payer and the claim status is updated in Medisoft.

10. If desired, a claim summary can be printed. This report lists each claim included in the claims file, including patient name, patient control number, dates of service, and total charges (see Figure 7-21).

7.8 SENDING ELECTRONIC CLAIM ATTACHMENTS

When a claim is sent electronically, an attachment that needs to accompany the claim, such as radiology films, must be referred to in the claim. In Medisoft, the EDI Report area within the Diagnosis tab of the Case dialog box is used to indicate to the payer when an attachment will accompany the claim and how the attachment will be transmitted (see Figure 7-22).

The EDI Notes box can be used for entering extra information for procedures and diagnoses that might be required by the patient's insurance carriers to process the electronic claim.

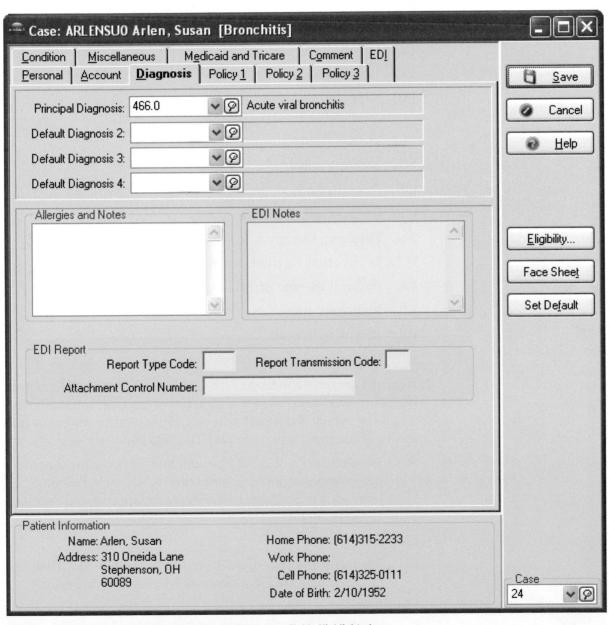

Figure 7-22 Diagnosis Tab with EDI Notes and EDI Report Fields Highlighted

The EDI Report section contains three boxes:

1. **Report Type Code** This box is used to record the report type code—a two-digit code that indicates the type of report being attached. For example, DG is the code for a diagnostic report. Other codes include

   77 Support data for verification. REFERRAL: use this code to indicate a completed referral form

   AS   Admission summary

   B2   Prescription

   B3   Physician order

   B4   Referral form

   CT   Certification

   DA   Dental models

   DG   Diagnostic report

   DS   Discharge summary

   EB   Explanation of benefits (coordination of benefits or Medicare secondary payer)

   MT   Models

   NN   Nursing notes

   OB   Operative note

   OZ   Support data for claim

   PN   Physician therapy notes

   PO   Prosthetics or orthotic certification

   PZ   Physical therapy certification

   RB   Radiology films

   RR   Radiology reports

   RT   Report of tests and analysis report

2. **Report Transmission Code** This box is used to record the report transmission code, a two-character code that indicates the means by which the report will be transmitted to the payer (for example, via mail, e-mail, or fax). Possible codes include

   AA   Available on request at provider site. This means that the paperwork is not being sent with the claim at this time. Instead, it is available to the payer (or appropriate entity) at its request.

   BM   By mail

   EL   Electronically only. Used to indicate that the attachment is being transmitted in a separate X12 functional group.

   EM   E-mail

   FX   By fax

3. Attachment Control Number This box contains the attachment's reference number (up to seven digits, assigned by the practice). This number is required if the transmission code is anything other than AA.

APPLYING YOUR SKILLS

4: REVIEWING CLAIMS

November 4, 2016
Using the List Only . . . feature, identify all claims for the insurance carrier EastOhio PPO. (*Note:* Do not include claims with a status of Done.)

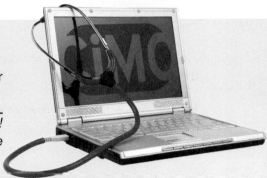

Remember to create a backup of your work before exiting Medisoft! To help you keep track of your work, name the backup file after the chapter you are working on, for example, StudentID-c7.mbk.

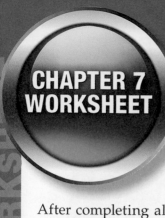

Name: _____ Date: _____

After completing all the exercises in the chapter, answer the following questions in the spaces provided.

1. *[LO 7.3]* Claims were created for which patients in Exercise 7-1?

   _____

2. *[LO 7.6]* After completing Exercise 7-1, what was listed in the Status 1 column for the claims created?

   _____

3. *[LO 7.5]* What transactions are listed on Lawana Brooks's insurance claim?

   _____

4. *[LO 7.6]* After completing Exercise 7-4, what is listed in the Status 1 column for the claims for John Fitzwilliams and Elizabeth Jones?

   _____

5. *[LO 7.5]* What transactions are listed on Lisa Wright's insurance claim?

   _____

7.1 Describe the role of claims in the billing cycle. Page 216	Once the services a patient has received from a provider have been entered into the practice management program, the next step is to create insurance claims. The insurance claim is the most important document for correct reimbursement. Claims communicate information about a patient's diagnosis and procedures and the charges to a payer.
7.2 Discuss the information contained in the Claim Management dialog box. Pages 216–220	The Claim Management dialog box contains a list of all claims created, and buttons used for editing claims, creating claims, printing/sending claims, reprinting claims, and deleting claims.
7.3 Demonstrate how to create claims in Medisoft. Pages 221–223	1. On the Activities menu, click Claim Management. The Claim Management dialog box is displayed. 2. Click the Create Claims button. 3. Enter dates in the Transaction Dates boxes, or leave the boxes blank to create claims for any date. When the program asks whether you want to change the date (because it is in the future), click the No button. 4. Enter the appropriate value(s) in the other fields as needed; remember that if a field is left blank, claims with any value in that field will be created. 5. When you have made your selections, click the Create button. The Create Claims box closes, and the new claims are listed in the Claim Management dialog box.

7.4 Describe how to locate a claim that has already been submitted. Pages 224–227	The List Only feature is used to locate a claim.
	1. Click the List Only . . . button in the Claim Management dialog box.
	2. In the List Only Claims That Match dialog box, complete the fields to filter claim selection by
	  - Chart number
	  - Claim created date
	  - Carrier status (all primary, secondary, etc.)
	  - Insurance carrier
	  - EDI receiver
	  - Billing method
	  - Claim status
	  - Billing date
	  - Batch number
	3. When you have made your selections, click Apply. The List Only Claims That Match dialog box closes, and the selected claim(s) are listed in the Claim Management dialog box.

7.5 Discuss how claims are edited in Medisoft. Pages 227–231	In the Claim Management dialog box, click the claim once to select it. With the claim selected, click the Edit button. Locate the information that requires editing in the tabs in the Claim dialog box. To save the changes, click the Save button.
7.6 Explain how to change the status of a claim. Pages 231–232	In the Claim Management dialog box, click the claim once to select it. With the claim selected, click the Change Status button. The Change Claim Status/Billing Method dialog box is displayed. Indicate whether you want to change the status for a batch of claims, or just for the selected claim. Click the appropriate fields to indicate the current status of the claim (Status From options) and the desired status (Status To options). If appropriate, make a selection in the For Carrier section at the bottom of the dialog box. Click the OK button to change the status.
7.7 List the steps required to submit electronic claims in Medisoft. Pages 232–236	1. Select Revenue Management > Revenue Management . . . on the Activities menu. 2. The Revenue Management main window opens. 3. Select Claims on the Process menu. 4. Select an EDI receiver. A list of claims ready to be sent is displayed. 5. Click Check Claims and select the EDI receiver. 6. Review claims that did not pass the edit. Correct the errors now or print an error report and fix the claims at a later time. 7. To continue with the ready-to-send claims, select Send, select Claims, and select the EDI receiver. Medisoft creates a claims file and displays a preview report. 8. The preview report checks the claims for ANSI errors. If any errors are found, the claims must be edited before they can be transmitted. Clicking the Remove Claims button removes the selected claim from the claims file. 9. Click the Send button to send the claims files. The file is transmitted to the payer and the claim status is updated in Medisoft. 10. If desired, a claim summary can be printed.
7.8 Describe how to add attachments to electronic claims. Pages 237–239	Information regarding claim attachments is entered in the EDI report section of the Diagnosis tab (within the Case folder). Fields include - Report Type Code - Report Transmission Code - Attachment Control Number

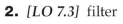

USING TERMINOLOGY

Define the terms below.

1. *[LO 7.1]* clean claims

_____

_____

2. *[LO 7.3]* filter

_____

_____

3. *[LO 7.2]* navigator buttons

_____

_____

CHECKING YOUR UNDERSTANDING

Answer the questions below in the space provided.

1. *[LO 7.4]* A claim needs to be submitted for John Fitzwilliams. How would you select only those claims pertaining to John Fitzwilliams?

_____

_____

2. *[LO 7.5]* If an error is found on a claim, how is it corrected?

_____

_____

3. *[LO 7.1]* What is meant by a "clean claim"?

_____

_____

4. *[LO 7.1]* What is HIPAA X12 837?

_____

_____

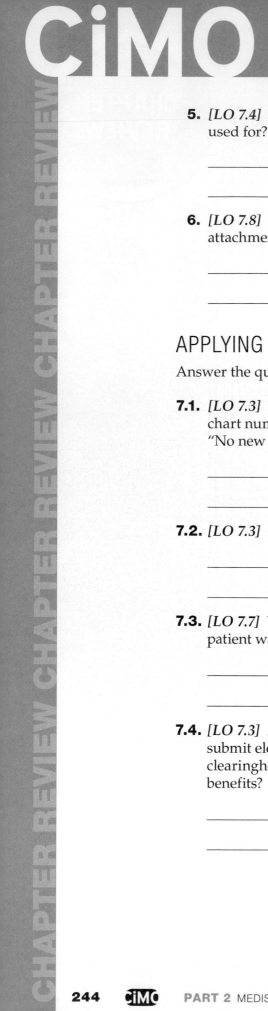

5. *[LO 7.4]* What is the List Only feature in the Claim Management dialog box used for?

_____

_____

6. *[LO 7.8]* In Medisoft, where is information about electronic claim attachments entered?

_____

_____

APPLYING YOUR KNOWLEDGE

Answer the questions below in the space provided.

7.1. *[LO 7.3]* You are asked to create a claim for Samuel Bell. After entering his chart number in the Create Claims dialog box, you receive the message "No new claims were created." Why were no claims created for Samuel Bell?

_____

_____

7.2. *[LO 7.3]* How would you create claims for one specific insurance carrier?

_____

_____

7.3. *[LO 7.7]* You are not sure whether an electronic claim for a particular patient was transmitted. How would you find out?

_____

_____

7.4. *[LO 7.3]* A new billing specialist in the office tells you it is less costly to submit electronic claims directly to insurance carriers without using a clearinghouse. Why do you think offices use clearinghouses? What are the benefits?

_____

_____

THINKING ABOUT IT

Answer the questions below in the space provided.

7.1. *[LO 7.1]* If claims were not created and transmitted, what would the consequence be?

_____

_____

7.2. *[LO 7.1]* Why is it important that claims be submitted soon after the patient's visit?

_____

_____

7.3. *[LO 7.1]* Why is it important that claims be submitted with complete and correct information?

_____

_____

AT THE COMPUTER

Answer the following questions at the computer.

7.1. *[LO 7.4]* How many claims were created on November 4, 2016?

_____

_____

7.2. *[LO 7.8]* What transactions were included on the October 28, 2016, claim for Sheila Giles?

_____

_____

Posting Insurance Payments and Creating Patient Statements

key terms

capitation payments

cycle billing

electronic remittance advice (ERA)

fee schedule

once-a-month billing

patient statement

payment schedule

remainder statements

standard statements

learning outcomes

When you finish this chapter, you will be able to:

8.1 Describe how an adjustment is calculated if the payer pays less than the provider's usual fee.

8.2 List the five steps for processing a remittance advice.

8.3 Demonstrate how to enter insurance payments.

8.4 Demonstrate how to apply insurance payments to charges.

8.5 Demonstrate how to enter capitation payments.

8.6 Demonstrate how to create patient statements.

8.7 Explain how statements are edited.

8.8 Demonstrate how to print patient statements.

what you need to know

To use this chapter, you need to know how to:

- Start Medisoft, use menus, and enter and edit text.
- Edit information in an existing case.
- Work with chart and case numbers.
- Select patients and cases for transaction entry.

8.1 THIRD-PARTY REIMBURSEMENT OVERVIEW

fee schedule a document that specifies the amount the provider bills for provided services

payment schedule a document that specifies the amount the payer agrees to reimburse the provider for a service

The amount a physician is reimbursed for a service depends on the patient's insurance benefits and the provider's agreement with the third-party payer. Providers establish a list of standard fees, known as a **fee schedule,** for procedures and services—this is the amount the provider bills the payer. Payers also develop a list of standard fees, but their **payment schedule** is based on a rate established in a contract with the provider. Most of the time, the amount the provider bills and the rate specified in the contract with the payer differ. The difference between the amount billed (the fee schedule) and the amount paid per contract (the payment schedule) is an adjustment that is entered in the billing area of the practice management program.

The following examples illustrate how reimbursement is calculated for an indemnity plan, a managed care plan, and a Medicare plan.

INDEMNITY PLAN EXAMPLE

In an indemnity plan, insurers often reimburse 80 percent of "reasonable charges," and the patient pays the remaining 20 percent.

Provider's usual fee	$100.00
Allowed charge	$100.00
Insurance payment	$80.00
Patient coinsurance	$20.00

In this example, the amount allowed by the payer is the same as the provider's charge. The payer reimburses at 80 percent, and the patient is responsible for the remaining 20 percent. The provider is paid for the entire billed amount; no adjustment is necessary.

MANAGED CARE EXAMPLE

Providers enter into contracts with managed care companies in which they agree to accept reduced fees for services. A managed care plan may require the patient to pay a fixed copayment.

Provider's usual fee	$100.00
Allowed charge	$90.00
Patient copayment	$20.00
Insurance payment	$70.00
Adjustment	$10.00

In this example, the provider charges $100.00. However, the provider's contract with the payer requires the provider to accept 90 percent of the usual and customary charge as full payment. This amount is known as the approved amount. The provider must enter an adjustment to write off the $10.00 difference between the amount charged and the amount approved per the contract. The patient pays a fixed copayment of $20.00, which is subtracted from the approved charge.

MEDICARE PARTICIPATING EXAMPLE

Medicare uses its own payment schedule, known as the Medicare Physician Fee Schedule (MPFS), which is updated annually. Providers who agree to participate in Medicare must accept the fee listed in the MPFS as payment in full. Medicare is responsible for paying 80 percent of this amount, and the patient is responsible for the other 20 percent (after a deductible has been met).

Provider's usual fee	$100.00
Medicare allowed charge	$64.00
Medicare pays 80 percent	$51.20
Patient pays 20 percent	$12.80
Adjustment	$36.00

In this example, the provider charges $100.00. The maximum allowed amount in the Medicare Fee Schedule is $64.00. The difference between $100.00 and $64.00 must be written off by the provider. Medicare pays 80 percent of the allowed amount, and the patient is billed for the remaining 20 percent, or $12.80.

Note: Providers who do not participate in the Medicare program may accept assignment on a claim-by-claim basis, but they are paid 5 percent less than providers who participate. Providers who do not participate and who do not accept assignment of a claim are subject to Medicare's limiting charge. This rule limits the amount a provider can charge to 115 percent of the fee listed in the Medicare nonparticipating fee schedule.

The chart displayed in Figure 8-1 contains the fee schedules for the providers and payers used in the exercises in this text/workbook. The information on the chart includes the following:

- **CPT code** The procedure code for the service provided
- **Provider's usual fee** The usual amount the provider bills for the service
- **Managed care allowed charge** The discounted fee specified by contract
- **Medicare allowed charge** The maximum fee a participating provider can collect for the service

CPT Code	Provider's Usual Fee	Managed Care Allowed	Medicare Allowed	CPT Code	Provider's Usual Fee	Managed Care Allowed	Medicare Allowed
12011	$202.00	$181.80	$148.70	90703	$29.00	$26.10	$14.30
29125	$99.00	$89.10	$61.21	93000	$84.00	$75.60	$25.72
29540	$121.50	$109.35	$40.50	92516	$210.00	$189.00	$59.32
50390	$551.00	$495.90	$101.47	93015	$401.00	$360.90	$103.31
71010	$91.00	$81.90	$26.77	96372	$40.00	$36.00	$18.74
71020	$112.00	$100.80	$34.71	96900	$39.00	$35.10	$16.42
71030	$153.00	$137.70	$45.25	99201	$66.00	$59.40	$35.58
73070	$102.00	$91.80	$27.06	99202	$88.00	$79.20	$63.28
73090	$99.00	$89.10	$27.44	99203	$120.00	$108.00	$94.28
73100	$93.00	$83.70	$26.37	99204	$178.00	$160.20	$133.56
73510	$124.00	$111.60	$32.56	99205	$229.00	$206.10	$169.28
73600	$96.00	$86.40	$26.37	99211	$36.00	$32.40	$20.68
80048	$50.00	$45.00	$11.20	99212	$54.00	$48.60	$37.36
80061	$90.00	$81.00	$18.72	99213	$72.00	$64.80	$51.03
82270	$19.00	$17.10	$4.54	99214	$105.00	$94.50	$80.15
82947	$25.00	$22.50	$5.48	99215	$163.00	$146.70	$116.96
82951	$63.00	$56.70	$16.12	99381	$210.00	$189.00	$100.27
83718	$43.00	$38.70	$11.44	99382	$218.00	$196.20	$108.13
84478	$29.00	$26.10	$8.04	99383	$224.00	$201.60	$106.00
85007	$21.00	$18.90	$4.81	99384	$262.50	$236.25	$115.30
85018	$13.00	$11.70	$3.31	99385	$247.50	$222.75	$115.30
85025	$13.60	$12.24	$10.79	99386	$267.00	$240.30	$135.69
85651	$24.00	$21.60	$4.96	99387	$298.50	$268.65	$147.13
86580	$25.00	$22.50	$6.86	99391	$165.00	$148.50	$76.39
87076	$75.00	$67.50	$11.29	99392	$184.50	$166.05	$85.69
87077	$60.00	$54.00	$11.29	99393	$192.00	$172.80	$84.63
87086	$51.00	$45.90	$11.28	99394	$222.00	$199.80	$93.56
87430	$29.00	$26.10	$16.01	99395	$204.00	$183.60	$94.63
87880	$24.00	$21.60	$16.01	99396	$222.00	$199.80	$104.64
90471	$15.00	$13.50	$17.82	99397	$236.00	$212.40	$115.37

Figure 8-1 Fee Schedule/Payment Schedule for Payers in Contract with the Family Care Center

8.2 REMITTANCE ADVICE (RA) PROCESSING

Once a claim has been received and accepted, it is processed, and the appropriate payment is determined. The payer then generates a remittance advice (RA) and sends it to the provider. A remittance advice lists patients, dates of service, charges, and the amount paid or denied by the insurance carrier. It contains payments for multiple claims for a number of different patients. A sample RA appears in Figure 8-2.

electronic remittance advice (ERA) an electronic document that lists patients, dates of service, charges, and the amount paid or denied by the insurance carrier

The RA may be sent in electronic format, called an **electronic remittance advice (ERA),** or in paper format. Although similar information is contained on an ERA and a paper RA, the ERA may offer additional data. The ERA that is mandated for use by HIPAA is called the ASC X12 835 Remittance Advice Transaction, or simply the 835. In addition to physicians, other health care providers receiving the 835 include hospitals, nursing homes, laboratories, and dentists.

① MICHAEL A. JONES, MD
414 ISLAND RD.
PAVE, OH 43068-1101

② PAGE: 1 OF 1
③ DATE: 01/13/2003
④ ID NUMBER: 010000482OH01

⑤ PATIENT: SMITH MARY ⑥ CLAIM: 99999999999 ⑦ ID. NO: 0001234567 ⑧ PLAN CODE: P-PAR ⑨ MFD. REC. NO: 0555-99

⑩ PROC CODE	⑪ FROM DATE	⑫ THRU DATE	⑬ TREAT-MENT	⑭ STATUS CODE	⑮ AMOUNT CHRGD	⑯ AMOUNT ALLWD	⑰ COPAY/ DEDUCT	⑱ COINS	⑲ OTHER REDUCT	⑳ AMOUNT APPRVD	㉑ PATIENT BALANCE
99213-00	01/13/03	01/13/03	1	A	55.00	54.00	.00	5.00	.00	49.00	5.00
93000-00	01/13/03	01/13/03	1	A	40.50	39.50	.00	.00	.00	39.50	.00
81000-00	01/13/03	01/13/03	1	A	8.00	5.85	.00	.00	.00	5.85	.00
CLAIM TOTALS					103.50	94.35	.00	5.00	.00	89.35	5.00

PATIENT: ALLEN ALLAN CLAIM: 89999999999 ID. NO: 0000234567 PLAN CODE: C2000 MFD. REC. NO: 0444-88

PROC CODE	FROM DATE	THRU DATE	TREAT-MENT	STATUS CODE	AMOUNT CHRGD	AMOUNT ALLWD	COPAY/ DEDUCT	COINS	OTHER REDUCT	AMOUNT APPRVD	PATIENT BALANCE
99201-00	02/17/03	02/17/03	1	A	90.00	82.00	.00	10.00	.00	63.80	10.00
CLAIM TOTALS					90.00	82.00	.00	10.00	.00	63.80	10.00

PATIENT: JAMES JAMES CLAIM: 79999999999 ID. NO: 0001034567 PLAN CODE: STATE MFD. REC. NO:

PROC CODE	FROM DATE	THRU DATE	TREAT-MENT	STATUS CODE	AMOUNT CHRGD	AMOUNT ALLWD	COPAY/ DEDUCT	COINS	OTHER REDUCT	AMOUNT APPRVD	PATIENT BALANCE
99214-00	01/07/03	01/07/03	1	A	101.00	58.00	.00	5.00	.00	68.00	5.00
CLAIM TOTALS					101.00	68.00	.00	5.00	.00	68.00	5.00

PAYMENT SUMMARY

TOTAL AMOUNT PAID	224.35
PRIOR CREDIT BALANCE	.00
CURRENT CREDIT DEFERRED	.00
PRIOR CREDIT APPLIED	.00
NEW CREDIT BALANCE	.00
NET DISBURSED	224.35

TOTAL ALL CLAIMS

AMOUNT CHARGES	294.50
AMOUNT ALLOWED	244.35
DEDUCTIBLE	.00
COPAY/COINS	20.00
OTHER REDUCTION	.00
AMOUNT APPROVED	224.35
PATIENT BALANCE	20.00
TOTAL CREDITS	.00

CHECK INFORMATION

NUMBER	00000XXXXXX
DATE	02/27/03
AMOUNT	224.35

㉒ STATUS CODES:
A - APPROVED   AJ - ADJUSTMENT   IP - IN PROCESS   R - REJECTED   V - VOID

Codes

1. Name and address of provider who rendered medical services.
2. Number of pages for the provider remittance.
3. Date the provider remittance was issued.
4. 13-digit identification number of provider who rendered medical services.
5. Name of the patient.
6. Claim number.
7. Identification number we assign to the claim.
8. Name of the member's benefit plan.
9. Number the provider's office has assigned to the patient; will be reflected only if submitted in box 26 of the red HCFA-1500 claim form.
10. Procedure code(s) describing medical services rendered.
11. Date on which medical services began.
12. Date on which medical services ended.
13. Number reflected in box 24g of the red HCFA-1500 claim form; describes the number of days or units related to the medical service.
14. The status of the claim; see box 22 for more information.
15. The amount charged by provider for performing the medical service(s).
16. The amount that we will pay.
17. The amount that has been applied to the member's deductible.
18. The amount of the copayment or the coinsurance for which the member is responsible.
19. Any plan-specific reduction for which the member may be financially responsible.
20. The amount that we will pay.
21. Any amount for which the member is financially responsible.
22. Describes the abbreviations of the status codes reflected in item 14.

Figure 8-2   Example of a Payer's Remittance Advice

Steps for Processing a Remittance Advice

1. Compare the RA to the original insurance claim. Make sure that all procedures listed on the claim are represented on the RA and that the CPT codes have not changed.

2. Review the payment amount against the expected amount.

3. Identify the reasons for denials or payment reductions; resubmit claim or appeal if necessary.

4. Post payment information for individual claims to the appropriate patient accounts.

5. Bill the patient's secondary health care plan (if appropriate).

In most cases, insurance carriers do not fully pay the amount billed by the provider. The provider bills according to the provider's fee schedule, while the payer's rate is determined by a contract with the provider. When the RA is reviewed, the billing specialist checks to see that the amount paid is the expected amount, per the provider's contract with the payer. If a payment is not as expected, the specialist must determine the reason for the discrepancy.

Charges may be denied by insurance carriers for a number of reasons. For example, a procedure may not be covered by the patient's plan, or a procedure or diagnosis may be coded incorrectly. If the reimbursement on an RA is lower than the amount expected, it is important to determine the reason and to take action to collect the correct amount. The problem could have originated in the provider's office, or it could have occurred during processing by the payer. When an error has been made in the provider's office, the billing staff member must correct the error in the billing software and resubmit the claim to the payer. If the error occurs during processing by the third-party payer, an appeal process may be started. Table 8-1 lists common errors that result in reduced or denied payments.

TABLE 8-1	Common Claim Errors
Remittance Advice Result	**Possible Reasons**
Reimbursement is made at a reduced rate.	• Clerical error was made. • Precertification or preapproval guidelines were not followed.
Reimbursement is denied.	• Clerical error was made. • Precertification or preapproval guidelines were not followed. • Insufficient documentation was provided to establish medical necessity. • All information required by payer was not included. • The wrong payer was billed.
Payment is not received.	• Claim is missing or lost in the system.
Multiple procedures were not paid.	• Payer either missed the additional procedures or grouped them with the primary procedure.

8.3 ENTERING INSURANCE PAYMENTS

In contrast to patient payments, which are entered in the Transaction Entry dialog box, insurance payments in Medisoft are entered in the Deposit List dialog box (see Figure 8-3). The Deposit List dialog box is opened by selecting Enter Deposits/Payments on the Activities menu or by clicking the Enter Deposits and Apply Payments short-cut button. The Deposit/Payments area of the program is very efficient for entering large insurance payments that must be split up and applied to a number of different patients.

THE DEPOSIT LIST DIALOG BOX

The Deposit List dialog box contains the following information:

Deposit Date   The program displays the current date (the Medisoft Program Date). The date can be changed by keying over the default date.

Show All Deposits   If this box is checked, all payments are displayed, regardless of the date entered.

Show Unapplied Only   If the Show Unapplied Only box is checked, only payments that have not been fully applied to charge transactions are displayed. If the box is not checked, all payments—both applied and unapplied—are listed.

Sort By   The Sort By drop-down list offers several choices for how payment information is listed. The default is sorting payments by date and description. Payments can also be sorted by other data fields (see Figure 8-4).

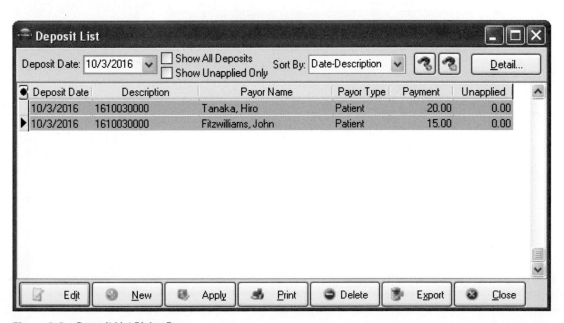

Figure 8-3   Deposit List Dialog Box

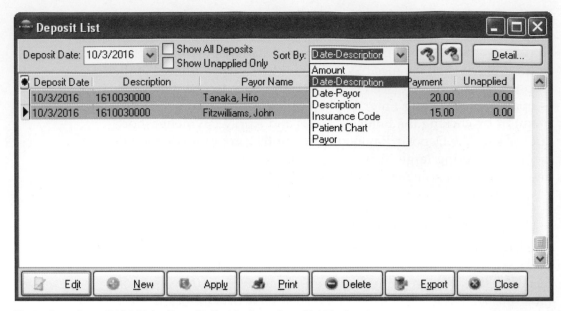

Figure 8-4   Deposit List Dialog Box with Sort By Drop-down List Displayed

Locate Buttons   The Locate and Locate Next buttons, indicated by the two magnifying glass icons, are used to search for a deposit.

Detail   To view a specific deposit in more detail, highlight the deposit, and click the Detail button. A dialog box opens with more information about the selected deposit (see Figure 8-5).

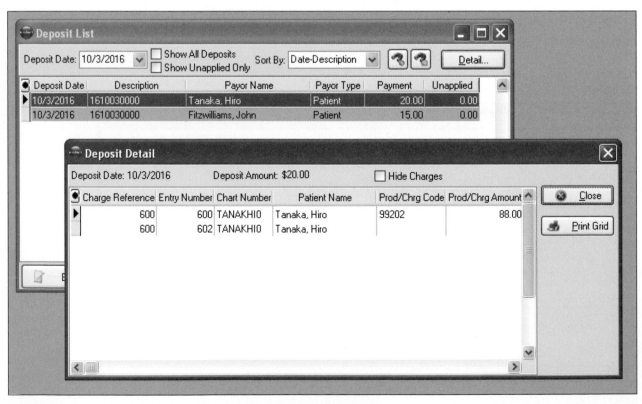

Figure 8-5   Deposit Detail Dialog Box with Deposit List Window in Background

In the middle section of the Deposit List window, information is listed for each deposit and payment, including the following:

Deposit Date   Lists the date of the deposit or payment.

Description   Displays whatever was entered in the Description or Check Number box in the Deposit dialog box. The Deposit dialog box is where new payments and deposits are recorded (see Figure 8-6). It is accessed by clicking the New button in the Deposit List dialog box.

Payor Name   Lists the name of the insurance carrier or individual who made the payment.

Payor Type   A classification column that lists whether the payment is an insurance payment, a patient payment, or a capitation payment. **Capitation payments** are made to physicians on a regular basis (such as monthly) for providing services to patients in a managed care insurance plan. In traditional insurance plans, physicians are paid based on the specific procedures they perform and the number of times the procedures are performed. Under a capitated plan, a flat fee is paid to the physician no matter how many times a patient receives treatment, up to the maximum number of treatments allowed per year. For example, a primary care physician with fifty patients may receive a payment of $2,500 per month for those patients, regardless of whether the physician has seen them during that month.

capitation payments payments made to physicians on a regular basis for providing services to patients in a managed care plan

Payment   Lists the amount of the payment.

Unapplied   Lists the amount of the deposit that has not been applied to a charge.

At the bottom of the Deposit List dialog box are buttons that perform the following actions:

Edit   Opens the highlighted payment or deposit for editing.

New   Opens the Deposit dialog box, where new payments and deposits are recorded.

Apply   Applies payments to specific charge transactions.

Print   Sends a command to print the deposit list.

Delete   Deletes the highlighted transaction.

Export   Exports the data in either Quicken or QuickBooks program formats.

Close   Exits the Deposit List dialog box.

THE DEPOSIT DIALOG BOX

When the New button is clicked in the Deposit List dialog box, the Deposit dialog box appears (see Figure 8-6).

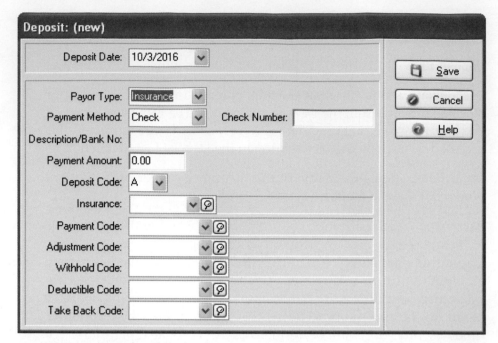

Figure 8-6   Deposit Dialog Box

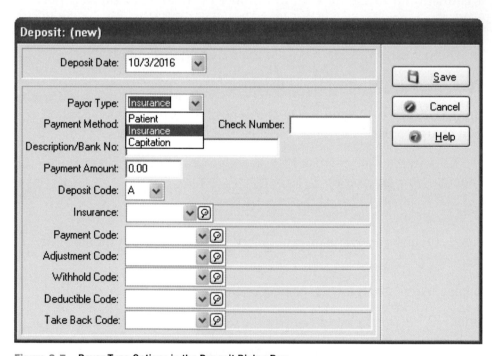

Figure 8-7   Payor Type Options in the Deposit Dialog Box

The Deposit dialog box contains the following fields:

Deposit Date   The program's current date is displayed by default and must be changed if it is not the date of the deposit.

Payor Type   The drop-down options in this box indicate whether the payer is an insurance carrier, a capitation plan, or a patient (see Figure 8-7). Some of the boxes at the bottom of the Deposit dialog box change based on the selection in this box. If Insurance is selected, the dialog box is as illustrated in Figure 8-6. If Capitation is selected, all the boxes below Insurance disappear. If Patient is chosen, the boxes listed below Deposit Code become Chart Number, Payment Code, Adjustment Code, and Copayment Code.

Payment Method   This box lists whether the payment is check, cash, credit card, or electronic.

Check Number   If payment is made by check, the number of the check is entered in this box.

Description/Bank No.   This box can be used to enter a description of the payment, if desired.

Payment Amount   The total amount of the payment is entered in this box.

Deposit Code   This field can be used by practices to sort deposits according to user-defined categories.

Insurance   The insurance carrier that is making the payment is selected.

Payment Code, Adjustment Code, Withhold Code, Deductible Code, and Take Back Code   The appropriate codes for the insurance carrier are selected.

Once all the information has been entered and checked for accuracy, the deposit is saved by clicking the Save button (see Figure 8-8). When the deposit entry is saved, the Deposit dialog box closes, and the Deposit List dialog box reappears, with the new deposit listed (see Figure 8-9).

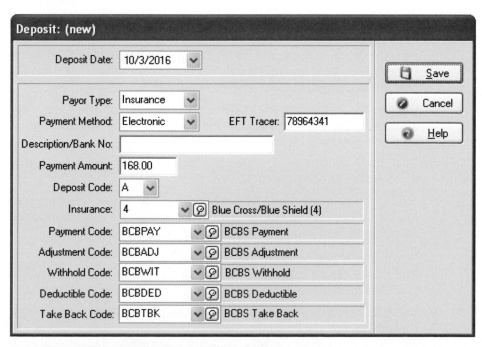

Figure 8-8   Deposit Dialog Box with Information Entered

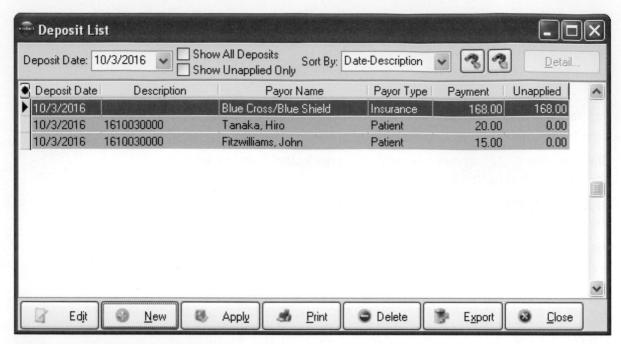

Figure 8-9 Deposit List Dialog Box with Deposit Entered

| EXERCISE 8-1 | ENTERING A DEPOSIT: CHAMPVA |

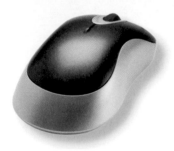

Using Source Document 8, enter the payment received from John Fitzwilliams's insurance carrier for services provided on September 6, 2016. Note that John is guarantor for his daughter Sarah, so her charges and payments are included on the remittance advice.

Date: October 3, 2016

1. Start Medisoft and restore the data from your last work session.

2. Change the Medisoft Program Date to October 3, 2016.

3. Click Enter Deposits/Payments on the Activities menu. The Deposit List dialog box is displayed. Verify that 10/3/2016 is displayed in the Deposit Date box, and that the two check boxes—Show All Deposits and Show Unapplied Only—are not checked.

4. Change the entry in the Sort By box to Date-Payor. Click No in response to the message about changing the date. Compare your screen to Figure 8-10.

5. Click the New button. The Deposit dialog box is displayed. Verify that the Deposit Date is 10/3/2016.

6. Since this is a payment from an insurance carrier, confirm that Insurance is selected in the Payor Type box. If it is not, change the selection in the Payor Type box to Insurance.

7. Accept the default entry (Check) in the Payment Method box.

8. Enter **214778924** in the Check Number box, and press Tab twice. (The Description/Bank No. field can be left blank.)

9. Enter the amount of the payment (**28.02**) in the Payment Amount box. Press Tab.

10. Accept the default entry (A) in the Deposit Code box. Press Tab.

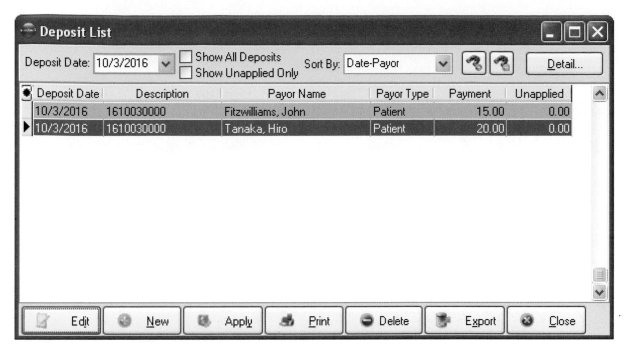

Figure 8-10   Deposit List with 10/3/2016 in Deposit Date Field and Date-Payor Selected in the Sort By Field

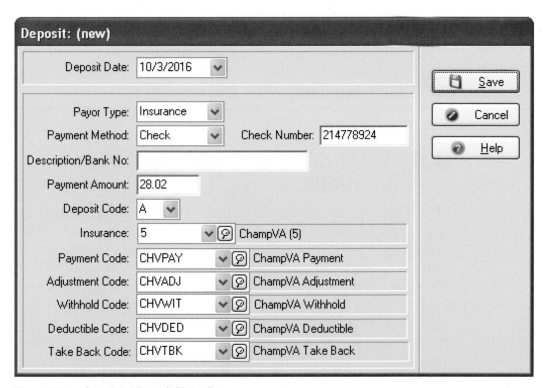

Figure 8-11   Completed Deposit Dialog Box

11. Select the insurance carrier that is making the payment (5—ChampVA) from the Insurance drop-down list. Medisoft automatically enters the defaults for ChampVA in the Payment, Adjustment, Withhold, Deductible, and Take Back Code boxes. Confirm that your screen looks the same as Figure 8-11 before going on to the next step.

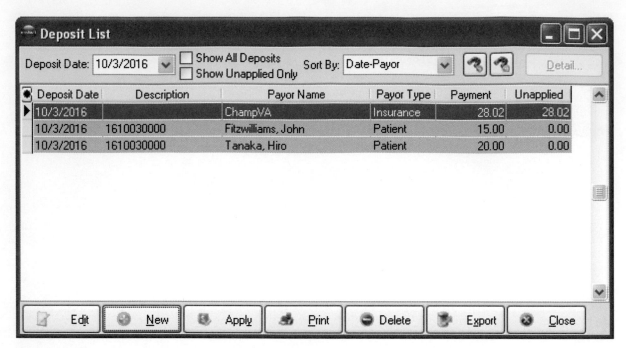

Figure 8-12   Deposit List Dialog Box with New Deposit Entered

12. Click the Save button to save the entry.

13. The Deposit List box reappears. The insurance payment appears in the list of deposits (see Figure 8-12).

✓ **You have completed Exercise 8-1.**

8.4 APPLYING INSURANCE PAYMENTS TO CHARGES

After a deposit has been entered, the next step is to apply the payment to the applicable transactions for each patient listed on the RA using the Apply Payment/Adjustments to Charges dialog box. To apply a deposit, the payment is highlighted in the Deposit List dialog box and the Apply button is clicked. The Apply Payment/ Adjustments to Charges dialog box opens (see Figure 8-13).

The top section of the dialog box contains information about the payer, the patient, and the amount of the payment that is unapplied.

The upper-left corner of the dialog box displays the payer's name in bold type, and it is also listed in the Ins 1 field. In Figure 8-13, the payer is Blue Cross and Blue Shield. The patient who has a transaction listed on the remittance advice is selected from the drop-down list in the For box.

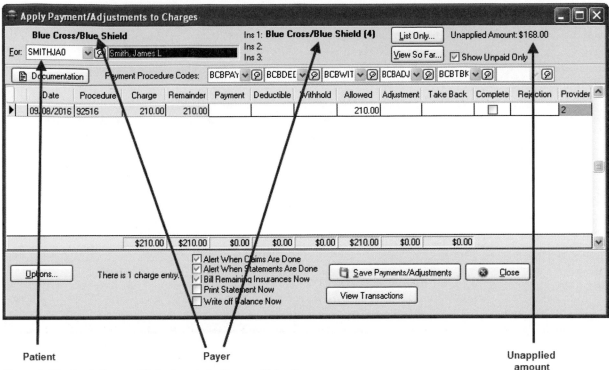

Figure 8-13 Apply Payment/Adjustments to Charges Dialog Box

The upper-right area of the dialog box lists the amount of the deposit that has not yet been applied (Unapplied Amount).

Note: If a patient is selected who does not have coverage with the insurance carrier that is making the deposit, a Select Payor window opens (see Figure 8-14) with the message that the payer does not match any case for the patient. Clicking the Cancel button closes the dialog box.

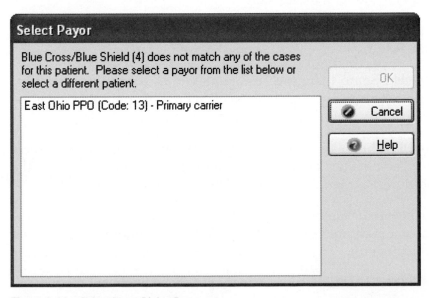

Figure 8-14 Select Payor Dialog Box

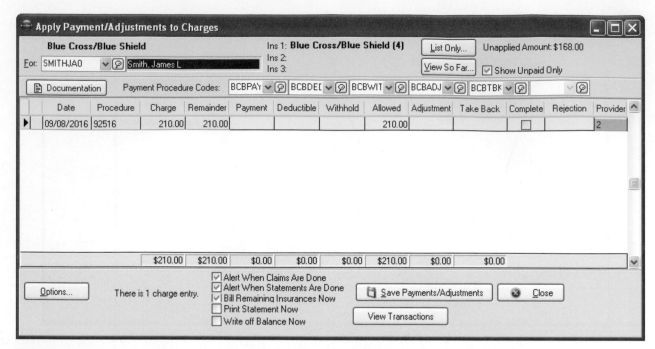

Figure 8-15 Apply Payment/Adjustments to Charges Dialog Box with Payment Entry Area Highlighted Yellow

The middle section of the Apply Payment/Adjustments to Charges dialog box is where payments are entered and applied (see Figure 8-15).

Date, Procedure, Charge, Remainder   These fields show the date of service, procedure code, charge amount, and amount remaining for each transaction, as already entered in the database. This information cannot be edited in the dialog box.

Payment   The amount of the payment for this procedure is entered. The program automatically makes this a negative sum, so it is not necessary to enter a minus sign.

Deductible   If applicable, enter the amount of the deductible listed on the RA.

Withhold   Some insurance companies may withhold money for multiple charges and then pay out all at once. If applicable, enter the withholding amount in this field.

Allowed   This is the amount allowed by the payer for this procedure. These values are located in the Allowed Amounts tab of the Procedure/Payment/Adjustment dialog box (see Figure 8-16).

Adjustment   The amount entered here is the charge amount minus whatever is entered in the Allowed field. This amount is calculated by the program.

Take Back   This field contains only positive adjustment amounts. It is provided for situations in which the insurance company overpays on one charge and then indicates that the overpayment should be

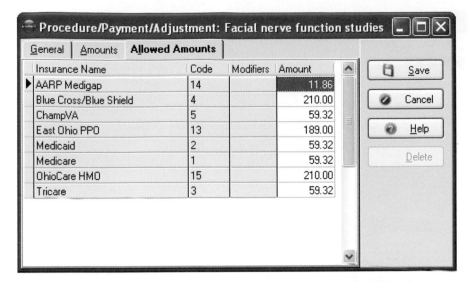

Figure 8-16   Allowed Amounts Tab in the Procedure/Payment/Adjustment Dialog Box

applied as a payment for another transaction. Most times, the take back should be applied to the same charge that had the overpayment.

Complete   The program places a check in this box to indicate that the payer's responsibility is complete for this transaction.

Rejection   If desired, a rejection message from the RA can be entered.

Provider   This field lists the provider assigned to the transaction.

Figure 8-17 shows an Apply Payment/Adjustments to Charges dialog box with a payment entered.

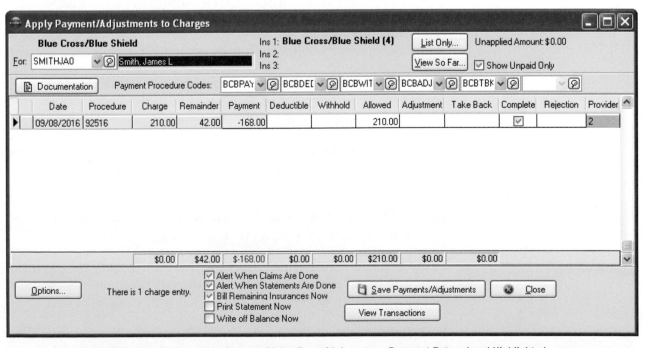

Figure 8-17   Apply Payment/Adjustments to Charges Dialog Box with Insurance Payment Entered and Highlighted

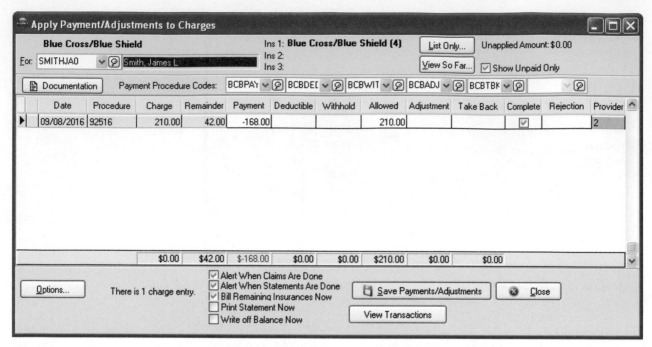

Figure 8-18 Apply Payment/Adjustments to Charges Dialog Box with Save Payments/Adjustments Button Highlighted

The lower third of the Apply Payment/Adjustments to Charges dialog box contains several options that affect claims and statements (see Figure 8-18).

Options The Options . . . button is used to change the default settings for patient payment application codes.

Alert When Claims Are Done This field determines whether a message appears as notification that a claim is done for a payer.

Alert When Statements Are Done This field determines whether a message appears as notification that a statement is done for a patient.

Bill Remaining Insurances Now If this box is checked, claims for any secondary or tertiary payer associated with the claim are created when the current insurance payment is saved.

Print Statement Now If a check mark appears in this box, the program creates a patient statement when the current insurance payment is saved.

Write Off Balance Now This field allows patient remainder balances to be written off from within this window.

Save Payments/Adjustments Clicking this button saves the payment currently being applied. Once the payment is saved, another patient can be selected in the For field, or the dialog box can be closed.

View Transactions Clicking this button opens the Transaction Entry dialog box so that the selected patient's transactions can be viewed.

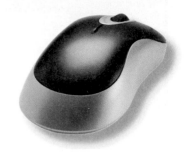

Using Source Document 8, apply the payment received from John Fitzwilliams's insurance carrier for services provided on September 6, 2016.

Date: October 3, 2016

1. Open the Deposit List dialog box, if it is not still open from Exercise 8-1.

2. With the CHAMPVA payment entry highlighted, click the Apply button. Click No in response to the message about changing the date. The Apply Payment/Adjustments to Charges dialog box appears. In the lower portion of the dialog box, make sure the first three check boxes are checked and the last two (Print Statement Now and Write off Balance Now) are unchecked.

3. Key **F** in the For box, and press Tab to select John Fitzwilliams, since a portion of this payment is for his account. All the charge entries for John Fitzwilliams that have not been paid in full are listed. Notice that the amount listed in the Unapplied box in the upper-right corner shows the full deposit amount, since nothing has been applied yet.

4. Refer to Source Document 8 to determine the first payment amount, which is for the 99211 procedure completed on 09/06/2016. Notice that the cursor is blinking in the Payment box for this charge. Enter **5.68** in the Payment box, and press Tab.

5. Medisoft automatically places a minus sign before the amount. Notice that once the payment is applied, the Complete box to the right of the dialog box is checked. This indicates that the transaction is complete for this payer. Also notice that the Unapplied amount has been reduced by $5.68. Press Tab to move through each column until you reach the end of the first row so that the program can update the amounts. When you tab past the end of row 1, notice that the amount in the Remainder column changes to 0.00 and the amount in the Adjustment column now displays −15.32.

6. Now enter the payment for the 84478 procedure charge. Enter **8.04** in the Payment box. Press Tab to move through each column until you reach the end of the first row so that the program can update the amounts. When you tab past the end of the row, the amount in the Remainder column changes to 0.00 and the amount in the Adjustment column now displays −20.96. Check your work against Figure 8-19.

7. Click the Save Payments/Adjustments button to save your entry. When you click this button, an Information dialog box displays the message that the claim has been marked "done" for the primary insurance. Click OK. The dialog box is cleared of the current transaction and is ready for a new transaction.

8. Now enter a payment for Sarah Fitzwilliams. Key **F** in the For box, and then locate her name in the drop-down list. Click on her chart number to display her data. Notice on the RA and in the Apply Payment/Adjustments to Charges dialog box that her $15.00 copayment was applied to the charge for procedure 90471, so that the procedure now has a 0.00 remainder balance. A zero payment from the insurance plan must be entered in the Payment column. Do this now and press Tab until the cursor is in the Payment column for the

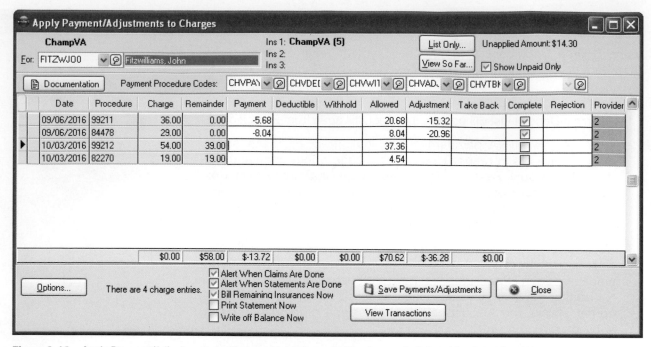

Figure 8-19 Apply Payment/Adjustments to Charges Dialog Box with Two Payments Entered for John Fitzwilliams

second charge. Now enter the payment for the procedure 90703, and again press Tab to the end of the line. Compare your screen to Figure 8-20.

9. Click the Save Payments/Adjustments button.

10. Click the Close button to exit the Apply Payment/Adjustments to Charges dialog box. The Deposit List box reappears. Notice that the unapplied amount for the CHAMPVA deposit is now 0.00.

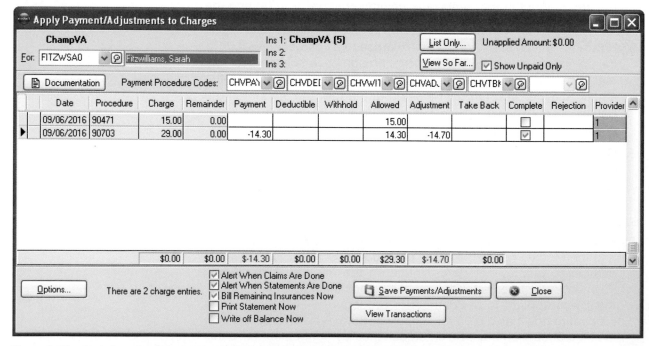

Figure 8-20 Apply Payment/Adjustments to Charges Dialog Box with One Payment Entered for Sarah Fitzwilliams

11. Without closing the Deposit List dialog box, open the Transaction Entry dialog box, select John Fitzwilliams, and scroll through the list of payments and adjustments at the bottom of the screen. In addition to the patient's copayment, there are two payments with corresponding adjustments, dated 10/3/2016. Payments entered in the Deposit List dialog box also appear in the Transaction Entry dialog box. In the Totals tab area of the dialog box, notice that there is still a balance of $58.00 due on Fitzwilliams's account, for his office visit on 10/3/2016.

12. Now select Sarah Fitzwilliams. The payment and corresponding adjustment from CHAMPVA appear in the Payments, Adjustments, and Comments section, and the Account Total balance in the Totals tab area is now 0.00.

13. Close the Transaction Entry dialog box.

 ☑ You have completed Exercise 8-2.

ENTERING A DEPOSIT AND APPLYING PAYMENTS: EAST OHIO PPO	EXERCISE 8-3

The medical office has just received an ERA from East Ohio PPO (see Source Document 9). The total amount of the electronic funds transfer (EFT) is $450.60. This amount includes payments for a number of patients. Enter the insurance carrier payment, and apply it to the appropriate patients. (*Note:* Source Document 9 consists of two pages.)

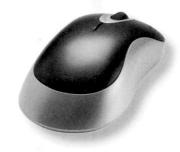

Date: October 3, 2016

1. Verify that the entry in the Deposit Date box in the Deposit List dialog box is 10/3/2016.

2. Click the New button. (If a message about changing the date appears, click No and press the New button again.) The Deposit dialog box is displayed.

3. Select Insurance in the Payor Type box.

4. Select Electronic in the Payment Method box, since this payment was sent electronically to the practice's bank account. Notice the Check Number box becomes an EFT Tracer box. Press Tab twice.

5. Enter the ERA ID number, **00146972**, in the Description/Bank No. box.

6. Enter **450.60** in the Payment Amount box, and press Tab.

7. Accept the default entry in the Deposit Code box.

8. Select 13—East Ohio PPO in the Insurance box. Medisoft automatically completes the Payment, Adjustment, Withhold, Deductible, and Take Back Code boxes.

9. Click the Save button.

10. The payment entry appears in the Deposit List dialog box.

11. Now apply the payment to the specific transaction charges.

12. With the East Ohio PPO line highlighted, click the Apply button. The Apply Payment/Adjustments to Charges dialog box is displayed.

13. Key **A** in the For box, and press Tab to select Susan Arlen.

14. Locate the charge on the ERA for procedure code 99212 on 09/5/2016. Key the amount of the payment, **28.60**, in the Payment box, and press Tab. Notice that Medisoft automatically checks the Complete box, since Susan Arlen has only one insurance carrier (there is no payment forthcoming from any other carrier, so the charge is complete). Tab through to the end of the line to have Medisoft update the adjustment amount and the new remainder amount.

15. Click the Save Payments/Adjustments button and then click the OK button when the Information box appears, reporting that the claim has been marked "done." The data for Susan Arlen that were visible in the Apply Payment/Adjustments to Charges dialog box are cleared, and the dialog box is ready for the next payment or adjustment. Notice also that the amount listed in the Unapplied column for East Ohio PPO has been reduced by the amount of the Arlen payment.

16. Now enter the payment for the next patient listed on the ERA, Herbert Bell.

17. Key **BE** in the For box, and press Tab to select Herbert Bell.

18. Enter the payment of **12.40** in the Payment box for the 99211 charge on 09/5/2016. Tab to the end of the line.

19. Click the Save Payments/Adjustments button, and then click the OK button.

20. Key **BELLSAM** in the For box, and press Tab to select Samuel Bell.

21. Enter the payment of **28.60** in the Payment box for the 99212 charge on 09/5/2016. Tab to the end of the line.

22. Click the Save Payments/Adjustments button, and then click the OK button.

23. Continue to apply the insurance payments for Janine Bell, Jonathan Bell, and Sarina Bell using the information on Source Document 9. Click the Save Payments/Adjustments button after you complete the payment entries for each patient. When you have applied all the payments, the amount in the Unapplied box for the East Ohio PPO payment should be 0.00.

24. Close the Apply Payment/Adjustments to Charges dialog box.

 You have completed Exercise 8-3.

EXERCISE 8-4

ENTERING A DEPOSIT AND APPLYING PAYMENTS: BLUE CROSS AND BLUE SHIELD

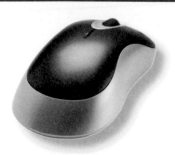

The medical office has just received an ERA from Blue Cross and Blue Shield (see Source Document 10). The total amount of the remittance is $214.40. This amount includes payments for a number of patients. Enter the insurance carrier payment for each patient. You will need to enter a zero payment on a charge for Sheila Giles, as one of her procedures was denied.

Date: November 3, 2016

1. In the Deposit List dialog box, change the date in the Deposit Date box to 11/3/2016, and press the Tab key. A Confirm box is displayed,

stating that the date entered is in the future, and asking if you want to change it. Click the No button to keep the new date.

2. Click the New button again.

3. Select Insurance in the Payor Type box. Press Tab.

4. Change the entry in the Payment Method box to Electronic.

5. Enter the ERA ID number, **001234**, in the Description/Bank No. box.

6. Enter **214.40** in the Payment Amount box. Press Tab.

7. Accept the default entry in the Deposit Code box. Press Tab.

8. Select 4—Blue Cross/Blue Shield in the Insurance box. Medisoft automatically completes the Payment, Adjustment, Withhold, Deductible, and Take Back Code boxes.

9. Click the Save button.

10. The payment entry appears in the Deposit List dialog box.

11. Now apply the payment to the specific transaction charges.

12. With the Blue Cross/Blue Shield line highlighted, click the Apply button. The Apply Payment/Adjustments to Charges dialog box is displayed.

13. Key **GI** in the For box to select Sheila Giles, and then press Tab.

14. Three charges are listed. Locate the charge for procedure code 99213 on 10/28/2016. Key the amount of the payment, **57.60**, in the Payment box, and press Tab. Medisoft automatically checks the Complete box, since Sheila Giles has only one insurance carrier (no payment is forthcoming from any other carrier, so the charge is complete). Continue pressing the Tab key until the amount listed in the Remainder column changes to $14.40.

15. Now enter the payment for the next procedure listed on the ERA— 71010. (*Note:* The order of procedures is different on the ERA than it is in the Apply Payment/Adjustments to Charges window. Be sure to apply the payment to the correct procedure.) Remember to click the Tab key until the amount in the Remainder column changes.

16. Look again at Source Document 10. Notice that the amount paid for the final procedure, 87430, is $0.00. Read the note listed to determine why the charge was not paid. This denial of payment must be entered in Medisoft so that the practice billing staff will be aware that Sheila Giles is responsible for the entire amount of that charge, $29.00.

17. Click in the Payment box for the charge for procedure 87430. Enter **0**, and press Tab. Notice that the amount listed in the Remainder column is the full amount of the charge, $29.00. The charge has also been marked as complete, since the insurance carrier is not responsible for the remainder amount.

18. Click the Save Payments/Adjustments button. An Information box is displayed, indicating that the claim has been marked "done" for the primary insurance. Click the OK button.

19. Close the Apply Payment/Adjustments to Charges dialog box; then, without closing the Deposit List dialog box, open the Transaction Entry dialog box.

20. Locate Sheila Giles's upper respiratory infection case. In the Charges area, notice that two of the charges appear in an aqua color, which indicates that they have been partially paid. The charge that was denied by the insurance carrier—87430—is still in gray, indicating that no payment has been made.

21. Now look at the Account Total in the Totals tab area in the Transaction Entry dialog box. Sheila Giles is listed as being responsible for paying $61.60, which breaks down as follows:

Code	Charge Amount	Patient Responsible for
99213	$72.00	$14.40 (20% of charge)
71010	$91.00	$18.20 (20% of charge)
87430	$29.00	$29.00 (100% of charge)
Totals	**$192.00**	**$61.60**

22. Close the Transaction Entry dialog box.

23. Back in the Deposit List dialog box, make sure the Blue Cross/Blue Shield line is still highlighted, and click the Apply button. You are returned to the Apply Payment/Adjustments to Charges dialog box with the Unapplied Amount for the Blue Cross/Blue Shield payment displayed as $84.00. Enter the payments for the second patient listed on Source Document 10, Jill Simmons.

24. Key **S** in the For box, and press Tab to select Jill Simmons.

25. Enter the payment of **43.20** in the Payment box for the 99212 charge on 10/28/2016. Tab to the end of the row.

26. Enter the other payment for Jill Simmons. Then notice that the amount listed in the Unapplied area is now 0.00, indicating that the entire payment has been entered.

27. Click the Save Payments/Adjustments button, and then click OK.

28. Close the Apply Payment/Adjustments to Charges dialog box.

29. The Deposit List dialog box reappears and the amount in the Unapplied column is now zero.

☑ **You have completed Exercise 8-4.**

8.5 ENTERING CAPITATION PAYMENTS

Capitation payments are entered in the Deposit List dialog box. To indicate a capitation payment, Capitation is selected from the Payor Type drop-down list in the Deposit window (see Figure 8-21).

When a capitation payment is entered in Medisoft, the payment is not applied to the charges of individual patients. Under capitated plans, the insurance carrier pays the practice a set fee to cover all the insured patients who elect to use the practice. This designated payment is made regardless of whether any of the patients visit the practice, or how often they visit. However, the charges in each patient's account

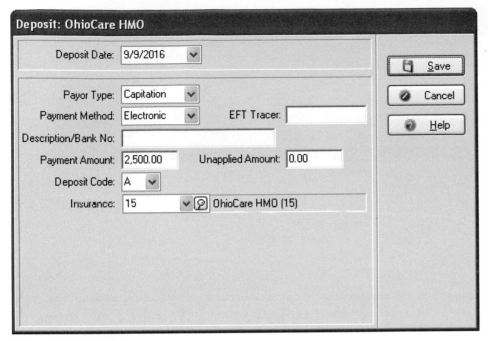

Figure 8-21 Deposit Dialog Box for a Capitation Payment

who have used the practice during the month covered by the capitation payment still must be adjusted to a zero balance to indicate that the insurance company has met its obligation (through the capitation payment) and that the patient has also done so (by paying a copayment at the time of the office visit).

In order to adjust the patient accounts of those covered by the capitated plan, a second deposit is entered as an insurance payment with a zero amount (see Figure 8-22).

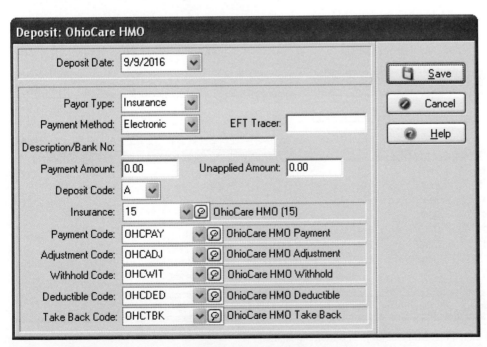

Figure 8-22 Deposit Dialog Box with a Zero Payment Amount

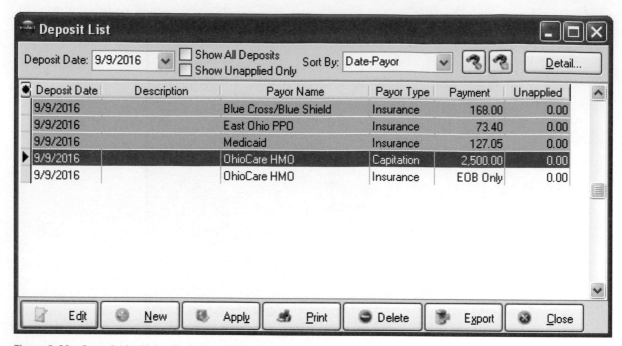

Figure 8-23   Deposit List Dialog Box with a Capitation Payment and a Zero Insurance Payment Entered

Once the zero amount deposit is saved, the deposit appears in the Deposit List window (see Figure 8-23). The Payment column lists "EOB Only," since there is no payment associated with the zero amount deposit.

The next step is to locate patients who have claims during the month covered by the capitation payment. This is accomplished using the List Only . . . button in the Claim Management dialog box (see Figure 8-24).

When the List Only . . . button is clicked, the List Only Claims That Match dialog box appears. The List Only Claims That Match dialog

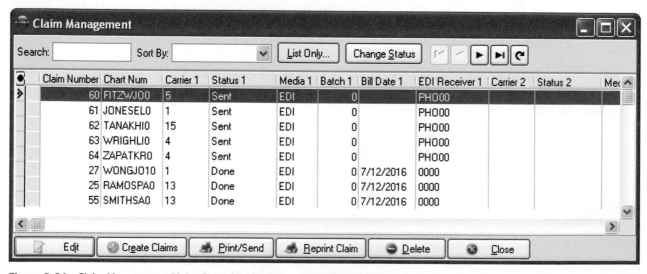

Figure 8-24   Claim Management Dialog Box with List Only . . . Button Highlighted

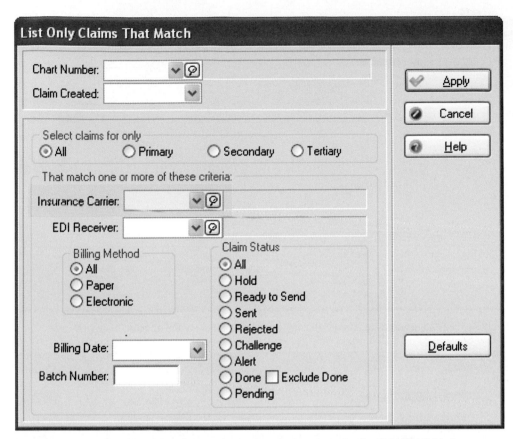

Figure 8-25 List Only Claims That Match Dialog Box with Insurance Carrier Field Highlighted

box (see Figure 8-25) provides an option for searching for claims by insurance carrier. Using this option, patients with active capitated claims from a given carrier can be identified.

Once patients have been identified, the Claim Management dialog box is closed, and the Deposit List dialog box is opened. The identified patient accounts must be adjusted to a zero balance in the Apply Payment/Adjustments to Charges dialog box.

To apply the zero payment amount to these patient accounts, select the line for the deposit and click the Apply button. In the Apply Payment/Adjustments to Charges dialog box, select the chart number of each patient covered by the zero payment, and enter an adjustment equal to the outstanding balance (see Figure 8-26). In the example in Figure 8-26, the amount in the Remainder column is $34.00. This is the amount that must be entered in the Adjustment column to take the account to a zero balance. Figure 8-27 shows the dialog box after the $34.00 adjustment has been applied. Notice that the amount in the Remainder column is now zero. This procedure must be followed for each patient who has transactions during the time period covered by the capitation payment.

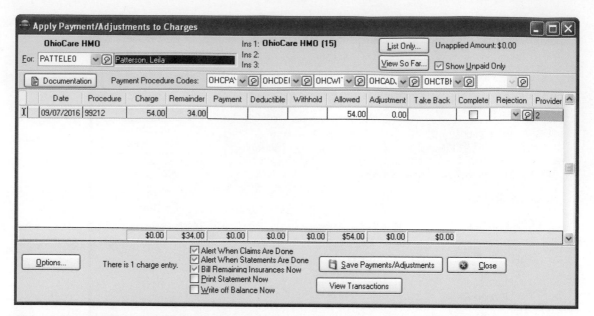

Figure 8-26 Apply Payment/Adjustments to Charges Dialog Box with Capitated Patient Account Displayed

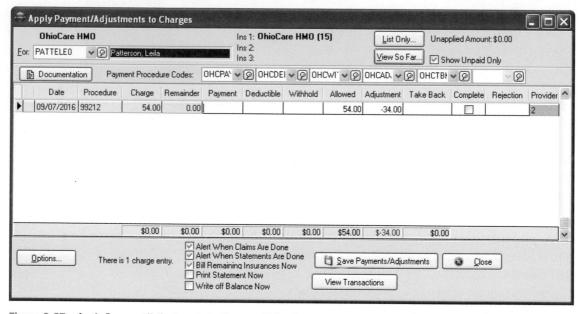

Figure 8-27 Apply Payment/Adjustments to Charges Dialog Box After the Patient Account Is Adjusted to a Zero Balance

EXERCISE 8-5   ENTERING A CAPITATION PAYMENT

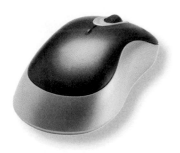

Using Source Document 11, enter a capitation payment from OhioCare HMO for the month of October 2016. The total amount of the electronic funds transfer is $2,500.00.

Date: November 3, 2016

1. In the Deposit List dialog box, confirm that the Deposit Date box is 11/3/2016. If it is not, change it to 11/3/2016. Click the New button. (If a Confirm box appears with a message about entering a future date, click No, and then click the New button again.) The Deposit dialog box appears.

2. In the Payor Type box, select Capitation. Press Tab.

3. Select Electronic in the Payment Method box. Press Tab twice.

4. Key **001006003** in the Description/Bank No. box. This is the ID number that is listed on the ERA. Press Tab.

5. Key **2500** in the Payment Amount box, and press Tab.

6. Accept the default entry of A in the Deposit Code box. Press Tab.

7. Click 15—OhioCare HMO in the Insurance drop-down list.

8. Click the Save button.

9. The Deposit List window reappears, displaying the payment just entered. As mentioned above, unlike other insurance payments, capitation payments are not applied to individual charges. However, amounts do need to be adjusted in the patient accounts. The next two exercises provide practice. First a zero amount payment is entered in the Deposit List dialog box. Then the zero amount payment is used to adjust the active accounts for capitated patients to a zero balance. **CiMO**

 You have completed Exercise 8-5.

ENTERING A ZERO AMOUNT PAYMENT — EXERCISE 8-6

Enter a zero payment amount deposit for OhioCare HMO.

Date: November 3, 2016

1. In the Deposit List dialog box, click the New button. The Deposit dialog box appears.

2. In the Payor Type box, select Insurance. Press Tab.

3. Select Electronic in the Payment Method box.

4. Verify that 0.00 is the amount displayed in the Payment Amount box.

5. Accept the default entry of A in the Deposit Code box.

6. Click 15—OhioCare HMO in the Insurance drop-down list.

7. Click the Save button. The Deposit List dialog box reappears with the zero amount payment displayed. **CiMO**

 You have completed Exercise 8-6.

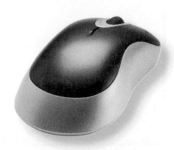

ADJUSTING A CAPITATED ACCOUNT — EXERCISE 8-7

Using the List Only Claims That Match option in Claim Management, locate the OhioCare HMO patients who visited the practice in October 2016, as these are the patients with active capitated accounts. Then, in the Apply Payment/Adjustments to Charges dialog box, enter any adjustments needed to zero out their accounts.

Date: November 3, 2016

1. Without closing the Deposit List dialog box, open the Claim Management dialog box by selecting Claim Management on the Activities menu.

2. Click the List Only . . . button.

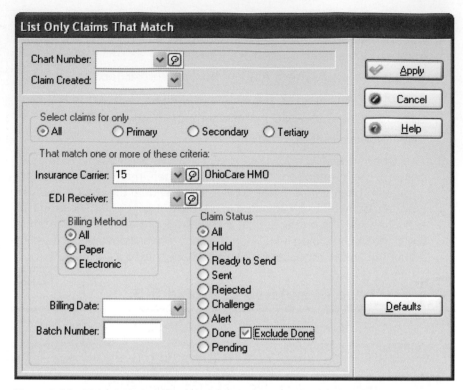

Figure 8-28   List Only Claims That Match Dialog Box with 15—OhioCare HMO Selected

3. In the List Only Claims That Match dialog box, select 15—OhioCare HMO in the Insurance Carrier drop-down list. In the Claim Status options, make sure the All button is selected, and the Exclude Done check box is checked to exclude claims that have already been paid (see Figure 8-28).

4. Click the Apply button. The Claim Management window appears with the capitated claim listed. In this case, there is only one capitated claim. Check your screen against Figure 8-29.

5. Use the Edit button and click the Transactions tab to view the details of the claim, verifying that any transactions listed took place in

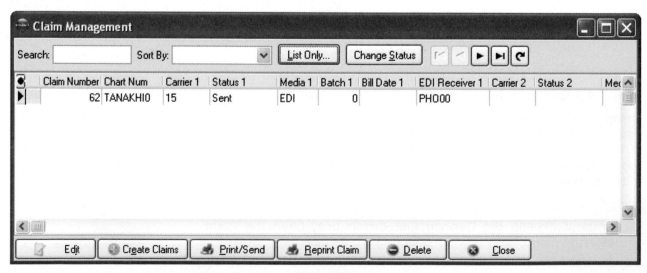

Figure 8-29   Claim Management Dialog Box with OhioCare HMO Patient Listed

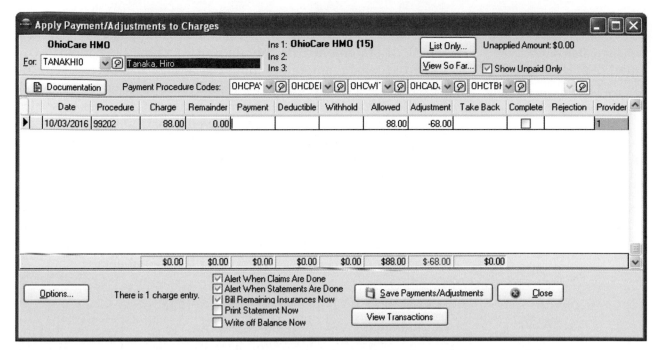

Figure 8-30   Apply Payment/Adjustments to Charges Dialog Box After Account Has Been Adjusted to a Zero Balance

October 2016. Make a note of the patient's name, and close the Claim dialog box and the Claim Management dialog box.

6. You are returned to the Deposit List dialog box. Select the OhioCare HMO deposit that has EOB Only listed in the Payment column, and click the Apply button.

7. Select the capitated patient in the For field, and press Tab.

8. Notice there is only one procedure on the claim. To enter the correct amount for the adjustment, identify the amount in the Remainder column, and enter an equal amount in the Adjustment column. Press Tab repeatedly, until the remainder amount changes to zero. Your screen should look like Figure 8-30.

9. Click the Save Payments/Adjustments button. To verify that the account has been adjusted to a zero balance, click the View Transactions button at the bottom of the dialog box. Key *TA* in the Chart box, press Tab, and then press OK when the two message boxes appear to display Tanaka's transaction information. Notice that the adjustment has been made and the account has a zero balance. When finished viewing the data, close the Transaction Entry dialog box.

10. You are back in the Apply Payment/Adjustments to Charges dialog box. If there were other OhioCare HMO patients with capitated claims in October, you would use the For field to display their information and repeat the process for each patient's account, entering an adjustment for each transaction line that had a remainder amount.

11. Close the Apply Payment/Adjustments to Charges dialog box.

12. Close the Deposit List dialog box.   **CiMO**

☑ **You have completed Exercise 8-7.**

8.6 CREATING STATEMENTS

patient statement a list of the amount of money a patient owes, the procedures performed, and the dates the procedures were performed

A **patient statement** lists the amount of money a patient owes, organized by the amount of time the money has been owed, the procedures performed, and the dates the procedures were performed. Patient statements are created after an insurance claim has been filed and a remittance advice has been received. A patient statement is sent to collect the balance on an account that is the patient's responsibility. This may include coinsurance charges and charges for procedures that were not covered by the insurance company.

Statements are created using the Statement Management feature, which is listed on the Activities menu. Just as Claim Management provides a range of options for billing insurance carriers, Statement Management offers multiple choices for billing patients.

STATEMENT MANAGEMENT DIALOG BOX

The Statement Management dialog box is displayed by clicking Statement Management on the Activities menu or by clicking the Statement Management shortcut button on the toolbar (see Figure 8-31). The dialog box lists all statements that have already been created (see Figure 8-32). In this dialog box, several actions can be performed: existing statements can be reviewed and edited, new statements can be created, the status of existing statements can be changed, and statements can be printed.

Figure 8-31
Statement Management Shortcut Button

Stmt # The Stmt # column lists the statement number, which is generated by the program in sequential order.

Guarantor In the Statement Management dialog box, guarantors rather than patients are listed because statements are created only

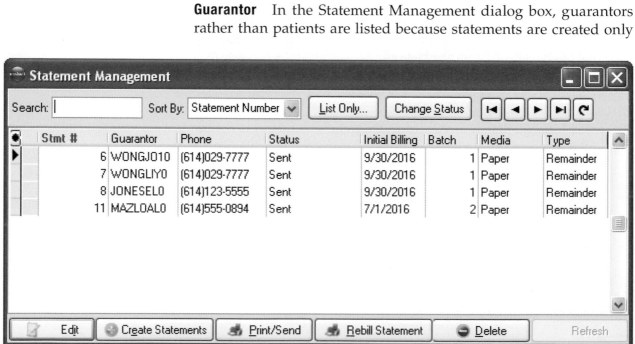

Figure 8-32 Statement Management Dialog Box

for those financially responsible for accounts. For example, if a patient's father is the guarantor, a statement is created for the patient's father, not for the patient. In the Statement Management dialog box, the statement is listed under the father's chart number. If the man is also guarantor on his wife's account, his chart number will appear twice in the Statement Management window. When statements are printed, however, all transactions for the guarantor's child and wife are billed on one statement.

Phone   The Phone column lists guarantors' phone numbers.

Status   The status assigned to each statement depends on whether the statement has been billed and whether the account has a zero balance:

- **Ready to Send** Transactions that have not been billed
- **Sent** Transactions that have been billed but not fully paid
- **Done** Transactions that have been billed and fully paid

Medisoft assigns status based on:

Initial Billing   The date the statement was initially sent appears in the Initial Billing column. If a statement has been sent more than once, the most recent date is shown in the Billing Date field located in the General tab of the Statement dialog box, which is used for editing statements.

Batch   The batch number assigned by Medisoft is displayed.

Media   The format for the statement, either paper or electronic, is designated.

Type   The type of statement, either Standard or Remainder, is listed.

CREATE STATEMENTS DIALOG BOX

The Create Statements dialog box is where information is entered that determines which statements are generated (see Figure 8-33).

The following filters can be applied in the Create Statements dialog box:

Transaction Dates   A range of dates is entered to select transactions that occur within those dates. The dates can be entered directly by keying in the boxes, or they can be selected from the calendar that appears when the drop-down arrow is clicked. To create statements for all available transactions, leave both date boxes blank.

Chart Numbers   In the Chart Numbers boxes, the starting and ending chart numbers for which statements will be created are entered. If the boxes are left blank, all chart numbers will be included.

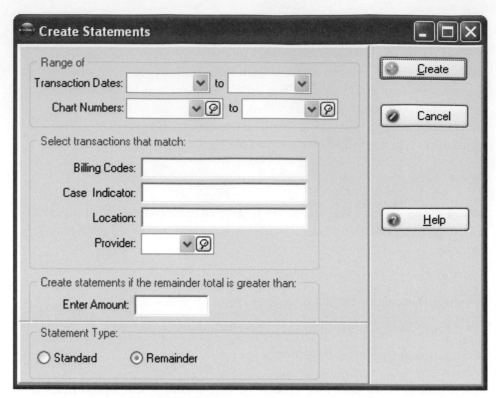

Figure 8-33   Create Statements Dialog Box

Select Transactions That Match   The options in this portion of the dialog box provide filters for creating statements for billing codes, case indicators, locations, and provider. In all instances except provider, commas must be placed between entries if more than one code is entered.

Create Statements If The Remainder Total Is Greater Than . . . Enter Amount   The dollar amount entered in this box is the minimum outstanding balance required for a statement to be created. For example, if 5.00 is entered in this box, the program will not create statements for accounts with balances below $5.00. If this field is left blank, statements will be created for all accounts, regardless of the balances.

standard statements
statements that show all charges regardless of whether the insurance has paid on the transactions

remainder statements
statements that list only those charges that are not paid in full after all insurance carrier payments have been received

Statement Type   **Standard statements** show all available charges regardless of whether the insurance has paid on the transactions. **Remainder statements** list only those charges that are not paid in full after all insurance carrier payments have been received. Once a statement type is selected, the setting remains in effect until the other type of statement is selected.

After all selections are complete in the Create Statements dialog box, clicking the Create button instructs the program to generate statements. (*Note:* If you click the Create button and no statements can be created, the following message appears: "No new statements were created." Click OK to close the dialog box that contains the message.)

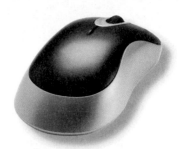

Create remainder statements for all patients with last names beginning with the letters *H* through *S*. *Note:* Be sure to enter *SYZMAM* instead of just *S* to select all patients whose last names begin with the letter *S*.

Date: October 28, 2016

1. Verify that the Medisoft Program Date is October 28, 2016. Select Statement Management on the Activities menu. The Statement Management dialog box appears. Verify that the Sort By field is set to Statement Number.

2. Click the Create Statements button. The Create Statements dialog box is displayed.

3. Enter the chart numbers that will select all patients with last names beginning with *H* through *S*. Note that you will need to select Michael Syzmanski in the second Chart Numbers field to include all patients with last names beginning with the letter *S*.

4. Be sure the Statement Type field is set to Remainder. If it is not, click the Remainder button. Check your work against Figure 8-34, and then click the Create button to generate statements.

5. A message appears stating the number of statements that have been created (see Figure 8-35).

6. Click the OK button. Change the entry in the Sort By field to Statement Number, if it is not already listed. Any new statements that were created are added to the list of statements in the Statement Management dialog box, with a Ready to Send status (see Figure 8-36).

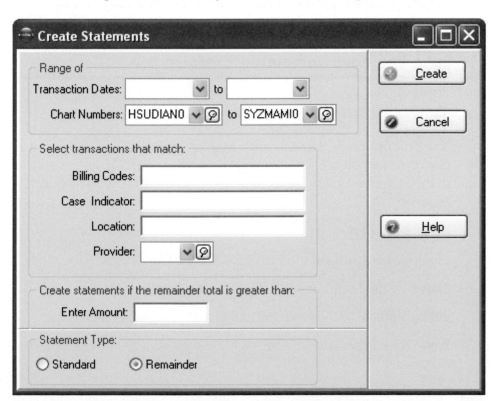

Figure 8-34 Create Statements Dialog Box with Selections Made

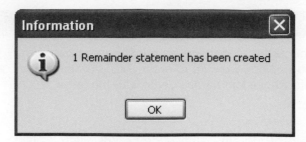

Figure 8-35 Information Box Indicating the Number of Statements Created

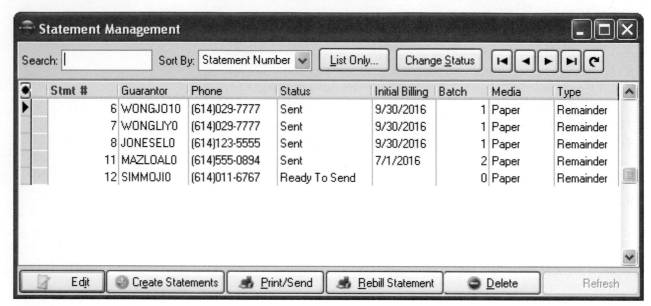

Figure 8-36 Statement Management Dialog Box with New Statement Created for Jill Simmons

 You have completed Exercise 8-8.

8.7 EDITING STATEMENTS

The Edit button in the Statement Management dialog box is used to perform edits on account statements (see Figure 8-37). The three tabs in the Statement dialog box contain important information about the statement.

GENERAL TAB

The following information is located in the General tab:

Status   These buttons indicate the current status of the statement.

Billing Method   The statement can be either paper or electronic.

Type   The Type field indicates whether the statement is standard or remainder.

Initial Billing Date   The Initial Billing Date is the date the statement was first created.

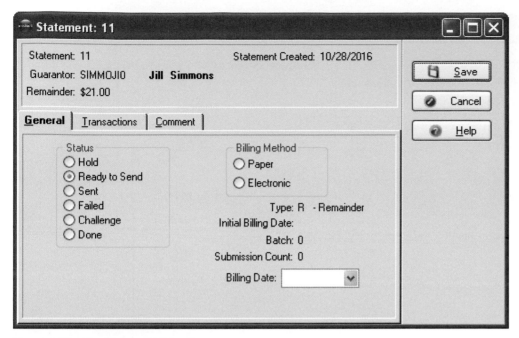

Figure 8-37 The Statement Dialog Box

Batch   The batch number assigned to the statement appears.

Submission Count   This entry shows how many times a statement has been sent or printed.

Billing Date   The most current billing date is displayed.

TRANSACTIONS TAB

The Transactions tab lists the transactions placed on the statement (see Figure 8-38). The buttons at the bottom of the tab are used to

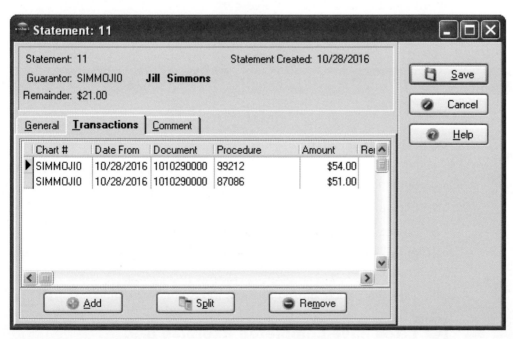

Figure 8-38 Transactions Tab

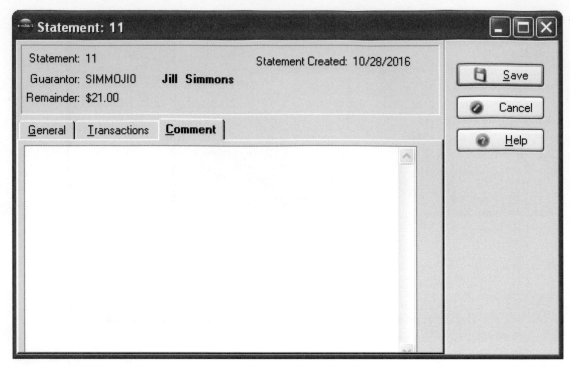

Figure 8-39   Comment Tab

add transactions to the statement, split transactions, or remove transactions from the statement.

COMMENT TAB

The Comment tab provides a place to include notes about the statement (see Figure 8-39).

EXERCISE 8-9   **REVIEWING A STATEMENT**

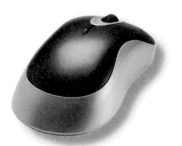

Review the statement created in Exercise 8-8.

Date: October 28, 2016

1. If it is not already highlighted, click on the statement created for Jill Simmons in Exercise 8-8 to highlight it.

2. Click the Edit button.

3. Review the information in the General tab.

4. Click on the Transactions tab to see the transactions that are on the statement.

5. Click the Cancel button to close the Statement dialog box.

 You have completed Exercise 8-9.

8.8 PRINTING STATEMENTS

Once statements have been created, the next step is to send them to a printer or to transmit them electronically. When the Print/Send button is clicked, the Print/Send Statements dialog box is displayed (see Figure 8-40). This dialog box lists options for choosing the type of statement that will be created—Paper or Electronic. Paper statements are printed and mailed by the practice. Electronic statements are sent electronically to a processing center, which prints and mails them.

The Exclude Billed Paid Entries box designates whether transactions that have been billed and paid are left out of the statement processing.

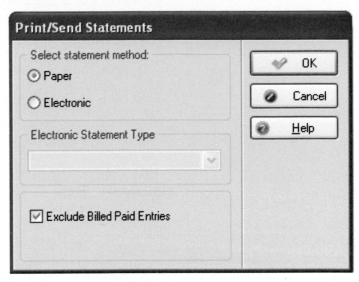

Figure 8-40   Print/Send Statements Dialog Box

When the Paper button is selected and the OK button clicked, the Open Report dialog box appears (see Figure 8-41).

SELECTING A FORMAT

The report selected in this dialog box must match the type of statement selected in the Statement Type field of the Create Statements

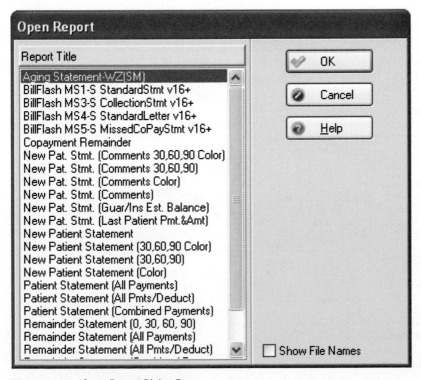

Figure 8-41   Open Report Dialog Box

dialog box—either Standard or Remainder. If Remainder was checked, statements will print only if one of the five Remainder Statement report formats is selected in the Open Report window:

1. Remainder Statement (0, 30, 60, 90)

2. Remainder Statement (All Payments)

3. Remainder Statement (All Pmts/Deduct)

4. Remainder Statement (Combined Payments)

5. Remainder Statement-WZ(SM)

Likewise, for Standard statements to print, one of the other patient statement report formats on the list must be chosen, such as Patient Statement (All Payments).

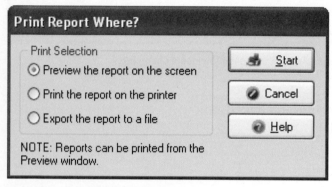

Figure 8-42   Print Report Where? Dialog Box

After selecting the report format, click the OK button to display the Print Report Where? dialog box, which asks whether to preview the report on screen, send the report directly to the printer, or export the report to a file format (see Figure 8-42).

Once the Start button is clicked, the Data Selection Questions dialog box appears (see Figure 8-43).

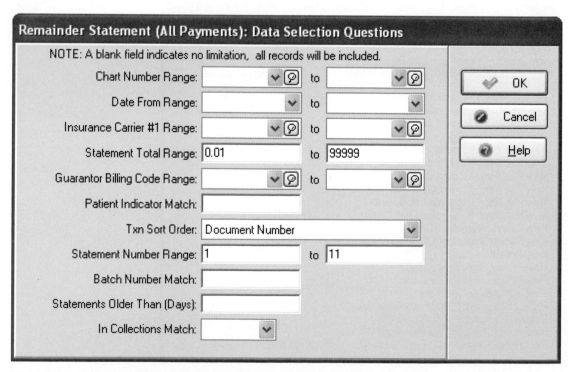

Figure 8-43   Remainder Statement (All Payments): Data Selection Questions Dialog Box

SELECTING THE FILTERS AND PRINTING THE STATEMENTS

The fields in the Data Selection Questions dialog box are used to filter statement selections. For example, to print statements for a certain group of patients, entries are made in the Chart Number Range field. In **once-a-month billing**, all statements are printed and mailed at once. Many practices use cycle billing instead. In a **cycle billing** system, patients are divided into groups, and statement printing and mailing is staggered throughout the month. For example, statements for guarantors whose last names begin with the letters *A* to *G* are mailed on the first of the month; those with last names that begin with *H* to *S* are mailed on the eighth of the month, and so on.

In addition to the Chart Number Range filter, other available filters include

Date From Range   Statements within a range of dates.

Insurance Carrier #1 Range   Statements for a range of insurance carriers.

Statement Total Range   Statements for guarantors with a balance within a specified range.

Guarantor Billing Code Range   Statements for a range of guarantors assigned billing codes (from the Other Information tab in the Patient/Guarantor dialog box).

Patient Indicator Match   Statements for patients assigned a particular patient indicator (from the Other Information tab in the Patient/Guarantor dialog box).

Txn Sort Order   Transactions can be listed on the statement by Date of Service (Date From), Document Number, or Entry Number.

Statement Number Range   Statements for a range of statement numbers (assigned by Medisoft).

Batch Number Match   Statements in a particular batch (assigned by Medisoft).

Statements Older Than (Days)   Statements that are older than a specified number of days.

In Collections Match   Statements for accounts that are in collections.

If no changes are made to the default entries in the Data Selection Questions dialog box, all statements that have a status of Ready to Send or Sent are included in the batch. To avoid printing statements with a Sent status, and to only print those with a Ready to Send status, a zero is entered in the Batch Number Match field. All statements that are Ready to Send have a batch number of zero. Figure 8-44 displays a sample remainder statement.

once-a-month billing a type of billing in which statements are mailed to all patients at the same time each month

cycle billing a type of billing in which statement printing and mailing is staggered throughout the month

Family Care Center			
285 Stephenson Boulevard			
Stephenson, OH 60089			
(614)555-0000			

Statement Date	Chart Number	Page
10/28/2016	SIMMOJI0	1

Make Checks Payable To:

Jill Simmons
30 Arbor Way
Stephenson, OH 60089

Family Care Center
285 Stephenson Boulevard
Stephenson, OH 60089
(614)555-0000

Date of Last Payment: 11/3/2016	Amount: -84.00	Previous Balance:	0.00

Patient:	Jill Simmons		Chart Number: SIMMOJI0		Case:	Urinary tract infection

Dates	Procedure	Charge	Paid by Primary	Paid By Guarantor	Adjustments	Remainder
10/28/16	99212	54.00	-43.20		0.00	10.80
10/28/16	87086	51.00	-40.80		0.00	10.20

Amount Due
21.00

Figure 8-44 Sample Remainder Statement

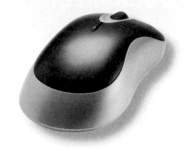

Print remainder statements for all patients with last names beginning with the letter *H* and ending with the letter *S*. *Note:* Be sure to enter *SYZMAM* instead of just *S* to select all patients whose last names begin with the letter *S*. *Note:* If you do not have access to a printer, manually change the statement status to Sent using the method you used to change claim status in Chapter 7.

Date: October 28, 2016

1. Click the Print/Send button in the Statement Management dialog box. The Print/Send Statements dialog box is displayed.

2. Select Paper as the statement method. Verify that the Exclude Billed Paid Entries box is checked. Click the OK button.

3. In the Open Report dialog box that appears, select Remainder Statement (All Payments). Click the OK button.

4. In the Print Report Where? dialog box, choose the option to preview the report on screen. Click the Start button. The Data Selection Questions dialog box is displayed.

5. In the Chart Number Range boxes, enter the chart numbers that will select all patients with last names beginning with *H* through *S*. In the Batch Number Match field, key *0*, so that only statements with a Ready to Send status will be printed. Click the OK button.

6. Scroll down through the statement displayed in the Preview Report window. Click the Print button. After printing, close the Preview window.

7. Notice that Jill Simmons's statement now has a status of Sent. Close the Statement Management dialog box. **CiMC**

 You have completed Exercise 8-10.

APPLYING YOUR SKILLS

5: ENTER INSURANCE PAYMENTS

October 28, 2016
Using Source Document 12, enter the payment information from the remittance advice, and apply payments to the patient's account.

APPLYING YOUR SKILLS

6: CREATE STATEMENTS

October 28, 2016
Create remainder statements for all patients with last names beginning with *T* through the end of the alphabet. Print the statements just created.

Remember to create a backup of your work before exiting Medisoft! To help you keep track of your work, name the backup file after the chapter you are working on, for example, StudentID-c8.mbk.

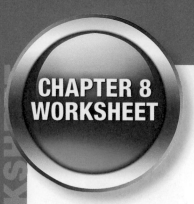
Name: _____ Date: _____

After completing all the exercises in the chapter, answer the following questions in the spaces provided.

1. *[LO 8.4]* What is the amount the insurance carrier paid for procedure 99211 for John Fitzwilliams on 9/6/2016?

   _____

2. *[LO 8.4]* What is the amount the insurance carrier paid for procedure 99211 for Herbert Bell on 9/5/2016?

   _____

3. *[LO 8.4]* What is the amount the insurance carrier paid for procedure 90471 for Sarah Fitzwilliams on 9/6/2016?

   _____

4. *[LO 8.4]* What is listed as the Last Payment Amount on Herbert Bell's account after the East Ohio PPO payments were entered on 10/3/2016 (Transaction Entry dialog box)?

   _____

5. *[LO 8.4]* What is the remaining balance on Sheila Giles's account after the Blue Cross and Blue Shield payments were entered on 11/3/2016?

   _____

6. *[LO 8.4]* What is listed as the Last Payment Amount on John Fitzwilliams's account after the CHAMPVA payments were entered on 10/3/2016 (Transaction Entry dialog box)?

   _____

7. *[LO 8.4]* What is listed as the Last Payment Amount on Sheila Giles's account after the Blue Cross and Blue Shield payments were entered on 11/3/2016 (Transaction Entry dialog box)?

   _____

8. *[LO 8.6]* A statement was created for which patient(s) in Exercise 8-8?

   _____

9. *[LO 8.4]* What is the amount of the Blue Cross and Blue Shield payment for procedure 71020 for Lisa Wright on 10/3/2016 (Transaction Entry dialog box)?

   _____

10. *[LO 8.8]* What is listed as the amount due on Lisa Wright's statement created in Applying Your Skills Exercise 6?

   _____

8.1 Describe how an adjustment is calculated if the payer pays less than the provider's usual fee. Pages 248–250	If the provider enters into a contract with the payer and agrees to accept reduced fees, the difference between what the provider bills and the contracted discount is recorded as an adjustment.
8.2 List the five steps for processing a remittance advice. Pages 250–252	1. Compare the RA to the original insurance claim to be sure that all procedures listed on the claim are represented on the RA and that the CPT codes have not changed. 2. Review the payment amount against the expected amount. 3. Identify the reasons for denials or payment reductions; resubmit claim or appeal if necessary. 4. Post payment information for individual claims to the appropriate patient accounts. 5. Bill the patient's secondary health care plan if appropriate.
8.3 Demonstrate how to enter insurance payments. Pages 253–260	1. Click Enter Deposits/Payments on the Activities menu. The Deposit List dialog box is displayed. 2. Confirm that the correct date is displayed in the Deposit Date box. 3. Click the New button. The Deposit dialog box is displayed. 4. Verify that the desired date is in the Deposit Date field. 5. Select Insurance in the Payor Type box. 6. Select the appropriate entry in the Payment Method box. 7. Complete the Check Number box if entering a check or the EFT Tracer box if entering an electronic payment. 8. Enter the ERA ID number or other number as appropriate in the Description/Bank No. field. 9. Enter the amount of the payment in the Payment Amount box. 10. Accept the default entry (A) in the Deposit Code box. 11. Select the insurance carrier from the Insurance drop-down list. The program automatically completes the remaining fields. 12. Click the Save button to save the entry.

8.4 Demonstrate how to apply insurance payments to charges. Pages 260–270	1. Click Enter Deposits/Payments on the Activities menu. The Deposit List dialog box is displayed. 2. Confirm that the correct date is displayed in the Deposit Date box. 3. In the list of deposits, click once on the payment that will be applied. The Apply Payment/Adjustments to Charges dialog box appears. 4. In the For box, select the first patient listed on the remittance advice. 5. Locate the first charge, enter the payment in the Payment column, and press Tab to the end of the first row. Follow the same steps for each procedure charge for that patient. 6. Click the Save Payments/Adjustments button. An Information dialog box displays the message that the claim has been marked "done" for the primary insurance. Click OK. If there are additional patients for whom the payment should be applied, repeat the procedure for each patient. 7. When all payments have been applied, click the Close button.
8.5 Demonstrate how to enter capitation payments. Pages 270–277	1. Click Enter Deposits/Payments on the Activities menu. The Deposit List dialog box is displayed. 2. Confirm that the correct date is displayed in the Deposit Date box. 3. Click the New button. The Deposit dialog box is displayed. 4. Verify that the desired date is displayed in the Deposit Date box. 5. Select Capitation in the Payor Type box. 6. Select the appropriate entry in the Payment Method box. 7. Complete the Check Number box if entering a check or the EFT Tracer box if entering an electronic payment. 8. Enter the ERA ID number or other number as appropriate in the Description/Bank No. field. 9. Enter the amount of the payment in the Payment Amount box. 10. Accept the default entry (A) in the Deposit Code box. 11. Select the insurance carrier from the Insurance drop-down list. 12. Click the Save button to save the entry, and close the Deposit dialog box. 13. To adjust patient accounts to zero, use the List Only option in the Claim Management dialog box to identify patients insured by the capitated plan who have claims for the period covered by the capitation payment. 14. Back in the Deposit List dialog box, select the capitated deposit that has EOB Only listed in the Payment column, and click the Apply button.

	15. In the For field, select the first capitated patient that was identified in Step 13, and press Tab.
	16. Locate the amount listed in the Remainder column, and enter an equal amount in the Adjustment column. Press tab repeatedly, until the remainder amount changes to zero.
	17. Continue this procedure for all patients identified in Step 13. When finished, click the Save Payments/Adjustments button.
8.6 Demonstrate how to create patient statements. Pages 278–282	1. Select Statement Management on the Activities menu. The Statement Management dialog box appears.
	2. Click the Create Statements button. The Create Statements dialog box is displayed.
	3. Enter the appropriate dates in the Transaction Dates fields.
	4. Enter the chart numbers of the appropriate patients, or leave these fields blank to select all patients.
	5. Set the Statement Type field to Standard or Remainder.
	6. Click the Create button to generate statements. A message appears stating the number of statements that have been created. Click the OK button.
8.7 Explain how statements are edited. Pages 282–285	1. Select Statement Management on the Activities menu.
	2. Click once on the statement to be edited.
	3. Click the Edit button.
	4. Review the information in the three tabs of the Statement dialog box and make changes as necessary.
	5. Click the Save button to save your changes.
8.8 Demonstrate how to print patient statements. Pages 286–289	1. Click the Print/Send button in the Statement Management dialog box. The Print/Send Statements dialog box is displayed.
	2. Select the statement method (paper or electronic). Click the OK button.
	3. In the Open Report dialog box that appears, select Remainder Statement (All Payments). Click the OK button.
	4. In the Print Report Where? dialog box, choose the option to print the reports on the printer. Click the Start button. The Data Selection Questions dialog box is displayed.
	5. In the Chart Number Range boxes, enter the chart numbers that will select the appropriate patients.
	6. Make other selections in the Data Selection Questions dialog box, if appropriate. When finished, click the OK button.
	7. The statements are sent to the printer.
	8. Close the Statement Management dialog box.

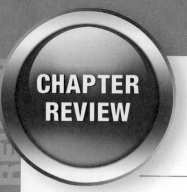

CHAPTER REVIEW

USING TERMINOLOGY

Match the terms on the left with the definitions on the right.

_____ **1.** *[LO 8.5]* capitation payments

_____ **2.** *[LO 8.8]* cycle billing

_____ **3.** *[LO 8.2]* electronic remittance advice (ERA)

_____ **4.** *[LO 8.1]* fee schedule

_____ **5.** *[LO 8.8]* once-a-month billing

_____ **6.** *[LO 8.6]* patient statement

_____ **7.** *[LO 8.1]* payment schedule

_____ **8.** *[LO 8.6]* remainder statements

_____ **9.** *[LO 8.6]* standard statements

a. A list of the amount of money a patient owes, organized by the amount of time the money has been owed, the procedures performed, and the dates the procedures were performed.

b. A type of billing in which patients are divided into groups and statement printing and mailing is staggered throughout the month.

c. A document that specifies the amount the provider will be paid for each procedure.

d. Statement that shows all charges regardless of whether the insurance has paid on the transactions.

e. Payments made to physicians on a regular basis (such as monthly) for providing services to patients in a managed care insurance plan.

f. An electronic document that lists patients, dates of service, charges, and the amount paid or denied by the insurance carrier.

g. A document that specifies the amount the payer agrees to pay the provider for a service, based on a contracted rate of reimbursement.

h. A type of billing in which statements are mailed to all patients at the same time each month.

i. Statements that list only those charges that are not paid in full after all insurance carrier payments have been received.

CHECKING YOUR UNDERSTANDING

Answer the questions below in the space provided.

1. *[LO 8.3]* Why is it easier to enter large insurance payments in the Deposit List dialog box than in the Transaction Entry dialog box?

_____

_____

2. *[LO 8.4]* When all payments on a remittance advice have been successfully entered and applied to charges, what should appear in the Unapplied box in the upper-right corner of the Deposit List dialog box?

_____

_____

3. *[LO 8.5]* Why do charges need to be adjusted for patients who are covered under a capitated insurance plan?

_____

_____

4. *[LO 8.6]* If a practice did not want to create statements for patients with an account balance of less than $5.00, how would this be done?

_____

_____

APPLYING YOUR KNOWLEDGE

Answer the questions below in the space provided.

8.1. *[LO 8.3, 8.4]* Randall Klein calls. He would like to know whether Medicare has paid any of the charges for his September office visit. How would you look up this information in Medisoft?

_____

_____

8.2. *[LO 8.6]* Why do many practices send out remainder statements rather than standard statements?

_____

_____

THINKING ABOUT IT

Answer the questions below in the space provided.

8.1. *[LO 8.1]* Why is it important to understand the differences among different types of health plans?

_____

_____

8.2. *[LO 8.5]* What would happen if a capitated patient account was not adjusted to a zero balance?

_____

_____

8.3. *[LO 8.2]* What is the purpose of reviewing a remittance advice before entering payments and adjustments?

_____

_____

8.4. *[LO 8.2]* If payments and adjustments listed on a remittance advice were not posted and applied to patients' accounts, what would the consequence be?

_____

_____

8.5. *[LO 8.6]* If statements were not created and mailed to patients, what would the consequence be?

_____

_____

AT THE COMPUTER

Answer the following questions at the computer.

8.1. *[LO 8.6]* What is the total amount that John Fitzwilliams paid in copayments in September 2016? (*Hint:* Include his daughter Sarah in the calculation.)

_____

_____

8.2. *[LO 8.4, 8.6]* On September 9, 2016, $168.00 was received from Blue Cross and Blue Shield as payment for James Smith's facial nerve function studies performed on September 8, 2016. On September 27, James Smith paid $52.00 as his portion of the visit. Assuming he has met his deductible for the year, and that he is responsible for 20 percent of covered charges, did he pay the correct amount? How much should he have paid?

_____

_____

chapter
9

Creating
Reports

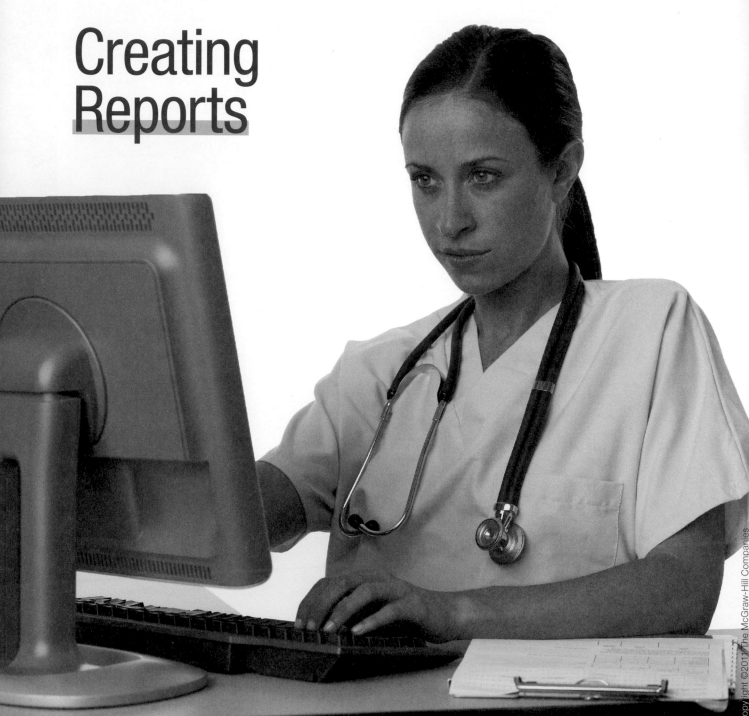

key terms

aging report
day sheet
insurance aging report
patient aging report
patient day sheet
patient ledger
payment day sheet
practice analysis report
procedure day sheet
selection boxes

learning outcomes

When you finish this chapter, you will be able to:

9.1 List the three types of reports available in Medisoft.

9.2 Describe how to select data to be included in a Medisoft report.

9.3 Distinguish between patient, procedure, and payment day sheets.

9.4 Demonstrate how to create a practice analysis report.

9.5 Demonstrate how to create a patient ledger report.

9.6 Demonstrate how to create a standard patient list report.

9.7 Describe how to use Medisoft Reports to create a report.

9.8 Explain how aging reports are used in a medical practice.

9.9 Explain how to access Medisoft's built-in custom reports.

9.10 Demonstrate how to open a report for editing in Medisoft's Report Designer.

what you need to know

To use this chapter, you need to know how to:

- Start Medisoft, use menus, and enter and edit text.
- Work with chart numbers and codes.

9.1 TYPES OF REPORTS IN MEDISOFT

Reports are an important tool in managing a medical office. They provide useful information about the day-to-day operations in the practice. Providers and office managers ask for different reports at different times. Some managers want to see daily reports of each day's transactions, while others want to see reports on particular patients' accounts on a weekly or bimonthly basis.

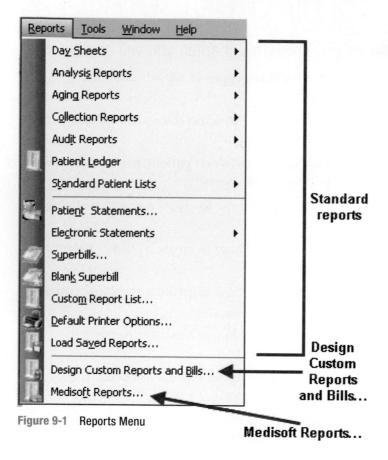

Medisoft® offers several options for creating reports, all of which can be accessed via the Reports menu (see Figure 9-1). These options include

- Standard reports
- Medisoft Reports …
- Design Custom Reports and Bills …

Standard reports include many of the basic reports used by a medical office, such as day sheets, practice analysis reports, and patient ledgers. Medisoft Reports, new in Version 16 of the software, include over a hundred reports not included in the standard reports. Finally, custom reports are created and modified using the Medisoft Report Designer program. In this chapter, you will learn about some of the reports used throughout the billing process, and you will gain experience creating all three types of reports.

Figure 9-1   Reports Menu

SELECTING PRINT OPTIONS

In Medisoft, the process of creating a report begins with selecting a report from the Reports menu. When a report is selected, a dialog box appears with options to preview the report on the screen, send it to a printer, or export it to a file (see Figure 9-2).

If the preview option is selected, the report will be displayed in a Print Preview window. This window, common to all reports, provides options for viewing or printing a report (see Figure 9-3). The buttons on the Print Preview toolbar control how a report is displayed on the screen and how to move from page to page within a report (see Figure 9-4).

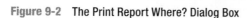

Figure 9-2   The Print Report Where? Dialog Box

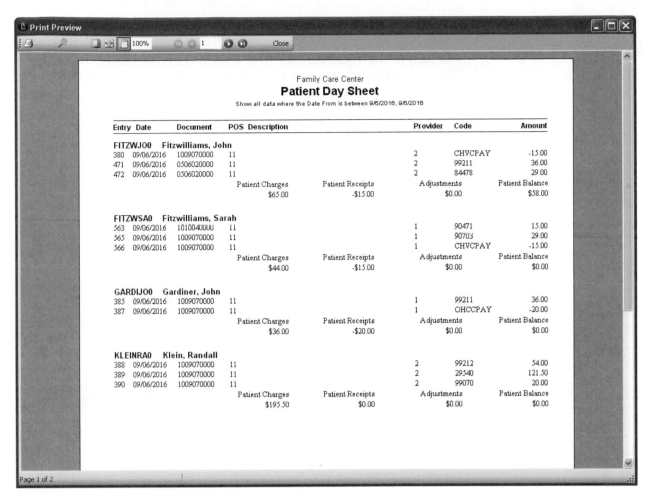

Figure 9-3   Print Preview Window

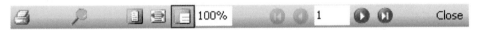

Figure 9-4   Buttons on Print Preview Toolbar

Print   The Print button is used to print the report.

Search Data   The Search Data button performs a case-sensitive text search in the report displayed in the preview window.

Window Display   The next three buttons are used to change the display of the report, which makes locating specific information in it easier. From left to right, the choices are whole page, page width, and percentage. A percentage can be entered in place of 100 percent for zooming in or out of the report.

Navigate   Four triangle buttons, two on the left and two on the right, are used to move through pages of a multipage report. The First Page button, farthest on the left, moves to the beginning of a report. The Prior Page button moves to the page that precedes the one currently displayed. The bar between the two sets of triangle buttons indicates the number of the current page. To the right of the bar are the other two triangle buttons. The Next Page button moves to the page following the current one. The Last Page button moves to the end of a report. If a button is dimmed, it means that there are no more pages in the direction indicated by the triangle. If a button is bright blue, there is an additional page or pages in the report.

Close　　This command is used to close the Print Preview window.

9.2 SELECTING DATA FOR A REPORT

Once a selection is made in the Print Report Where? dialog box and the Start button is clicked, the Search dialog box is displayed. This dialog box is used to select the range of data that will be included in the report (see Figure 9-5). While the exact contents of the Search box vary from report to report, the way selections are made does not change. Once you learn how to use the Search dialog box, you can create any report.

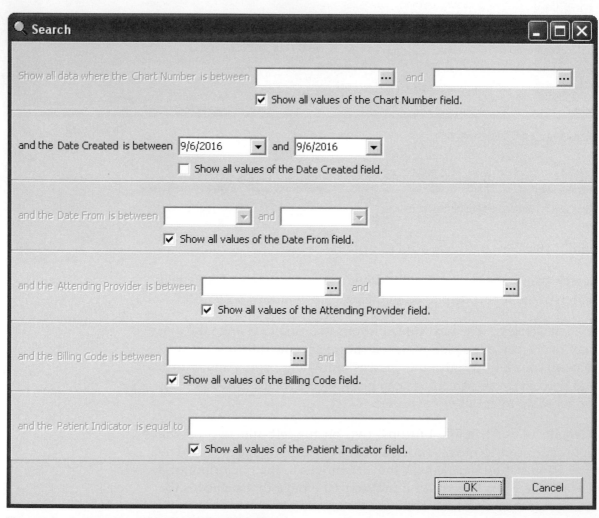

Figure 9-5　Search Dialog Box for Patient Day Sheet Report

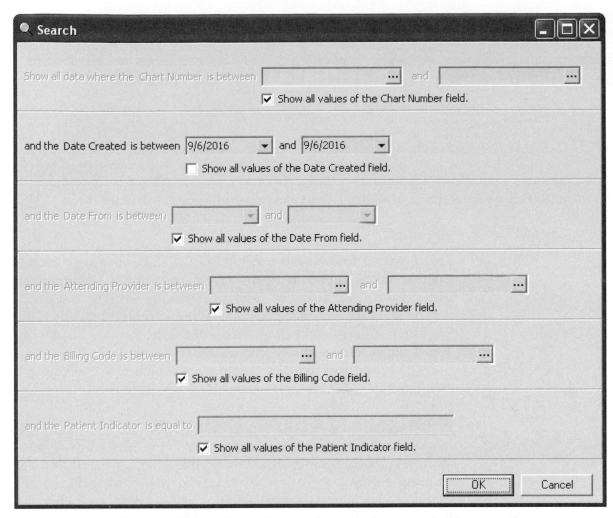

Figure 9-6   Search Dialog Box for Patient Day Sheet Report with Selection Boxes Highlighted in Yellow

The Search dialog box contains a number of fields called selection boxes. Some reports have one selection box in a Search box, while others, such as the Patient Day Sheet Search box in Figures 9-5 and 9-6, have many. The **selection boxes** determine what data are included in the report.

Some selection boxes use a drop-down list for entering data; others use a button with three dots (see Figures 9-7a and 9-7b).

selection boxes fields within the Search dialog box that are used to select the data that will be included in a report

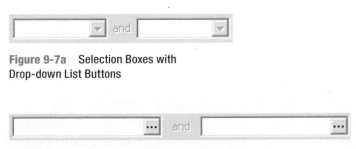

Figure 9-7a   Selection Boxes with Drop-down List Buttons

Figure 9-7b   Selection Boxes with Lookup Buttons

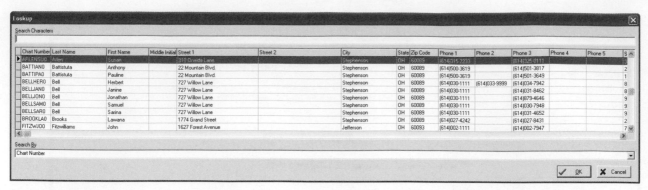

Figure 9-8 The Lookup Dialog Box That Is Displayed When the Lookup Button in the Chart Number Selection Box Is Clicked

This button is known as a Lookup button, since clicking it causes the Lookup dialog box to be displayed. You already know how to use a drop-down list. The Lookup button is similar to a drop-down list; however, instead of displaying a limited list, when the Lookup button is clicked, a Lookup dialog box opens displaying a full list of choices from the database for that field (see Figure 9-8). When you click an item in the dialog box (for example, a chart number), that item is automatically inserted into the selection box.

Beneath each selection box or set of boxes in the Search box, there is an option labeled Show all values of the _____ field. If you are printing a report and want all values for the field included (for example, all patients), you will need to make sure this box is checked. If instead you want only some of the values included (for example, only patients with last names beginning with the letter *H*), you will need to make entries in the selection boxes. Clicking one of the selection boxes automatically removes the check mark from the Show all values box.

In the Patient Day Sheet Search box pictured in Figures 9-5 and 9-6, selections can be made to include some or all of the following data:

Chart Number (Show all data where the Chart Number is between)   In the two Chart Number boxes, a range of chart numbers for patients is entered. If a report on just one patient is needed, that patient's chart number is entered in both boxes. If a report on all patients is needed, a check mark must remain in the Show all values of the Chart Number field box.

Date Created (and the Date Created Range is between)   The Date Created entries refer to the actual dates the information was entered in the computer. The date created may or may not be the same as the date a transaction took place. For example, suppose transactions from Friday, October 1, are entered in Medisoft on Monday morning, October 4. In this example, the Date Created value is the date the transaction was entered—October 4. The transaction date is the date on which the patient was in the office—October 1.

By default, Medisoft enters the Windows System Date in both Date Created boxes. The Windows System Date is today's date—the day you are sitting at your computer working on the exercises in this chapter. *Note:* **In the exercises in this chapter, always click to place a check mark in the Show all values of the Date Created field box.** If you do not show all values, because the exercises take place in the future (2016), the program will not find all the data it needs to create the report, and no report will be created.

Date From (and the Date From is between)   The Date From entries refer to the actual dates of the transactions. If the day sheet report is for September 5, 2016, then 9/5/2016 is entered in both fields. At the beginning of each exercise, these fields must be changed to the date listed before step 1 of the exercise.

Note: There are two ways of changing dates in the Search dialog box. You can use the keyboard to enter the numbers and slashes. For example, January 1, 2016, would be keyed as 1/1/2016. The other way of entering dates is to use the pop-up calendar. The pop-up calendar is displayed when you click the down arrows at the right side of the box that contains the date (see Figure 9-9). Once this calendar is visible, clicking the month in the blue banner at the top of the calendar displays a list of the months (see Figure 9-10). Clicking any month in the list changes the calendar to that month. Clicking the year in the blue banner displays a list of years. Clicking any year in the list changes the calendar to that year (see Figure 9-11). The day is changed by clicking the desired day in the calendar below the blue banner.

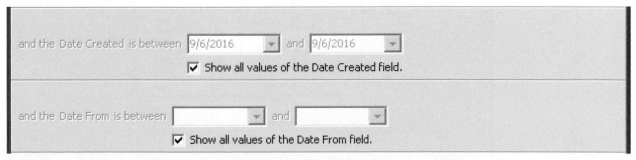

Figure 9-9   Down Arrows (Highlighted in Yellow) Used to Display the Pop-up Calendar

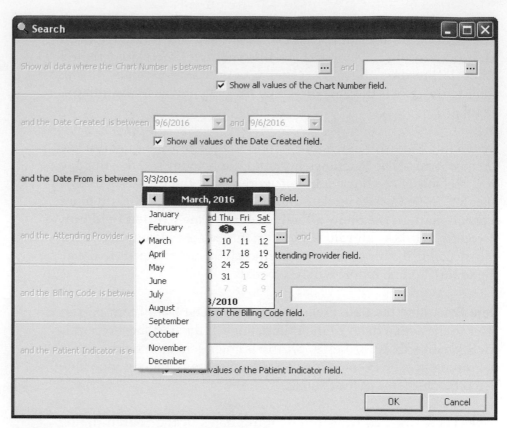

Figure 9-10 List of Months in the Pop-up Calendar

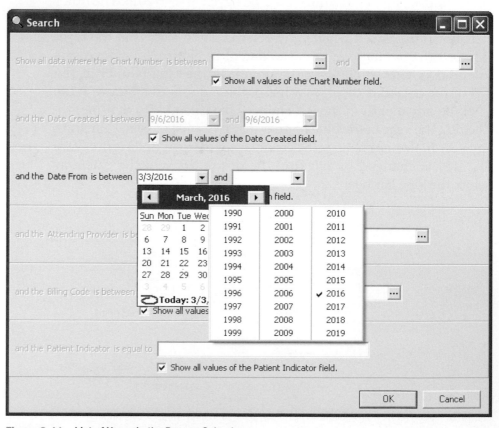

Figure 9-11 List of Years in the Pop-up Calendar

Attending Provider (and the Attending Provider is between)   A range of codes for the attending providers is entered in the Attending Provider fields.

Billing Code (and the Billing Code is between)   If the practice uses Medisoft's Billing Code feature, codes can be entered in this box to select only those patients with the designated billing codes.

Patient Indicator (and the Patient Indicator is equal to)   If the practice has assigned a Patient Indicator code to each patient, an entry can be made to select only those patients who match a specific code.

9.3 DAY SHEETS

A **day sheet** is a standard report that provides information on practice activities for a twenty-four-hour period. In Medisoft, there are three types of day sheet reports: patient day sheets, procedure day sheets, and payment day sheets. Options to view or print the three types of day sheets are located on the Reports menu, within the Day Sheets submenu (see Figure 9-12).

day sheet a report that provides information on practice activities for a twenty-four-hour period

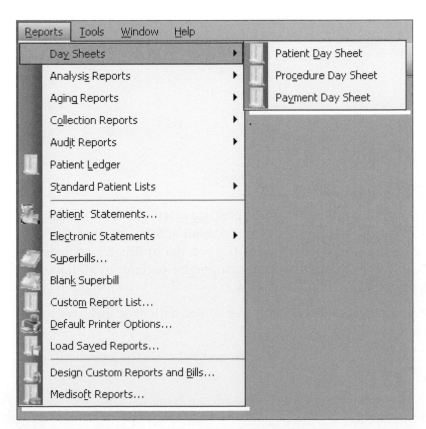

Figure 9-12   Reports Menu with Day Sheets Submenu Displayed

Family Care Center
Patient Day Sheet
Show all data where the Date From is between 9/6/2016, 9/6/2016

Entry	Date	Document	POS	Description	Provider	Code	Amount
FITZWJO0	**Fitzwilliams, John**						
380	09/06/2016	1009070000	11		2	CHVCPAY	-15.00
471	09/06/2016	0506020000	11		2	99211	36.00
472	09/06/2016	0506020000	11		2	84478	29.00

Patient Charges	Patient Receipts	Adjustments	Patient Balance
$65.00	-$15.00	$0.00	$58.00

Entry	Date	Document	POS	Description	Provider	Code	Amount
FITZWSA0	**Fitzwilliams, Sarah**						
563	09/06/2016	1010040000	11		1	90471	15.00
565	09/06/2016	1009070000	11		1	90703	29.00
566	09/06/2016	1009070000	11		1	CHVCPAY	-15.00

Patient Charges	Patient Receipts	Adjustments	Patient Balance
$44.00	-$15.00	$0.00	$0.00

Entry	Date	Document	POS	Description	Provider	Code	Amount
GARDIJO0	**Gardiner, John**						
385	09/06/2016	1009070000	11		1	99211	36.00
387	09/06/2016	1009070000	11		1	OHCCPAY	-20.00

Patient Charges	Patient Receipts	Adjustments	Patient Balance
$36.00	-$20.00	$0.00	$0.00

Entry	Date	Document	POS	Description	Provider	Code	Amount
KLEINRA0	**Klein, Randall**						
388	09/06/2016	1009070000	11		2	99212	54.00
389	09/06/2016	1009070000	11		2	29540	121.50
390	09/06/2016	1009070000	11		2	99070	20.00

Patient Charges	Patient Receipts	Adjustments	Patient Balance
$195.50	$0.00	$0.00	$0.00

Figure 9-13a Page 1 of a Patient Day Sheet Report

PATIENT DAY SHEET

patient day sheet a summary of patient activity on a given day

At the end of the day, a medical practice often prints a **patient day sheet,** which is a summary of the patient activity on that day (see Figures 9-13a and 9-13b). Medisoft's version of this report lists the procedures for a particular day, grouped by patient, in alphabetical order by chart number. It includes

- Procedures performed for a particular patient or group of patients

- Charges, receipts, adjustments, and balances for a particular patient or group of patients

- A summary of a practice's charges, payments, and adjustments

Family Care Center
Patient Day Sheet
Show all data where the Date From is between 9/6/2016, 9/6/2016

Entry Date	Document	POS Description	Provider	Code	Amount
		Total # Patients	4		
		Total # Procedures	8		
		Total Procedure Charges	$340.50		
		Total Product Charges	$0.00		
		Total Inside Lab Charges	$0.00		
		Total Outside Lab Charges	$0.00		
		Total Billing Charges	$0.00		
		Total Charges	$340.50		
		Total Insurance Payments	$0.00		
		Total Cash Copayments	$0.00		
		Total Check Copayments	-$50.00		
		Total Credit Card Copayments	$0.00		
		Total Patient Cash Payments	$0.00		
		Total Patient Check Payments	$0.00		
		Total Credit Card Payments	$0.00		
		Total Receipts	-$50.00		
		Total Credit Adjustments	$0.00		
		Total Debit Adjustments	$0.00		
		Total Insurance Debit Adjustments	$0.00		
		Total Insurance Credit Adjustments	$0.00		
		Total Insurance Withholds	$0.00		
		Total Adjustments	$0.00		
		Net Effect on Accounts Receivable	$290.50		

Figure 9-13b   Page 2 of a Patient Day Sheet Report

PRINTING A PATIENT DAY SHEET   EXERCISE 9-1

Print a patient day sheet report for October 3, 2016.

Date: October 3, 2016

Note: It is not necessary to change the Medisoft Program Date before each exercise in this chapter as Medisoft uses the Windows System Date as the default date when creating reports. You will, however, need to enter the date(s) listed at the beginning of each exercise in the date range boxes as you create each report.

1. Start Medisoft and restore the data from your last work session.

2. On the Reports menu, click Day Sheets and then Patient Day Sheet. The Print Report Where? dialog box appears.

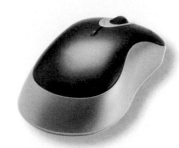

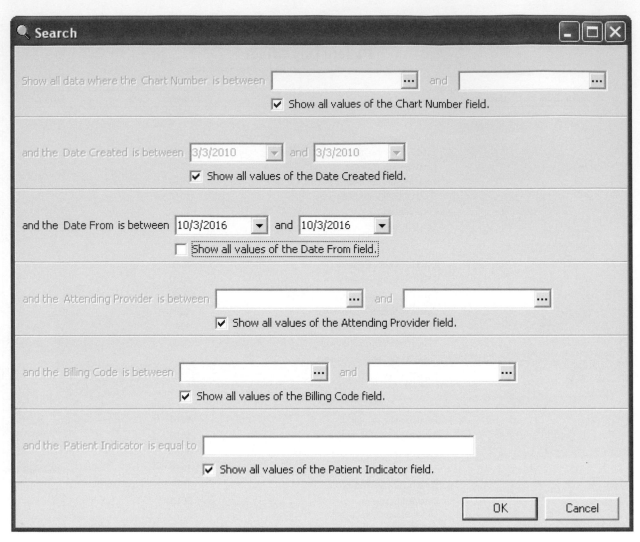

Figure 9-14   Search Dialog Box with Entries

3. Accept the default selection to preview the report on screen. Click the Start button. The Search dialog box is displayed.

4. Leave the Chart Number fields blank.

5. Today's date—that is, the date on which you are working on this exercise—will likely appear in both Date Created boxes. Make sure to check the box labeled Show all values of the Date Created field. This will clear the current Date Created range boxes to include all dates for this field.

6. Click in the first Date From box, and then enter **_10/3/2016_** in both Date From boxes, or use the pop-up calendar to change the date to October 3, 2016. Leave all other fields in the Search box blank. This will select data for all patients and attending providers for October 3, 2016. Your screen should look like the dialog box in Figure 9-14.

7. Click the OK button. The patient day sheet report is displayed in the Print Preview window (see Figure 9-15).

8. If necessary, use the scroll bar to view additional entries on the first page of the report.

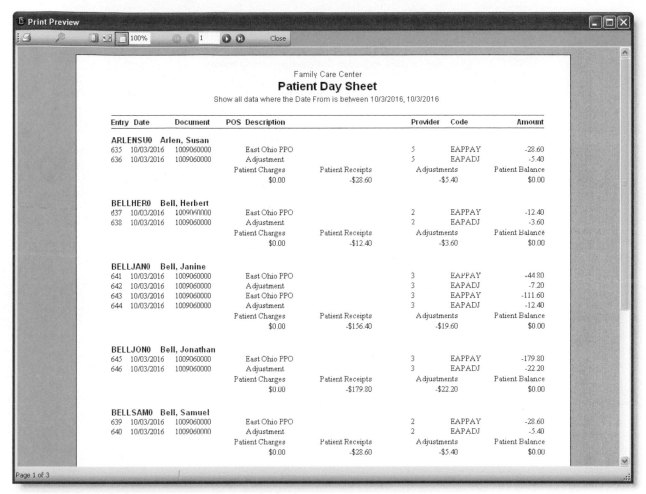

Entry	Date	Document	POS	Description		Provider	Code	Amount
ARLENSU0	**Arlen, Susan**							
635	10/03/2016	1009060000		East Ohio PPO		5	EAPPAY	-28.60
636	10/03/2016	1009060000		Adjustment		5	EAPADJ	-5.40
		Patient Charges		Patient Receipts		Adjustments		Patient Balance
		$0.00		-$28.60		-$5.40		$0.00
BELLHER0	**Bell, Herbert**							
637	10/03/2016	1009060000		East Ohio PPO		2	EAPPAY	-12.40
638	10/03/2016	1009060000		Adjustment		2	EAPADJ	-3.60
		Patient Charges		Patient Receipts		Adjustments		Patient Balance
		$0.00		-$12.40		-$3.60		$0.00
BELLJAN0	**Bell, Janine**							
641	10/03/2016	1009060000		East Ohio PPO		3	EAPPAY	-44.80
642	10/03/2016	1009060000		Adjustment		3	EAPADJ	-7.20
643	10/03/2016	1009060000		East Ohio PPO		3	EAPPAY	-111.60
644	10/03/2016	1009060000		Adjustment		3	EAPADJ	-12.40
		Patient Charges		Patient Receipts		Adjustments		Patient Balance
		$0.00		-$156.40		-$19.60		$0.00
BELLJON0	**Bell, Jonathan**							
645	10/03/2016	1009060000		East Ohio PPO		3	EAPPAY	-179.80
646	10/03/2016	1009060000		Adjustment		3	EAPADJ	-22.20
		Patient Charges		Patient Receipts		Adjustments		Patient Balance
		$0.00		-$179.80		-$22.20		$0.00
BELLSAM0	**Bell, Samuel**							
639	10/03/2016	1009060000		East Ohio PPO		2	EAPPAY	-28.60
640	10/03/2016	1009060000		Adjustment		2	EAPADJ	-5.40
		Patient Charges		Patient Receipts		Adjustments		Patient Balance
		$0.00		-$28.60		-$5.40		$0.00

Family Care Center
Patient Day Sheet
Show all data where the Date From is between 10/3/2016, 10/3/2016

Page 1 of 3

Figure 9-15 The Print Preview Window with the First Page of the Patient Day Sheet for 10/3/2016

9. Notice at the top of the Print Preview window that the triangle next to the number 1 is bright blue. This indicates that there is more than one page in the report. Click the triangle just to the right of 1 to advance to the second page of the report.

10. Follow the same procedure to view the third page of the report.

11. Click the Print button, and then click the OK button to print the report.

12. Click the red Close box at the top right of the window to exit the Print Preview window. **CiMC**

☑ **You have completed Exercise 9-1.**

PROCEDURE DAY SHEET

A **procedure day sheet** lists all procedures performed on a particular day and gives the dates, patients, document numbers, places of service, debits, and credits relating to them (see Figure 9-16). Procedures are listed in numerical order.

procedure day sheet a report that lists all the procedures performed on a particular day, in numerical order

Procedure Day Sheet

Show all data where the Date From is between 9/6/2016, 9/6/2016

Entry	Date	Chart	Name	Document	POS	Debits	Credits
29540							
389	9/6/2016	KLEINRA0	Klein, Randall	1009070000	11	121.50	
		Total of 29540		Quantity: 1		$121.50	$0.00
84478							
472	9/6/2016	FITZWJO0	Fitzwilliams, John	0506020000	11	29.00	
		Total of 84478		Quantity: 1		$29.00	$0.00
90471							
563	9/6/2016	FITZWSA0	Fitzwilliams, Sarah	1010040000	11	15.00	
		Total of 90471		Quantity: 1		$15.00	$0.00
90703							
565	9/6/2016	FITZWSA0	Fitzwilliams, Sarah	1009070000	11	29.00	
		Total of 90703		Quantity: 1		$29.00	$0.00
99070							
390	9/6/2016	KLEINRA0	Klein, Randall	1009070000	11	20.00	
		Total of 99070		Quantity: 1		$20.00	$0.00
99211							
471	9/6/2016	FITZWJO0	Fitzwilliams, John	0506020000	11	36.00	
385	9/6/2016	GARDIJO0	Gardiner, John	1009070000	11	36.00	
		Total of 99211		Quantity: 2		$72.00	$0.00
99212							
388	9/6/2016	KLEINRA0	Klein, Randall	1009070000	11	54.00	
		Total of 99212		Quantity: 1		$54.00	$0.00
CHVCPAY							
380	9/6/2016	FITZWJO0	Fitzwilliams, John	1009070000	11		-15.00
566	9/6/2016	FITZWSA0	Fitzwilliams, Sarah	1009070000	11		-15.00
		Total of CHVCPAY		Quantity: 2		$0.00	-$30.00
OHCCPAY							
387	9/6/2016	GARDIJO0	Gardiner, John	1009070000	11		-20.00
		Total of OHCCPAY		Quantity: 1		$0.00	-$20.00
				Total of Codes:		$340.50	-$50.00
				Balance:		$290.50	

Figure 9-16   Procedure Day Sheet

Procedure day sheets are printed by clicking Day Sheets and then Procedure Day Sheet on the Reports menu. The same Search dialog box used for a patient day sheet is displayed, except that a range of procedure codes rather than patients can be selected. A procedure day sheet will be generated only for data that meet the selection criteria. If any box is left blank, all values are included in the report. The report can be previewed on the screen, printed, or exported to a file.

PAYMENT DAY SHEET

payment day sheet a report that lists all payments received on a particular day, organized by provider

A **payment day sheet** lists all payments received on a particular day, organized by provider (see Figure 9-17). It is printed by clicking Day

Family Care Center
Payment Day Sheet
Show all data where the Date From is between 9/6/2016, 9/6/2016

Entry	Date	Document	Description	Chart	Code	Amount
1		**Yan, Katherine**				
566	9/6/2016	1009070000		FITZWSA0	CHVCPAY	-15.00
387	9/6/2016	1009070000		GARDIJO0	OHCCPAY	-20.00
			Count: 2		**Provider Total**	-$35.00
2		**Rudner, John**				
380	9/6/2016	1009070000		FITZWJO0	CHVCPAY	-15.00
			Count: 1		**Provider Total**	-$15.00

Report Totals

Total # Payments		3
Total Payments	-50.00	

Figure 9-17   Payment Day Sheet

Sheets and then Payment Day Sheet on the Reports menu. The same Search dialog box is displayed, but with fewer data fields.

A payment day sheet will be generated only for data that meet the selection criteria. If any box is left blank, all values for that box are included in the report. Again, the report can be previewed on the screen, printed, or exported to a file.

9.4 ANALYSIS REPORTS

Medisoft includes a number of standard reports that provide information about practice finances. These reports are known as analysis reports. The Analysis Reports submenu is shown in Figure 9-18. The following paragraphs provide a description of each report. Not all reports can be created in student exercises because data have not been sent to insurance carriers and patients.

BILLING/PAYMENT STATUS REPORT

The billing/payment status report lists the status of all transactions that have responsible insurance carriers, showing who has paid

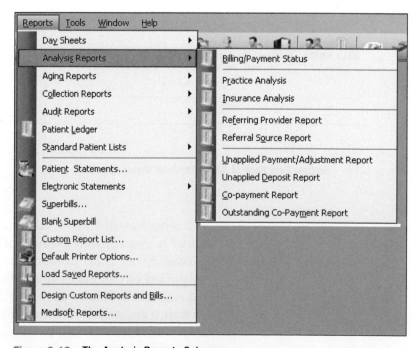

Figure 9-18   The Analysis Reports Submenu

Billing/Payment Status Report

Show all data where the Date From is between 10/1/2016, 10/31/2016

Date	Document	Procedure	Amount	Policy 1	Policy 2	Policy 3	Guarantor	Adjustments	Balance
ARLENSU0	**Susan Arlen (614)315-2233**								
Case 24	1: East Ohio PPO			(419)444-1505					
	2:								
	3:								
							Patient Balance:		0.00
BATTIAN0	**Anthony Battistuta (614)500-3619**								
Case 25	1: Medicare			(215)599-0000					
	2:								
	3:								
10/27/2016	1009280000	99212	54.00	10/31/2016	0.00*	0.00*	Not Billed	0.00	54.00
10/27/2016	1009280000	82947	25.00	10/31/2016	0.00*	0.00*	Not Billed	0.00	25.00
							SubTotal:		79.00
					Unapplied Payments and Adjustments:				0.00
							Case Balance:		79.00
							Patient Balance:		79.00
BATTIPA0	**Pauline Battistuta (614)500-3619**								
							Patient Balance:		0.00
BELLHER0	**Herbert Bell (614)030-1111**								
Case 21	1: East Ohio PPO			(419)444-1505					
	2:								
	3:								
							Patient Balance:		0.00
BELLJAN0	**Janine Bell (614)030-1111**								
Case 22	1: East Ohio PPO			(419)444-1505					
	2:								
	3:								
							Patient Balance:		0.00
BELLJON0	**Jonathan Bell (614)030-1111**								
Case 4	1: East Ohio PPO			(419)444-1505					
	2:								
	3:								
							Patient Balance:		0.00
BELLSAM0	**Samuel Bell (614)030-1111**								
Case 19	1: East Ohio PPO			(419)444-1505					
	2:								
	3:								
							Patient Balance:		0.00

Figure 9-19a   Sample First Page of Billing/Payment Status Report

and who has not been billed (see Figures 9-19a and 9-19b). The report is in a column format sorted first by chart number and then by case. Every chart number listed shows a patient balance and any unapplied payments or unapplied adjustments. An asterisk (*) next to a number indicates that the payer has made a complete payment for that transaction. Information in this report can be used by practices to determine whether billing charges can be applied to a patient account.

Family Care Center
Billing/Payment Status Report
Show all data where the Date From is between 10/1/2016, 10/31/2016

Date	Document	Procedure	Amount	Policy 1	Policy 2	Policy 3	Guarantor	Adjustments	Balance
ZAPATKR0	Kristin Zapata (614)033-0044								
Case 60	1:	Blue Cross/Blue Shield		(614)024-9000					
	2:								
	3:								
10/3/2016	1610030000	NSFFEE	35.00	Not Billed	0.00*	0.00*	Not Billed	0.00	35.00

SubTotal:	35.00
Unapplied Payments and Adjustments:	247.50
Case Balance:	282.50
Patient Balance:	282.50
Report Balance:	$1,320.50

Figure 9-19b Sample Last Page of Billing/Payment Status Report

PRACTICE ANALYSIS REPORT

Medisoft's **practice analysis report** analyzes the revenue of a practice for a specified period of time, usually a month or a year (see Figures 9-20a and 9-20b). The report can be used to generate medical

practice analysis report a report that analyzes the revenue of a practice for a specified period of time

Family Care Center
Practice Analysis
Show all data where the Date From is between 9/1/2016, 9/30/2016

Code	Description	Amount	Units	Average	Cost	Net
02	Patient payment, check	-299.50	2	-149.75	0.00	-299.50
29540	Strapping, ankle	121.50	1	121.50	0.00	121.50
50390	Aspiration of renal cyst by needle	551.00	1	551.00	0.00	551.00
73510	Hip x-ray, complete, two views	124.00	1	124.00	0.00	124.00
84478	Triglycerides test	29.00	1	29.00	0.00	29.00
90471	Immunization administration	15.00	1	15.00	0.00	15.00
90703	Tetanus injection	29.00	1	29.00	0.00	29.00
92516	Facial nerve function studies	210.00	1	210.00	0.00	210.00
93000	Electrocardiogram--ECG with interpre	84.00	1	84.00	0.00	84.00
99070	Supplies and materials provided	20.00	1	20.00	0.00	20.00
99201	OF--new patient, minimal	66.00	1	66.00	0.00	66.00
99211	OF--established patient, minimal	144.00	4	36.00	0.00	144.00
99212	OF--established patient, low	324.00	6	54.00	0.00	324.00
99213	OF--established patient, detailed	216.00	3	72.00	0.00	216.00
99214	OF--established patient, moderate	105.00	1	105.00	0.00	105.00
99394	Preventive est., 12-17 years	222.00	1	222.00	0.00	222.00
AARPAY	AARP Payment	-19.57	3	-6.52	0.00	-19.57
BCBDED	BCBS Deductible	0.00	1	0.00	0.00	0.00
BCBPAY	BCBS Payment	-168.00	2	-84.00	0.00	-168.00
CHVCPAY	ChampVA Copayment	-30.00	2	-15.00	0.00	-30.00
EAPADJ	East Ohio PPO Adjustment	-12.60	2	-6.30	0.00	-12.60
EAPCPAY	East Ohio PPO Copayment	-160.00	8	-20.00	0.00	-160.00
EAPPAY	East Ohio PPO Payment	-73.40	2	-36.70	0.00	-73.40
MCDADJ	Medicaid Adjustment	-479.95	2	-239.97	0.00	-479.95
MCDCPAY	Medicaid Copayment	-10.00	1	-10.00	0.00	-10.00
MCDPAY	Medicaid Payment	-127.05	2	-63.52	0.00	-127.05
MEDADJ	Medicare Adjustment	-212.73	6	-35.46	0.00	-212.73
MEDPAY	Medicare Payment	-209.42	7	-29.92	0.00	-209.42
OHCADJ	OhioCare HMO Adjustment	-50.00	2	-25.00	0.00	-50.00
OHCCPAY	OhioCare HMO Copayment	-40.00	2	-20.00	0.00	-40.00

Figure 9-20a Page 1 of Practice Analysis Report

Family Care Center
Practice Analysis
Show all data where the Date From is between 9/1/2016, 9/30/2016

Code	Description	Amount	Units	Average	Cost	Net
			Total Procedure Charges			$2,260.50
			Total Global Surgical Procedures			$0.00
			Total Product Charges			$0.00
			Total Inside Lab Charges			$0.00
			Total Outside Lab Charges			$0.00
			Total Billing Charges			$0.00
			Total Insurance Payments			-$597.44
			Total Cash Copayments			$0.00
			Total Check Copayments			-$240.00
			Total Credit Card Copayments			$0.00
			Total Patient Cash Payments			$0.00
			Total Patient Check Payments			-$299.50
			Total Credit Card Payments			$0.00
			Total Debit Adjustments			$0.00
			Total Credit Adjustments			$0.00
			Total Insurance Debit Adjustments			$0.00
			Total Insurance Credit Adjustments			-$721.28
			Total Insurance Withholds			$0.00
			Net Effect on Accounts Receivable			$402.28
			Practice Totals			
			Total # Procedures			50
			Total Charges			$4,049.00
			Total Payments			-$2,349.64
			Total Adjustments			-$731.14
			Accounts Receivable			$968.22

Figure 9-20b   Page 2 of Practice Analysis Report

practice financial statements. It can also be used for profit analysis. The summary at the end of the report breaks down the information into total charges, total payments and copayments, and total adjustments.

EXERCISE 9-2   PRINTING A PRACTICE ANALYSIS REPORT

Print a practice analysis report for October 2016.

Date: October 31, 2016

1. On the Reports menu, click Analysis Reports and then Practice Analysis. The Print Report Where? dialog box appears.

2. Select the option to print the report rather than preview it. Click the Start button. The Search dialog box is displayed.

3. Leave the Code 1 fields blank.

4. Make sure to check the box to show all values for the Date Created field.

5. Enter *10/1/2016* in the first Date From box, and *10/31/2016* in the second. This will select data for the month of October 2016.

6. Click the OK button. The Print dialog box for your printer appears.

7. In the Print dialog box, click OK again. The report will print.

 You have completed Exercise 9-2.

INSURANCE ANALYSIS

The insurance analysis report tracks charges, insurance payments received during a specified period, and copayments applied to accounts that include those procedures. It is usually printed at the end of the month. The amount listed as the outstanding balance displays the total charges, subtracting the full amount of the charge if the insurance payment was made.

REFERRING PROVIDER REPORT

The referring provider report enables a practice to determine the origins of revenue derived from providers who have referred patients to the practice. The report lists the percentage of total income that was generated by referring providers.

REFERRAL SOURCE REPORT

The referral source report tracks the source of referrals that are not from other medical offices or providers, such as referrals from established patients.

UNAPPLIED PAYMENT/ADJUSTMENT REPORT

The unapplied payment/adjustment report lists payments or adjustments that have not been fully applied. Information about the payment or adjustment includes the case, document number, posting date, code, code description, transaction amount, and unapplied amount.

UNAPPLIED DEPOSIT REPORT

The unapplied deposit report lists deposits that have unapplied amounts. The report includes the date, code, payer name, payer type, deposit amount, and unapplied amount.

CO-PAYMENT REPORT

This report lists patients who have copayment transactions. It shows the amount paid, how much was applied, and how much, if any, was left unapplied.

OUTSTANDING CO-PAYMENT REPORT

This report shows patients who have outstanding copayment transactions. The report shows the copayment amount expected, the actual amount paid, and the amount due.

9.5 PATIENT LEDGER REPORTS

patient ledger a report that lists the financial activity in each patient's account

A **patient ledger** lists the transaction details of a patient's account, including charges, payments, and adjustments (see Figures 9-21a and 9-21b). Like day sheets and analysis reports, the patient ledger report is one of the standard reports in Medisoft. The information it

Family Care Center
Patient Account Ledger
As of October 31, 2016
Show all data where the Date From is between 1/1/1980, 10/31/2016

Entry	Date	POS	Description	Procedure	Document	Provider	Amount
ARLENSU0	**Susan Arlen**			(614)315-2233			
	Last Payment: -28.60		On: 10/3/2016				
359	09/05/2016	11		99212	1009060000	5	54.00
361	09/05/2016	11		EAPCPAY	1009060000	5	-20.00
618	10/03/2016		#00146972 East Ohio PPO	EAPPAY	1009060000	5	-28.60
619	10/03/2016		Adjustment	EAPADJ	1009060000	5	-5.40
						Patient Total:	0.00
BATTIAN0	**Anthony Battistuta**			(614)500-3619			
	Last Payment: 0.00		On:				
425	10/27/2016	11		99212	1009280000	4	54.00
426	10/27/2016	11		82947	1009280000	4	25.00
						Patient Total:	79.00
BELLHER0	**Herbert Bell**			(614)030-1111			
	Last Payment: -12.40		On: 10/3/2016				
364	09/05/2016	11		EAPCPAY	1009060000	2	-20.00
362	09/05/2016	11		99211	1009060000	2	36.00
620	10/03/2016		#00146972 East Ohio PPO	EAPPAY	1009060000	2	-12.40
621	10/03/2016		Adjustment	EAPADJ	1009060000	2	-3.60
						Patient Total:	0.00
BELLJAN0	**Janine Bell**			(614)030-1111			
	Last Payment: -156.40		On: 10/3/2016				
368	09/05/2016	11		EAPCPAY	1009060000	3	-20.00
365	09/05/2016	11		99213	1009060000	3	72.00
366	09/05/2016	11		73510	1009060000	3	124.00
624	10/03/2016		#00146972 East Ohio PPO	EAPPAY	1009060000	3	-44.80
625	10/03/2016		Adjustment	EAPADJ	1009060000	3	-7.20
626	10/03/2016		#00146972 East Ohio PPO	EAPPAY	1009060000	3	-111.60
627	10/03/2016		Adjustment	EAPADJ	1009060000	3	-12.40
						Patient Total:	0.00
BELLJON0	**Jonathan Bell**			(614)030-1111			
	Last Payment: -179.80		On: 10/3/2016				
371	09/05/2016	11		EAPCPAY	1009060000	3	-20.00
369	09/05/2016	11		99394	1009060000	3	222.00
628	10/03/2016		#00146972 East Ohio PPO	EAPPAY	1009060000	3	-179.80
629	10/03/2016		Adjustment	EAPADJ	1009060000	3	-22.20
						Patient Total:	0.00
BELLSAM0	**Samuel Bell**			(614)030-1111			
	Last Payment: -28.60		On: 10/3/2016				
372	09/05/2016	11		99212	1009060000	2	54.00
374	09/05/2016	11		EAPCPAY	1009060000	2	-20.00
622	10/03/2016		#00146972 East Ohio PPO	EAPPAY	1009060000	2	-28.60
623	10/03/2016		Adjustment	EAPADJ	1009060000	2	-5.40
						Patient Total:	0.00

Figure 9-21a First Page of Patient Account Ledger Report

Family Care Center
Patient Account Ledger
As of October 31, 2016
Show all data where the Date From is between 1/1/1980, 10/31/2016

Entry	Date	POS	Description	Procedure	Document	Provider	Amount
ZAPATKR0	Kristin	Zapata		(614)033-0044			
	Last Payment: -247.50		On: 9/21/2016				
580	08/28/2016	11		99385	0803270000	1	247.50
582	09/10/2016		#456789 Blue Cross/Blue Shield	BCBPAY	0803270000	1	0.00
583	09/10/2016		Carrier 1 Deductible -$247.50	BCBDED	0803270000	1	0.00
584	09/21/2016	11		02	0807010000	1	-247.50
607	10/03/2016	11		NSFFEE	1610030000	1	35.00
608	10/03/2016	11	Returned Check	NSF	1610030000	1	247.50
						Patient Total:	282.50
						Ledger Total:	$1,284.62

Figure 9-21b Last Page of Patient Account Ledger Report

provides is especially useful when there is a question about a patient's account.

The patient account ledger report is created by clicking Patient Ledger on the Reports menu. The Print Report Where? dialog box is displayed. After the preview, print, or export selection is made, the Search dialog box is displayed, as it is with the other reports. It provides options to select by chart numbers, patient reference balances, dates, attending providers, billing codes, and patient indicators. A patient account ledger is generated only for data that meet the selection criteria.

PRINTING A PATIENT ACCOUNT LEDGER	EXERCISE 9-3

Print a patient account ledger for October 2016 for patients whose last names begin with the letters *R* through *Z*.

Date: October 1–October 31, 2016

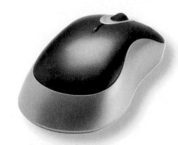

1. On the Reports menu, click Patient Ledger. The Print Report Where? dialog box is displayed.

2. Select the choice to send the report to the printer, and then click Start. The Search box is displayed.

3. In the selection area for Chart Number, rather than select all values of the Chart Number field, you will use the Lookup button to select a range of chart numbers. Click in the Show all values of the Chart Number field box to remove the check mark. Then click the Lookup button that is located to the right of the first Chart Number selection box (see Figure 9-22). A portion of the Lookup dialog box for the Chart Number fields is pictured in Figure 9-23.

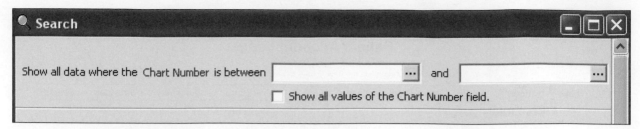

Figure 9-22   Chart Number Selection Boxes with Lookup Buttons Highlighted

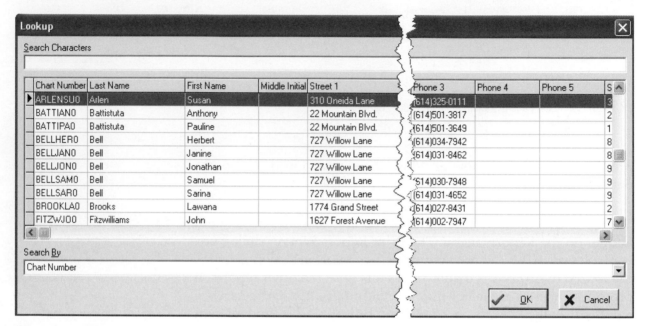

Figure 9-23   Lookup Dialog Box for Chart Number Selection Boxes

4. In the Search Characters field in the Lookup dialog box, key **R**. Notice that the program moves to RAMOSMA0, the first chart number that begins with the letter *R*. Click the OK button at the lower-right corner of the dialog box to accept the chart number selection. The Lookup box disappears, and you are returned to the Search dialog box. Notice that the chart number for the patient you selected in the Lookup box is now in the first Chart Number selection field.

5. Click the Lookup button in the second Chart Number selection field. The Lookup box appears. Key **Z** in the Search Characters box. The chart for Kristin Zapata is selected. Click the OK button to accept the selection.

6. Now you need to enter the dates. Click the first Date From field and enter **10/1/2016**.

7. Click the second Date From field and enter **10/31/2016**. Your Search box should look like Figure 9-24.

8. Click the OK button.

Figure 9-24   Search Dialog Box with Chart Number and Date From Selection Boxes Complete

9. The Print dialog box for your printer appears. Click OK.

10. The report is sent to the printer. **ciMO**

☑ **You have completed Exercise 9-3.**

9.6 STANDARD PATIENT LISTS

Medisoft includes several convenient reports for identifying patients by diagnosis or insurance carrier. These reports are accessed via the Standard Patient Lists submenu on the Reports menu (see Figure 9-25).

The Patient by Diagnosis report lists diagnosis code, chart number, patient name, age, attending provider, facility, and date of last visit. The Patient by Insurance Carrier report lists patients sorted by provider or facility, and then by their insurance carrier.

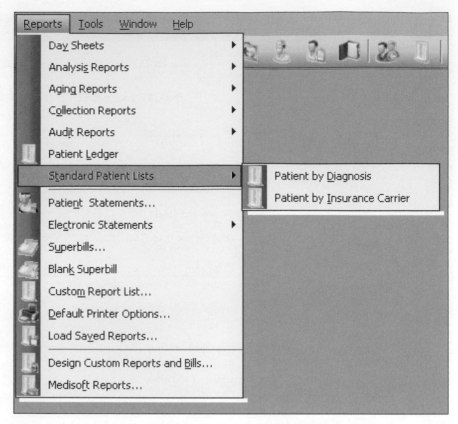

Figure 9-25 Reports Menu with Standard Patient Lists Submenu Displayed

| EXERCISE 9-4 | PRINTING A PATIENT BY INSURANCE CARRIER LIST |

Print a Patient by Insurance Carrier list for all patients in the practice.

Date: October 31, 2016

1. On the Reports menu, click Standard Patient Lists, and then Patient by Insurance Carrier. The Print Report Where? dialog box is displayed. Make the selection to send the report to the printer, and then click the Start button.

2. Accept the Show all values of the Code field entry in the Search box. Click the OK button.

3. The Print dialog box for your printer appears. Click OK.

4. The report is sent to the printer. **CiMC**

 You have completed Exercise 9-4.

9.7 NAVIGATING IN MEDISOFT REPORTS

The Medisoft Reports feature is new in Version 16. It does not replace existing reports, but instead provides access to over a hundred new reports. To start the Medisoft Reports feature, select Medisoft

Reports on the Reports menu (see Figure 9-26), or click the shortcut button on the toolbar (see Figure 9-27).

The Medisoft Reports application window features its own main window that contains menu items and a toolbar with shortcut buttons (see Figure 9-28).

The window is divided into two sections: an All Folders area and a Contents of All Folders area. The All Folders section displays the reports directory and the subfolders in the directory. The Contents of All Folders section lists the individual reports included in the folder that is selected in the All Folders list. In Figure 9-29, the Aging Power Pack folder is selected in All Folders, and the reports within the Aging Power Pack folder are listed in Contents of All Folders.

Above the All Folders and Contents of All Folders area, the Medisoft Reports window has its own menu bar, toolbar, and search area.

THE MEDISOFT REPORTS MENUS

The Medisoft Reports menus include File, View, and Help. The File menu, displayed in Figure 9-30, contains commands for creating a new folder, deleting a report, renaming a report, printing a report, previewing a report, importing a report from a file, exporting a report to a file, and closing the Medisoft Reports feature.

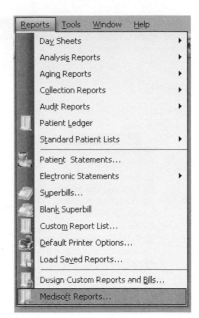

Figure 9-26 The Medisoft Reports Option on the Reports Menu

Figure 9-27 The Medisoft Reports Shortcut Button

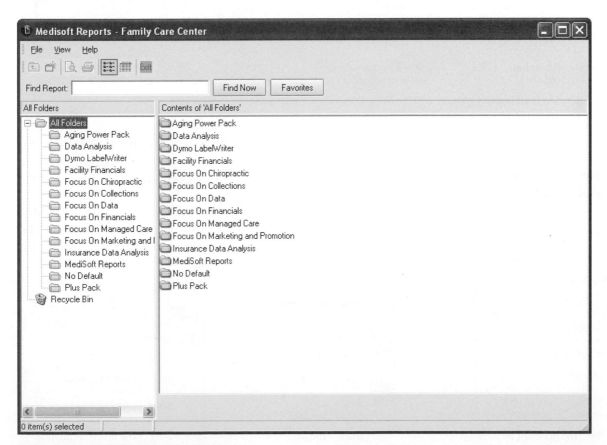

Figure 9-28 The Medisoft Reports Window

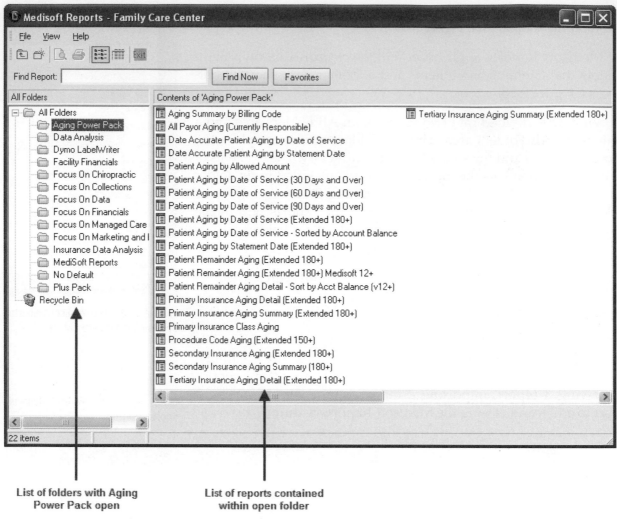

List of folders with Aging Power Pack open

List of reports contained within open folder

Figure 9-29 The Medisoft Reports Window with the Aging Power Pack Folder Selected

Commands on the View menu include options for displaying the toolbar and status bar, and whether to display the Contents of All Folders list of reports in List view or in Detail view (see Figure 9-31).

The Help menu contains entries for viewing help contents, navigating to Medisoft's website, viewing Medisoft Reports file location and path, and displaying the version of Medisoft Reports you are using. The Help menu is pictured in Figure 9-32.

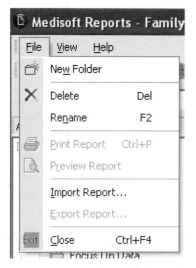

Figure 9-30 The Medisoft Reports File Menu

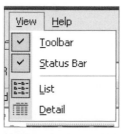

Figure 9-31 The Medisoft Reports View Menu

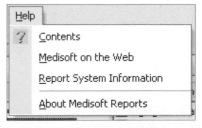

Figure 9-32 The Medisoft Reports Help Menu

THE MEDISOFT REPORTS TOOLBAR

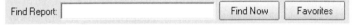

Figure 9-33 The Medisoft Reports Toolbar

Below the menu bar is a toolbar featuring shortcut buttons (see Figure 9-33). From left to right, these buttons are used for

- Moving up a folder level
- Creating a new folder
- Previewing a report
- Printing a report
- Displaying reports in a list
- Displaying report details
- Exiting the application

THE MEDISOFT REPORTS FIND BOX

Find Report:		Find Now	Favorites

Figure 9-34 The Medisoft Reports Find Report box

Below the toolbar are the Find Report box and the Find Now button, which are used for searching for specific reports, and the Favorites button, which displays reports marked as favorites (see Figure 9-34).

THE MEDISOFT REPORTS HELP FEATURE

To view descriptions of all the reports available in Medisoft Reports, select Contents on the Medisoft Reports Help menu. The Medisoft Reports window appears. In the left side of the window, under the Contents tab, click Reports Available from the Medisoft Reports window (see Figure 9-35). Scroll down the window for a full listing of the reports and their descriptions.

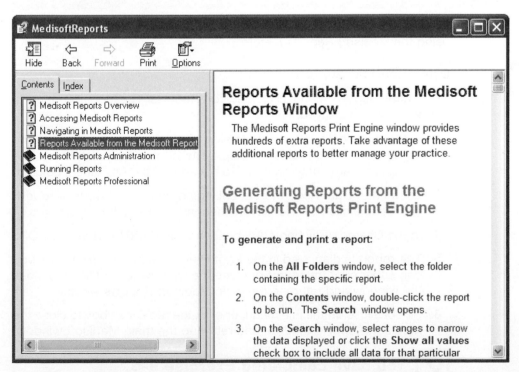

Figure 9-35 Contents of the Medisoft Reports Help File with Reports Available from the Medisoft Reports Window Selected

9.8 AGING REPORTS

aging report a report that lists the amount of money owed to the practice, organized by the amount of time the money has been owed

patient aging report a report that lists a patient's balance by age, date and amount of the last payment, and telephone number

insurance aging report a report that lists how long a payer has taken to respond to insurance claims

Aging reports are of particular importance to medical billing specialists. An **aging report** lists the amount of money owed to the practice, organized by the amount of time the money has been owed. Medical practices use aging reports to determine which accounts require follow-up to collect past-due balances. A **patient aging report** lists a patient's balance by age, date and amount of the last payment, and telephone number.

An **insurance aging report** shows how long a payer has taken to respond to each claim. This information is used to compare the response time with the terms of the practice's contract with the payer. For example, a practice may discover that a payer is routinely responding to claims ten days later than the claim turnaround time specified in the contract. In that case, the practice manager might review the situation with the payer's customer service manager and ask the payer to adhere to its guidelines.

Standard aging reports are contained on the Reports menu under the Aging Reports submenu. Additional aging reports are also contained in the Medisoft Reports feature. Refer back to Figure 9-29 to see the list of aging reports available in the Aging Power Pack folder of the Medisoft Reports feature. The exercise that follows provides practice in creating an aging report using the Medisoft Reports feature.

EXERCISE 9-5	PRINTING A PATIENT AGING REPORT

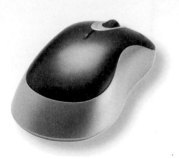

Print a patient aging report for the period ending September 30, 2016, using the Medisoft Reports feature.

Date: September 30, 2016

1. On the Reports menu, click Medisoft Reports. The Medisoft Reports window is displayed.

2. In the All Folders list on the left side of the window, double click the Aging Power Pack folder to display its contents. The contents are listed in the area of the window to the right of the All Folders column.

3. Locate the Date Accurate Patient Aging by Date of Service report, and double click it. After several seconds, a Search box appears.

4. In the Charges/Payments/Adj box, enter **9/30/2016**. Then click OK.

5. The report is displayed in the Print Preview window. From here, you can either print the report or close the window. Click Close to close the window and return to the main Medisoft Reports window.

6. Select Close on the File menu, or click the red Close box to close the Medisoft Reports window, and return to the main Medisoft window.

 You have completed Exercise 9-5.

9.9 CUSTOM REPORTS

In addition to its standard reports on the Reports menu and the reports in the Medisoft Report feature, Medisoft has a number of built-in custom reports, including

- Lists of addresses, billing codes, EDI receivers, patients, patient recalls, procedure codes, providers, and referring providers

- The CMS-1500 and Medicare CMS-1500 forms in a variety of printer formats

- Patient statements and walkout receipts

- Superbills (encounter forms)

The built-in custom reports, which were created in Medisoft using the Report Designer, are accessed via the Custom Report List option on the Reports menu (see Figure 9-36). When Custom Report List is clicked on the Reports menu, the Open Report dialog box is displayed (see Figure 9-37). When a new custom report is created, it is added to the list of custom reports displayed on the screen.

Listed under the heading Show Report Style, the Open Report dialog box contains eleven radio buttons that are used to control the list of reports displayed in the dialog

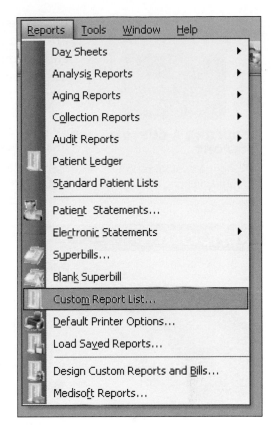

Figure 9-36 Custom Report List Option on the Reports Menu

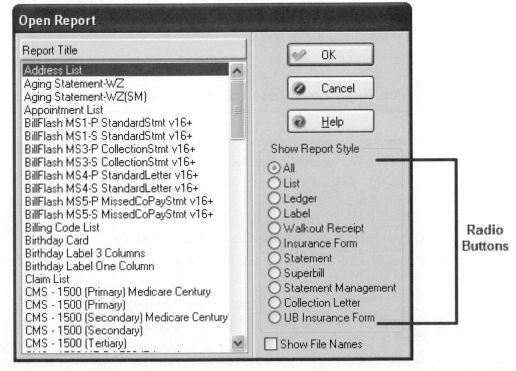

Figure 9-37 Open Report Dialog Box

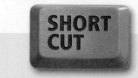

box. When the All radio button is clicked, all types of custom reports are listed in the dialog box. When one of the other radio buttons is clicked, only reports of that style are listed. For example, if the Insurance Form radio button is clicked, only reports that are insurance forms are listed.

To print a custom report, highlight the title of the report by clicking it, and then click the OK button. The same options that are available with standard reports for previewing the report on the screen, sending it directly to the printer, or exporting it to a file are available with reports created through the Custom Report List option.

EXERCISE 9-6 · PRINTING A LIST OF PATIENTS

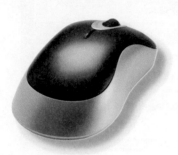

Print a list of all patients.

Date: July 31, 2016

1. On the Reports menu, click Custom Report List.
2. In the Show Report Style list, click the List radio button. Only list reports are displayed in the Open Report dialog box.
3. Select the Patient List report and click the OK button.
4. Accept the option to preview the report on the screen, and click the Start button. The Data Selection Questions dialog box appears.
5. Leave the Chart Number Range boxes blank to select all patients.
6. Click the OK button.
7. View the report on the screen. Notice that the computer's system date—the date you are doing the exercise—is displayed at the top of the report by default.
8. Send the report to the printer.
9. Exit the Preview Report window.

 You have completed Exercise 9-6.

EXERCISE 9-7 · PRINTING A LIST OF PROCEDURE CODES

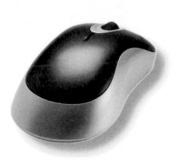

Print a list of all procedure codes in the database.

Date: July 31, 2016

1. On the Reports menu, click Custom Report List.
2. In the Show Report Style section of the dialog box, click the List radio button.
3. Select Procedure Code List. Click the OK button.
4. Click the radio button to preview the report on the screen. Click the Start button.
5. Leave the Code 1 Range boxes blank to select all procedure codes. Click the OK button.

6. View the report on the screen.

7. Send the report to the printer.

8. Exit the Preview Report window.

✓ **You have completed Exercise 9-7.**

9.10 USING REPORT DESIGNER

Medisoft comes with a built-in program, called the Medisoft Report Designer, that allows users to modify existing reports or create new reports to add to the custom report list. The program provides maximum flexibility and control over data in the report and over how the data are displayed. Formatting styles include list, ledger, statement, and insurance. A report can be created from scratch, or an existing report can be used as a starting point. Although the details of how to create new custom reports with the Report Designer are beyond the coverage of this text/workbook, Exercise 9-8 offers practice using the Report Designer to modify an existing report.

The Report Designer is accessed by clicking Design Custom Reports and Bills on the Reports menu. This action displays the Medisoft Report Designer window (see Figure 9-38).

Figure 9-38 **The Report Designer Window**

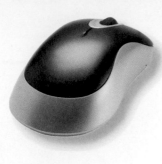

Using the Medisoft Report Designer, modify the Patient List report so that a work telephone number replaces a home telephone number in the report.

Date: July 31, 2016

1. On the Reports menu, click Design Custom Reports and Bills. The Report Designer window is displayed.

2. Click Open Report on the File menu. The Open Report dialog box is displayed.

3. Double click Patient List in the list. The Patient List report is displayed (see Figure 9-39).

4. Double click Phone, which appears between the two horizontal black lines near the top of the report, to select it. Then, double click Phone again to edit it. The Text Properties dialog box is displayed (see Figure 9-40).

5. Enter **Work Phone** in the Text box that currently reads "Phone." Be sure that the Auto Size button is checked, so the program will automatically resize the text box to accommodate the longer title.

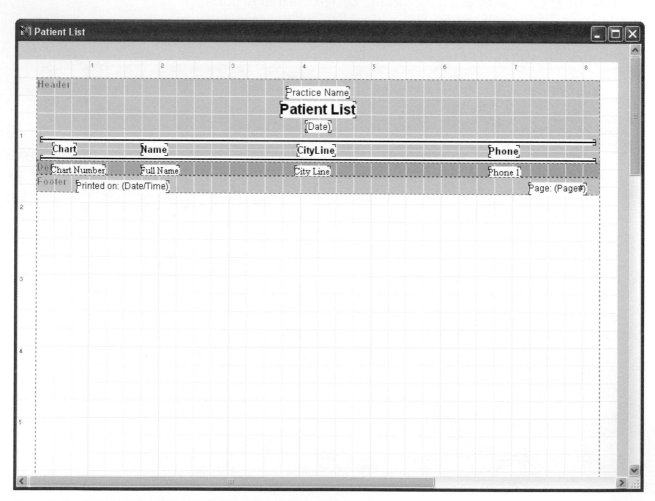

Figure 9-39 Patient List Report Open in Medisoft Report Designer

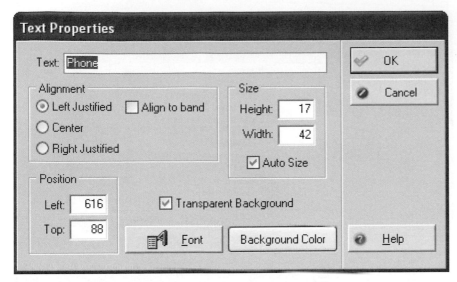

Figure 9-40   Text Properties Dialog Box

6. Click the OK button. Work Phone is displayed in the band where Phone used to be.

7. In the green band below the band in which Work Phone appears, click the Phone 1 box to select it. Then double click the Phone 1 box again to edit its contents. The Data Field Properties dialog box is displayed (see Figure 9-41).

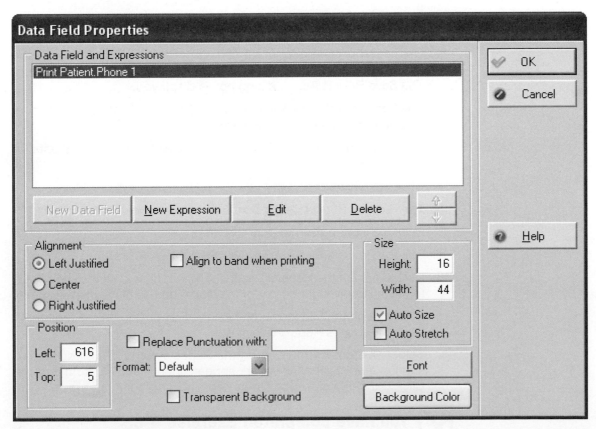

Figure 9-41   Data Field Properties Dialog Box

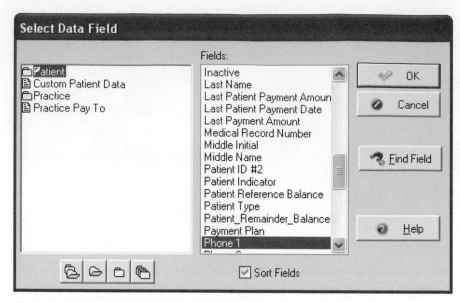

Figure 9-42 Select Data Field Dialog Box

8. The current data box, Print Patient.Phone 1, is active in the Data Field and Expressions box. Click the Edit button to change this box. The Select Data Field dialog box is displayed (see Figure 9-42).

9. In the Fields column, scroll down, highlight Work Phone, and click OK. The Data Field and Expressions box now lists Print Patient.Work Phone.

10. Be sure the Auto Size box is checked, and click the OK button. Work Phone is displayed where Phone 1 used to be.

11. On the Report Designer File menu, click Preview Report to save the file as a new report and see how the report will look when printed. The Save Report As . . . dialog box is displayed.

12. Key **Patient List—Work** in the Report Title box. Click the OK button. The Search dialog box is displayed.

13. Leave the Chart Number Range boxes blank to select all patients for the report.

14. Click the OK button.

15. The Preview Report dialog box is displayed, showing the report.

16. Click the Print button to print the report.

17. Exit the Preview Report window.

18. Click Close on the Report Designer File menu, or click the Close button in the upper-right corner of the dialog box, to close the report file.

19. Click Exit on the File menu, or click the Exit button on the toolbar, to leave Medisoft's Report Designer.

20. Select Custom Report List on the Reports menu. Scroll down and confirm that Patient List—Work appears in the list of custom reports. Click Cancel to close the Open Report dialog box.

✓ **You have completed Exercise 9-8.**

APPLYING YOUR SKILLS

7: PRINT A PATIENT DAY SHEET

September 6, 2016
Using Medisoft standard reports, print a patient day sheet for September 6, 2016.

APPLYING YOUR SKILLS

8: PRINT AN INSURANCE PAYMENT BY TYPE REPORT

September 1–September 30, 2016
Using Medisoft Reports, open the Plus Pack folder and locate the Insurance Payment by Type report to create a report for September 2016.

Remember to create a backup of your work before exiting Medisoft! To help you keep track of your work, name the backup file after the chapter you are working on, for example, StudentID-c9.mbk.

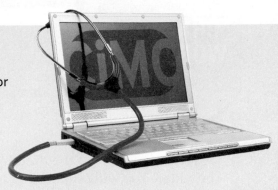

ELECTRONIC HEALTH RECORD EXCHANGE

Viewing Data Transfer Reports

In addition to the many standard reports available in Medisoft, the Communications Manager program provides reports on inbound and outbound data transfers to and from an electronic health record. Communications Manager is the program that makes it possible for Medisoft and an electronic health record to exchange information.

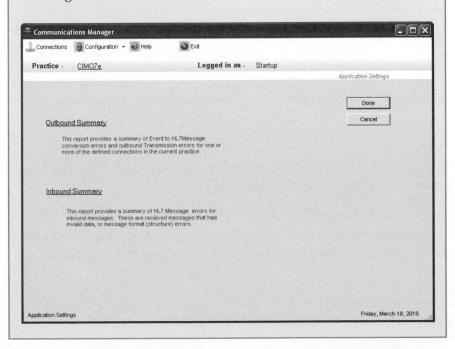

 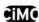

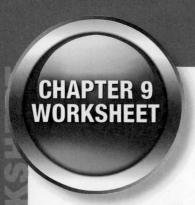

Name: _____ Date: _____

After completing all the exercises in the chapter, answer the following questions in the spaces provided. You will need to refer to your printouts of the reports created in the exercises to complete this worksheet.

1. *[LO 9.3]* In the patient day sheet created in Exercise 9-1, what is the total of the adjustments to Jonathan Bell's account?

   _____

2. *[LO 9.3]* In the patient day sheet created in Exercise 9-1, what is the patient's balance on John Fitzwilliams's account?

   _____

3. *[LO 9.4]* In the practice analysis report created in Exercise 9-2, what were the total procedure charges?

   _____

4. *[LO 9.5]* In the patient account ledger created in Exercise 9-3, what is Jill Simmons's patient total at the end of October?

   _____

5. *[LO 9.8]* In the Patient by Insurance Carrier report created in Exercise 9-4, how many patients are listed under Medicare?

   _____

6. *[LO 9.6]* In the Patient List report created in Exercise 9-6, what are the four columns of information displayed?

   _____

7. *[LO 9.9]* In the Procedure Code List created in Exercise 9-7, what is the description and charge for procedure code 99214?

   _____

8. *[LO 9.10]* According to the patient day sheet created in Applying Your Skills Exercise 7, how many procedures were performed on September 6, 2016?

   _____

9. *[LO 9.10]* According to the Insurance Payment by Type report created in Applying Your Skills 8, which type of insurance carrier plan paid the greatest amount to the Family Care Center?

   _____

10. *[LO 9.10]* According to the Insurance Payment by Type report created in Applying Your Skills 8, what percentage of the Family Care Center's payments came from Medicare during September 2016?

   _____

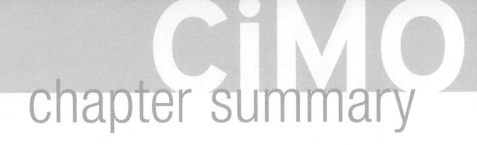

9.1 List the three types of reports available in Medisoft. Pages 300–302	1. Standard reports 2. Medisoft Reports 3. Custom reports
9.2 Describe how to select data to be included in a Medisoft report. Pages 302–307	Data for a report is selected in the Search dialog box. The Search dialog box contains one or more selection boxes. Entering data in the selection boxes causes the data in the report to be limited to the data selected. If all data are to be included, the Show all values of the _____ field is selected.
9.3 Distinguish between patient, procedure, and payment day sheets. Page 307–313	A patient day sheet lists patient transactions for a day, organized alphabetically by chart number. A procedure day sheet lists patient transactions by procedure code, and is sorted numerically, then alphabetically (for codes that begin with letters). A payment day sheet lists patient transactions by provider, ordered numerically by the code assigned to the provider in Medisoft.
9.4 Demonstrate how to create a practice analysis report. Pages 313–317	1. On the Reports menu, click Analysis Reports and then Practice Analysis. The Print Report Where? dialog box appears. 2. Select the desired option in the Print Report Where? dialog box. 3. Click the Start button. The Search dialog box is displayed. 4. Make the necessary entries in the following selection boxes: Code 1 Date Created Date From Attending Provider Place of Service 5. Click the OK button. If you elected to preview the report, the report will open in the Print Preview window. If you chose to print the report, the Print dialog box for your printer appears. Click OK to print the report.

9.5 Demonstrate how to create a patient ledger report. Pages 318–321	1. On the Reports menu, click Patient Ledger. The Print Report Where? dialog box appears.
	2. Select the desired option in the Print Report Where? dialog box.
	3. Click the Start button. The Search dialog box is displayed.
	4. Make the necessary entries in the following selection boxes:
	Chart Number
	Patient Reference Balance
	Date From
	Attending Provider
	Billing Code
	Patient Indicator
	5. Click the OK button. If you elected to preview the report, the report will open in the Print Preview window. If you chose to print the report, the Print dialog box for your printer appears. Click OK to print the report.
9.6 Demonstrate how to create a standard patient list report. Pages 321–322	1. On the Reports menu, click Standard Patient Lists. Select Patient by Diagnosis or Patient by Insurance Carrier from the submenu. The Print Report Where? dialog box appears.
	2. Select the desired option in the Print Report Where? dialog box.
	3. Click the Start button. The Search dialog box is displayed.
	4. For a Patient by Diagnosis report, make the necessary entries in the Diagnosis Code 1 selection box. For a Patient by Insurance Carrier report, make the necessary entry in the Code selection box.
	5. Click the OK button. If you elected to preview the report, the report will open in the Print Preview window. If you chose to print the report, the Print dialog box for your printer appears. Click OK to print the report.

9.7 Describe how to use Medisoft Reports to create a report. Pages 322–325	1. Select Medisoft Reports on the Reports menu. The Medisoft Reports window opens. 2. Locate the folder in the All Folders column that contains the report you want to create. 3. Double click the folder to see its contents. 4. In the list of reports that appears in the window to the right of the All Folders list, locate the report. 5. Double click the report. After several seconds, the Search dialog box appears. 6. Make the necessary entries in the selection boxes, and then click the OK button. 7. The report appears in the Print Preview window. 8. To send the report to the printer, click the Print button.
9.8 Explain how aging reports are used in a medical practice. Page 326	Medical practices use aging reports to determine which accounts require follow-up to collect past-due balances. Aging reports list the amount of money owed to the practice, sorted by the amount of time the money has been owed.
9.9 Explain how to access Medisoft's built-in custom reports. Pages 327–329	1. Click Custom Report List on the Reports menu. The Open Report dialog box appears. 2. Select the desired report from the list of reports, and click the OK button. 3. Select the option to preview or print the report, and then click the Start button. 4. Make the necessary entries in the Data Selection Questions dialog box and click OK. 5. The report appears in the Print Preview window or is sent to the printer.
9.10 Demonstrate how to open a report for editing in Medisoft's Report Designer. Pages 329–332	1. On the Reports menu, click Design Custom Reports and Bills. The Medisoft Report Designer window is displayed. 2. Click Open Report on the File menu. The Open Report dialog box is displayed. 3. Click to select a report in the list, and click the OK button, or simply double click the report title. 4. The report opens in Report Designer for editing.

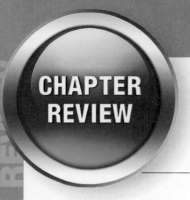

CHAPTER REVIEW

USING TERMINOLOGY

Match the terms on the left with the definitions on the right.

_____ **1.** *[LO 9.8]* aging report

_____ **2.** *[LO 9.3]* day sheet

_____ **3.** *[LO 9.8]* insurance aging report

_____ **4.** *[LO 9.8]* patient aging report

_____ **5.** *[LO 9.3]* patient day sheet

_____ **6.** *[LO 9.5]* patient ledger

_____ **7.** *[LO 9.3]* payment day sheet

_____ **8.** *[LO 9.4]* practice analysis report

_____ **9.** *[LO 9.3]* procedure day sheet

_____ **10.** *[LO 9.2]* selection boxes

a. A summary of the patient activity on a given day.

b. Fields within the Search dialog box that are used to filter the data that will appear in a report.

c. A report that lists the amount of money owed the practice, organized by the length of time the money has been owed.

d. A report that provides information on practice activities for a twenty-four-hour period.

e. A report that lists the financial activity in each patient's account, including charges, payments, and adjustments.

f. A report that lists a patient's balance by age, the date and amount of the last payment, and the telephone number.

g. A report that lists payments received on a given day, organized by provider.

h. A report that analyzes the revenue of a practice for a specified period of time, usually a month or a year.

i. A report that lists the procedures performed on a given day, listed in numerical order.

j. A report that lists how long a payer has taken to respond to insurance claims.

CHECKING YOUR UNDERSTANDING

Answer the questions below in the space provided.

1. *[LO 9.1]* What three types of report options are provided in Medisoft?

_____

_____

2. *[LO 9.3]* What is the difference between a patient day sheet and a procedure day sheet?

_____

_____

3. *[LO 9.2]* What is the name of the dialog box that provides options for selecting data to be included on a report?

_____

_____

4. *[LO 9.7]* How do you select a report in the Medisoft Reports program?

_____

_____

5. *[LO 9.1]* What are the three options in the Print Report Where? dialog box?

_____

_____

APPLYING YOUR KNOWLEDGE

Answer the questions below in the space provided.

9.1. *[LO 9.3]* One of the providers in a practice asks for a report of yesterday's transactions. How would this report be created?

_____

_____

9.2. *[LO 9.5]* A patient is unsure whether she mailed a check last month to pay an outstanding balance on her account. What standard report would you use to help answer her question?

_____

_____

THINKING ABOUT IT

Answer the questions below in the space provided.

9.1. *[LO 9.3]* If the office manager asked you for a list of procedure codes representing services performed on a particular day, what report would you create in Medisoft?

_____

_____

9.2. *[LO 9.8]* What would the consequences be if a medical practice did not produce patient aging reports on a regular basis?

_____

_____

AT THE COMPUTER

Answer the following question at the computer.

9.1. *[LO 9.3]* The office manager has asked you which procedure codes were used most often on October 28, 2016. Create a report that contains this information. Which procedure code was used most often? How many times was it used? What was the second most often used code? How many times was it used?

_____

_____

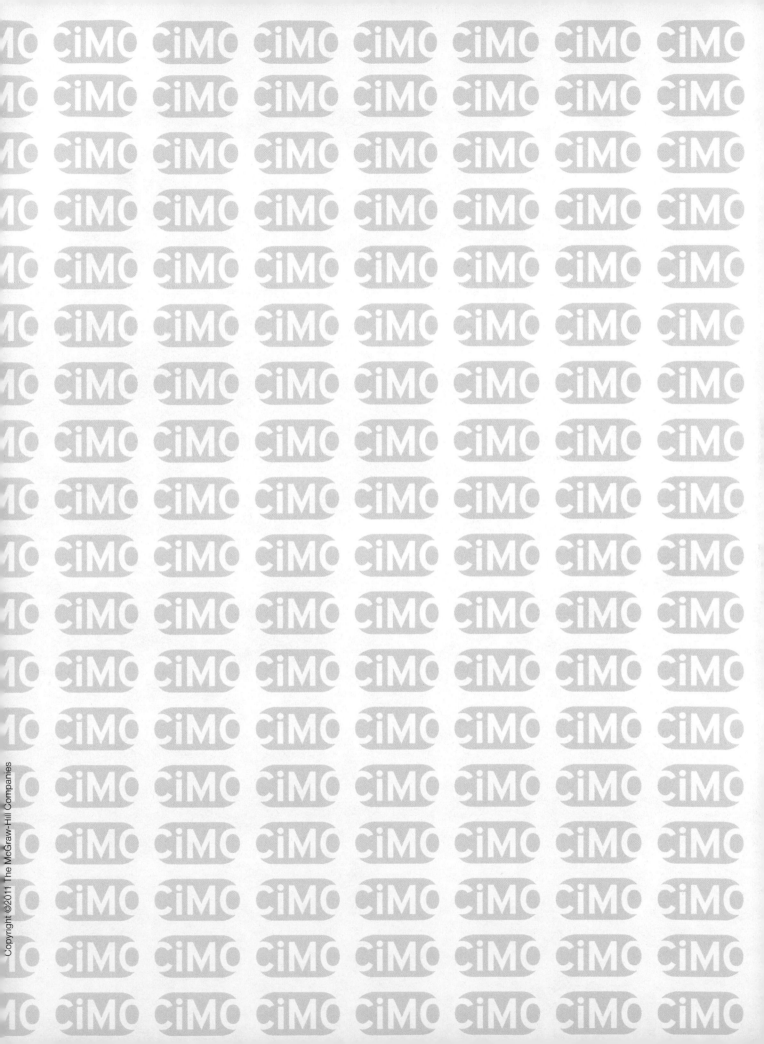

10

Collections in the Medical Office

key terms

collection agency

collection list

collection tracer report

payment plan

prompt payment laws

tickler

uncollectible account

write-off

learning outcomes

When you finish this chapter, you will be able to:

10.1 Explain the importance of prompt payment laws.

10.2 Summarize the importance of a financial policy in a medical office.

10.3 Identify the laws that regulate collections from patients.

10.4 Demonstrate how to post a payment from a collection agency.

10.5 Discuss the process of writing off uncollectible accounts.

10.6 Explain how to use a patient aging report to identify past-due accounts.

10.7 Demonstrate how to add an account to the collection list.

10.8 Demonstrate how to create a collection letter.

10.9 Demonstrate how to create a collection tracer report.

what you need to know

To use this chapter, you need to know how to:

- Start Medisoft, use menus, and enter and edit text.
- Work with chart numbers and codes.
- Create an aging report.

Receiving prompt payment for services is a critical factor in determining the financial success of a medical practice. Practices collect payments from patients and from insurance carriers. While most patients and health plans pay on time, there are some that do not. Members of the billing staff may be asked to work with patients and representatives of health plans to follow up on overdue accounts and unpaid claims. The goal of the follow-up is to resolve problems and collect payments.

10.1 LAWS GOVERNING TIMELY PAYMENT OF INSURANCE CLAIMS

In some instances, insurance carriers dispute claims. They may contend that patient care services were not medically necessary or that the method in which services were provided violated the payer-provider contract. When a carrier contests a claim or delays payment because more information is needed, providers frequently are not given notice in a timely manner. When further documentation is requested and the physician provides the information, an insurer or health plan can further delay payment by asking for additional information or clarification. Resubmitting rejected claims is a time-consuming process, resulting in increased practice expenses and more delay in payment.

prompt payment laws state laws that mandate a time period within which clean claims must be paid; if they are not, financial penalties are levied against the payer

Most states have enacted prompt payment laws to ensure that claims are paid in a timely manner. **Prompt payment laws** are state laws that mandate a time period within which clean claims must be paid and that call for financial penalties to be levied against late payers. (Clean claims are error-free claims that do not require additional documentation.) For example, under the New York Prompt Payment Law, when a managed care organization or insurance company fails to make payment on a clean claim within forty-five days of submission, the physician is entitled to receive interest on the late payment at the rate of 12 percent per year.

If a clean claim is not paid within the allotted time frame, the payer should be notified in writing that payment has not been received according to applicable prompt payment laws. Practices should also request written explanations for all claim delays, partial payments, and denials. If satisfaction is not achieved, the applicable state or federal regulatory agency may be notified of the violation.

10.2 THE IMPORTANCE OF A FINANCIAL POLICY

The average patient is now responsible for paying nearly 35 percent of medical bills, more than three times the amount paid by a patient in 1980, according to the Centers for Medicare and Medicaid Services (CMS). While most patients pay their bills on time, every practice has some patients who do not. Patients' reasons for not paying include

- Lack of insurance
- Lack of financial resources
- Significant medical costs
- Consumer-directed health plans with high out-of-pocket costs
- Lack of understanding that payment is their responsibility

The patient collection process begins with a clear financial policy and effective communications with patients about their financial responsibilities. When patients understand the charges and the practice's financial policy in advance, collecting payments is not usually problematic. As a result, it is important to have a written financial policy that spells out patients' responsibilities.

The financial policy of a medical practice explains how the practice handles financial matters. When new patients register, they should be given copies of the financial policy along with the practice's HIPAA privacy policies and patient registration material. The policy should tell patients how the practice handles

- Collecting copayments and past-due balances
- Setting up financial arrangements for unpaid balances
- Providing charity care or using a sliding scale for patients with low incomes
- Collecting payments for services not covered by insurance
- Collecting prepayment for services
- Accepting cash, checks, money orders, and credit cards

Figure 10-1 shows a sample financial policy of a medical practice.

Despite the practice's efforts to communicate the financial policy to all patients, some individuals still do not pay in full and on time. Medical insurance specialists are often responsible for some aspect of the collection process. Each practice sets its own procedures. Large bills have priority over smaller ones. Usually, an automatic reminder notice and a second statement are mailed when a bill has not been paid within thirty days after it was issued. Some practices phone a patient whose account is thirty days overdue. If the bill is not paid then, a series of collection letters is generated at intervals, each more stringent in tone and more direct in approach. Table 10-1 provides an example of one practice's collection timeline; different approaches are used in other practices. Some practices send all accounts that are past thirty days to an outside agency.

Financial Policy of
Any Medical Practice
Any Town, USA

Thank you for choosing Any Medical Practice for your health care needs. The following information is being provided to assist you in understanding our financial policies and to address the questions most frequently asked by our patients.

Account Responsibility
You are responsible for all charges incurred on your account. It is also your responsibility to make sure all information on your account is current and accurate. Incorrect information can cause payment delays, which may result in late fees being applied to your account. Many people are under the impression that it is up to the physician and staff to make sure that all charges are paid or covered by insurance. This is not the case. Please remember that the insurance contract is between you and the insurance company, not the physician. It is your responsibility to know what your contract covers and pays and to communicate this to physicians and staff. Therefore, you are responsible for charges incurred regardless of insurance coverage.

Insurance Billing
If you have medical insurance, we will be happy to bill your insurance carrier for you. As a courtesy we will also bill the carrier of any secondary insurance coverage that you may have. Any Medical Practice contracts with many insurance companies, but due to the fact that these companies have many different plans available, it is impossible for us to know if your specific plan is included. You will need to check with your insurance company in advance. Please remember that your insurance may not cover or pay all charges incurred. Any unpaid balance after insurance is your responsibility.

Copays
All copays are due at time of service. A $5.00 billing fee is assessed if your copay is not paid at time of service. This fee will not be waived. It is your responsibility to know whether your insurance requires you to pay a copay.

No Insurance
If you have no insurance, payment in full is expected at time of service, unless payment arrangements have been made prior to your visit.

Late Fees
All patient balances are to be paid in full within 60 days. This refers to balances after your insurance has paid. If you are unable to pay your balance in full within 60 days, please contact the business office to set up a payment plan. A late fee of $20.00 per month will be assessed on patient balances over 60 days.

Cash Only
If your account has been turned over to collection, it will also be changed to a cash-only account. This means that all services will need to be paid in full at time of service. A letter will be sent to inform you if your account has been changed to a cash-only basis.

Dishonored Checks
A $25.00 service charge will be assessed on all dishonored checks.

Payment Methods
Any Medical Practice accepts cash, personal checks, and the following credit cards: Visa, MasterCard, American Express, and Discover. Payments can be made at any reception area. For your convenience, an ATM machine is located in the lobby of the building.

Figure 10-1 A Sample Medical Practice Financial Policy

TABLE 10-1	Patient Collection Timeline
Amount Past Due	Action
30 days	Bill patient
45 days	Call patient regarding bill
60 days	Letter 1
75 days	Letter 2 and call
80 days	Letter 3
90 days	Turn over to collections

10.3 LAWS GOVERNING PATIENT COLLECTIONS

Collections from insurance carriers are considered business collections. Collections from patients, on the other hand, are consumer collections and are regulated by federal and state laws. The Fair Debt Collection Practices Act of 1977 and the Telephone Consumer Protection Act of 1991 regulate debt collections, forbidding unfair practices. General guidelines include the following:

- Do not call a patient before 8 A.M. or after 9 P.M.

- Do not make threats or use profane language.

- Do not discuss the patient's debt with anyone except the person who is responsible for payment. If the patient has a lawyer, discuss the problem only with the lawyer, unless the lawyer gives permission to talk with the patient.

- Do not use any form of deception or violence to collect a debt. For example, do not impersonate a law officer to try to force a patient to pay.

If the practice's printed or displayed payment policy covers adding finance charges on late accounts, it is acceptable to do so. The amount of the finance charge must comply with federal and state law.

USING PAYMENT PLANS

For large bills or special situations, some practices may offer payment plans to patients. A **payment plan** is an agreement between a patient and a practice in which the patient agrees to make regular monthly payments over a specified period of time. If no finance charges are applied to unpaid balances, this type of arrangement is between the practice and the patient, and no legal regulations apply. If, however, the practice adds finance charges and the payments are to be made in

payment plan an agreement between a patient and a practice in which the patient agrees to make regular monthly payments over a specified period of time

more than four installments, the arrangement is subject to the Truth in Lending Act, which is part of the Consumer Credit Protection Act. In this case, the practice notifies the patient in writing about the total amount, the finance charges (stated as a percentage), when each payment is due and the amount, and the date the last payment is due. The agreement must be signed by the practice manager and the patient.

10.4 WORKING WITH COLLECTION AGENCIES

collection agency an outside firm hired to collect on delinquent accounts

After a number of collection attempts that do not produce results, some practices use collection agencies to pursue large unpaid bills. A **collection agency** is an outside firm hired to collect on delinquent accounts. The agency that is selected should have a reputation for fair and ethical handling of collections.

When a patient's account is referred to an agency for collection, the medical insurance specialist no longer contacts the patient or sends statements. If a payment is received from a patient while the account is with the agency, the agency is notified. Collection agencies are often paid on the basis of the amount of money they collect. For example, a collection agency may keep 30 percent of the amount they collect.

When a payment is received from a collection agency, it must be posted to the patient's account. The agency provides a statement that shows which patient accounts have paid, and the amounts of the payments.

EXERCISE 10-1	POSTING A PAYMENT FROM A COLLECTION AGENCY

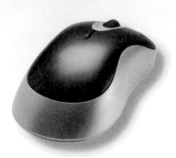

The practice has received a payment from a collection agency for Ali Mazloum's account. Per the Family Care Center's financial policy, the account was assigned to the agency once it was more than ninety days past due. The statement included with the payment indicates that the agency collected 50 percent of the amount owed, or $360.25, as payment in full. The agency then subtracted its fee of 25 percent ($90.06), leaving a payment to the provider of $270.19. Post this amount to the patient's account in Medisoft®.

Amount owed	$720.50
Amount collected	$360.25
Fees	$ 90.06
Net paid to provider	$270.19

Date: October 31, 2016

1. Start Medisoft and restore the data from your last work session.

2. Change the Medisoft Program Date to October 31, 2016, if it is not already set to that date.

3. On the Activities menu, click Enter Transactions. The Transaction Entry dialog box is displayed.

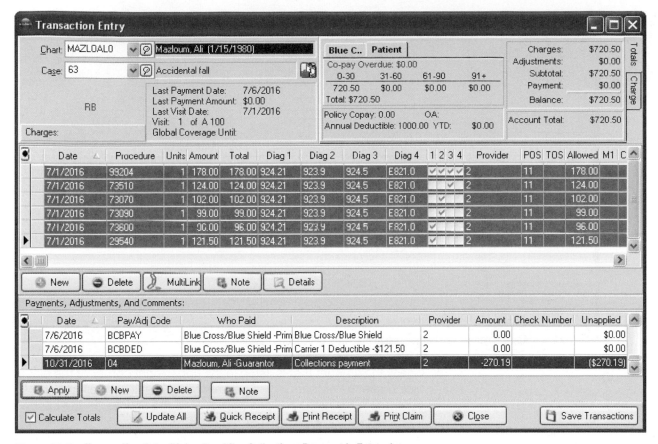

Figure 10-2 Transaction Entry Dialog Box After Collections Payment Is Entered

4. Key **M** in the Chart box, and then press Tab to select Ali Mazloum.

5. Verify that Accidental fall is active in the Case box.

6. In the Payments, Adjustments, and Comments section of the dialog box, click the New button.

7. Verify that the entry in the Date box is 10/31/2016.

8. Click in the Pay/Adj Code box, select the payment code 04—Patient pymt from collections as the payment code, and then press Tab.

9. Verify that Mazloum, Ali—Guarantor is listed in the Who Paid box.

10. Enter **Collections payment** in the Description field.

11. Enter the amount of the payment, **270.19**, in the Amount box, and then press Tab.

12. The Unapplied Amount box should read ($270.19).

13. Your screen should look like the dialog box in Figure 10-2.

14. Click the Apply button. The Apply Payment to Charges dialog box is displayed.

15. In the first line of charges, the amount owed is $178.00. Since the payment is for more than $178.00, you will enter $178.00 toward this charge and the remaining amount to the other charges. Enter **178.00** in the This Payment box for the first charge and press Enter.

Apply Payment to Charges

Payment From: G
For: Mazloum, Ali

Unapplied 0.00

Date From	Document	Procedure	Charge	Balance	Payor Total	This Payment
7/1/2016	1607010000	99204	178.00	0.00	-178.00	-178.00
7/1/2016	1607010000	73510	124.00	31.81	-92.19	-92.19
7/1/2016	1607010000	73070	102.00	102.00	0.00	0.00
7/1/2016	1607010000	73090	99.00	99.00	0.00	0.00
7/1/2016	1607010000	73600	96.00	96.00	0.00	0.00
7/1/2016	1607010000	29540	121.50	121.50	0.00	0.00

There are 6 charge entries.

Apply To Oldest | Close | Help

Figure 10-3 Apply Payment to Charges Dialog Box After Collections Payment Is Applied

16. Check the amount that is listed in the upper-right corner of the dialog box to see the amount of the payment that is still unapplied (–92.19). Enter the remaining unapplied amount to the charge on the second line. Check your work against Figure 10-3.

17. Click the Close button.

18. Click the Save Transactions button.

19. When a Date of Service Validation message appears, click Yes to save the transaction. Leave the Transaction Entry dialog box open.

☑ **You have completed Exercise 10-1.**

10.5 WRITING OFF UNCOLLECTIBLE ACCOUNTS

uncollectible account an account that does not respond to collection efforts and is written off the practice's expected accounts receivable

write-off a balance that has been removed from a patient's account

When all collection attempts have been exhausted and the cost of continuing to pursue the debt is higher than the total amount owed, the collection process is ended. Medical practices have policies on how to handle bills they do not expect to collect. Usually, the amount owed is called an **uncollectible account** or a bad debt, and it is written off the practice's expected accounts receivable. A **write-off** is a balance that has been removed from a patient's account.

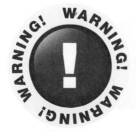

● In the Medicare and Medicaid programs, it is fraudulent to forgive or write off any payments that beneficiaries are responsible for, such as copayments and coinsurance, unless a rigid set of steps has been followed to verify the patient's financial situation. Similarly, it is fraudulent to discount services for other providers or their families, which was formerly a common practice.

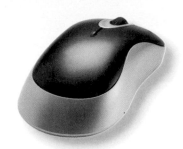

The collection agency accepted 50 percent of the amount owed from Ali Mazloum as payment in full. The practice manager has informed you that the remaining balance is to be written off, even though it is a significant amount.

Date: November 30, 2016

1. If it is not still open from Exercise 10-1, open the Transaction Entry dialog box and select Ali Mazloum's chart number.
2. Change the Medisoft Program Date to November 30, 2016.
3. Verify that Accidental fall is active in the Case box.
4. In the Payments, Adjustments, and Comments section of the dialog box, click the New button.
5. Verify that the entry in the Date box is 11/30/2016.
6. Click in the Pay/Adj Code box, select WRITEOFF—Write Off as the adjustment code, and press Tab.
7. Select Mazloum, Ali—Guarantor in the Who Paid box.
8. Enter the amount to be written off, **450.31**, in the Amount box and press Tab.
9. The Unapplied Amount box should read ($450.31). Check your work against Figure 10-4.
10. Click the Apply button. The Apply Adjustment to Charges dialog box is displayed.
11. Locate the Balance column. In the This Adjust. column, enter an amount equal to the amount in the Balance column for each outstanding charge.
12. When all the charges have been adjusted, click the Close button.

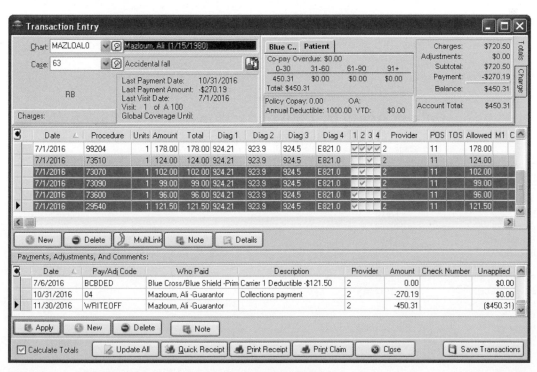

Figure 10-4   Transaction Entry Dialog Box After Write Off Is Entered

13. Confirm that amount listed in Account Total is $0.00.

14. Click the Save Transactions button. When the Date of Service Validation box appears, click Yes to save the transaction.

15. Close the Transaction Entry dialog box.

☑ **You have completed Exercise 10-2.**

10.6 USING A PATIENT AGING REPORT FOR COLLECTIONS

Medical practices frequently use practice management software to monitor collection activities. While specific collection features vary from program to program, common features used for this purpose include aging reports, collection lists, collection letters, and collection reports.

The aging report, which shows the status of each account over time, is an important tool in the collections process. For each account, an aging report shows the patient's chart number and name, and the amount of unpaid charges in each of these categories:

- Current: Up to 30 days

- Past: Thirty-one to 60 days

- Past: Sixty-one to 90 days

- Past: Ninety-one to 120 days

- Past: More than 121 days

Figure 10-5 shows a sample patient aging report created in Medisoft Reports.

Patient Aging by Date of Service
Family Care Center
Show all data where the Charges/Payments/Adj is on or before 9/30/2016

Chart	Name	0-30	31-60	61-90	91-120	121+	Total
ARLENSU0	Arlen, Susan	34.00					34.00
BELLHER0	Bell, Herbert	16.00					16.00
BELLJAN0	Bell, Janine	176.00					176.00
BELLJON0	Bell, Jonathan	202.00					202.00
BELLSAM0	Bell, Samuel	34.00					34.00
BELLSAR0	Bell, Sarina	52.00					52.00
FITZWJO0	Fitzwilliams, John	50.00					50.00
FITZWSA0	Fitzwilliams, Sarah	29.00					29.00
JONESEL0	Jones, Elizabeth	21.17	7.47				28.64
MAZLOAL0	Mazloum, Ali				720.50		720.50
WONGJO10	Wong, Jo	7.47		7.47			14.94
WONGLIY0	Wong, Li	4.14					4.14
Report Totals:		625.78	7.47	7.47	720.50	0.00	1,361.22

Figure 10-5 Sample Patient Aging Report

Review the patient aging report displayed in Figure 10-5. Using the information contained in the report, locate the patient account that is 61–90 days overdue. List the chart number, patient name, past-due amounts, and account balance below. This information will be used later on in Exercise 10-4 to create a tickler item for the practice's collection list.

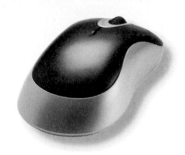

Chart #	Name	Past 31–60	Past 61–90	Past 91+	Total

You have completed Exercise 10-3.

10.7 ADDING AN ACCOUNT TO THE COLLECTION LIST

Once overdue accounts have been identified, the next step is to add collection items to a collection list. The **collection list** is designed to track activities that need to be completed as part of the collection process. Ticklers or collection reminders are displayed as collection list items. A **tickler** is a reminder to follow up on an account that is entered on the collection list.

In Medisoft, the selections for the Collection List feature are located on the Activities menu (see Figure 10-6).

USING THE COLLECTION LIST WINDOW

The Collection List dialog box displays ticklers that have already been entered into the database (see Figure 10-7). The information displayed in the dialog box depends on the dates entered in the Date boxes at the top-left corner of the window. For example, if the date in both boxes is 9/30/2016, only ticklers marked for follow-up on September 30, 2016, will be listed.

Options for controlling what appears in the Collection List window are at the top of the dialog box and include the following:

Date Items can be displayed for the current date, for a range of dates, or for all dates. By default, the current date (the Windows System Date) is used as the range of dates, and only those tickler items that are due on that date are displayed. To see all ticklers regardless of the date, click the Show All Ticklers box.

Show All Ticklers A check in this box results in the listing of all tickler items.

collection list a tool for tracking activities that need to be completed as part of the collection process

tickler a reminder to follow up on an account

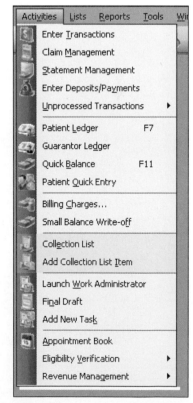

Figure 10-6 Collection List Options on the Activities Menu

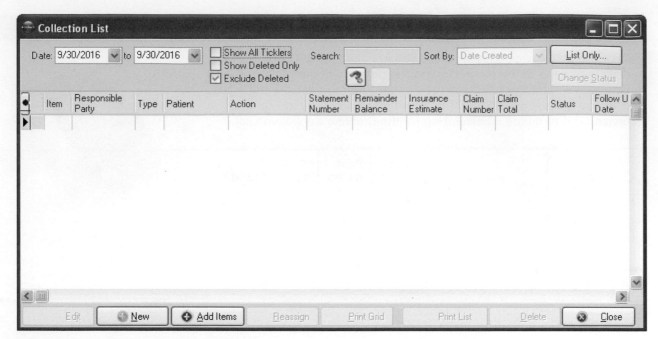

Figure 10-7   Collection List Dialog Box

Show Deleted Only   A check in this box displays only ticklers that have been deleted.

Exclude Deleted   A check in this box indicates that deleted ticklers are not displayed.

The Collection List dialog box contains the following information about each tickler item:

Item   This unique number identifying a tickler item is assigned automatically by the program.

Responsible Party   This field contains the chart number (patient/guarantor) or insurance code (insurance carrier) that identifies the responsible party for this item. By clicking a plus sign (+) that appears to the left of an entry, the field can be expanded to view more information about the responsible party. *Note:* The plus sign is only visible when a tickler has been entered.

When the responsible party is an insurance carrier, the following additional information appears (see Figure 10-8):

- Code
- Name
- Contact
- Phone
- City
- State
- Zip Code
- Group Number
- Policy Number

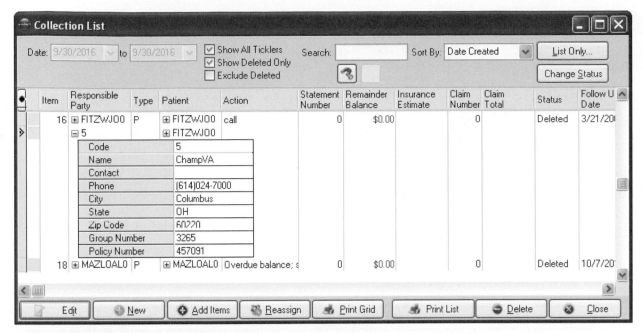

Figure 10-8   Additional Information Displayed When the Responsible Party Is an Insurance Carrier

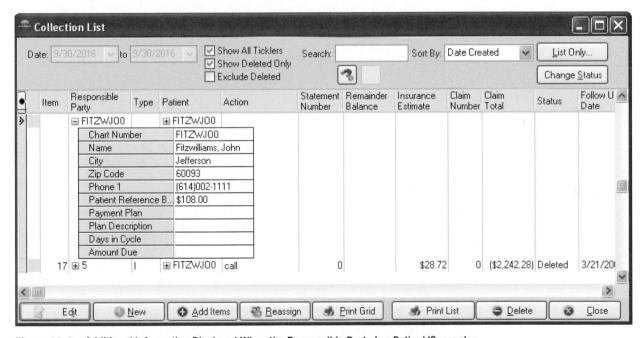

Figure 10-9   Additional Information Displayed When the Responsible Party Is a Patient/Guarantor

When the responsible party is a patient/guarantor, the following
additional information is displayed (see Figure 10-9):

- Chart Number
- Name
- City
- Zip Code
- Phone 1

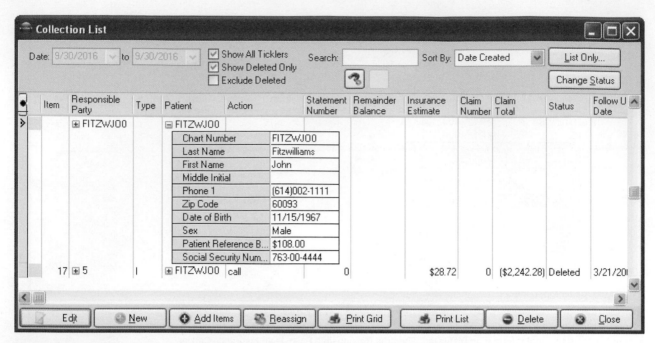

Figure 10-10 Additional Information Available in the Patient Field of the Collection List Dialog Box

- Patient Reference Balance
- Payment Plan
- Plan Description
- Days in Cycle
- Amount Due

Type The type is either a *P* for Patient or an *I* for Insurance. If the type is *P*, the responsible party is a patient. If the type is *I*, the responsible party is the insurance carrier.

Patient This field contains the patient chart number for this tickler. Clicking the plus sign (+) expands it to show more information on the patient (see Figure 10-10).

The additional information displayed includes

- Chart Number
- Last Name
- First Name
- Middle Initial
- Phone 1
- Zip Code
- Date of Birth
- Sex
- Patient Reference Balance
- Social Security Number

Other information in the Collection List dialog box includes the following:

Action This field lists the action required. To see all of the text entered for this field, double click in the field. This opens a window showing the complete text entry.

Statement Number If the tickler is for a patient, the statement number is listed.

Remainder Balance If the responsible type is Patient, the balance reported is the patient's balance as listed in Transaction Entry. If the responsible type is Insurance, the balance reported is an estimated balance for the patient's specified carrier. This is the balance at the time the tickler is created. This balance does not refresh when payments are made to the patient's account. To manually update the amounts, the tickler must be edited and saved again.

Insurance Estimate This field displays an estimate of the amount of payment expected from the insurance carrier.

Claim Number If the tickler is for an insurance carrier, the claim number is listed in this column.

Claim Total If the tickler is for an insurance carrier, the total amount of charges on the claim is listed here.

Status The entries in the field are Open, Resolved, and Deleted.

Follow Up Date This is the date the tickler will appear on the collection list.

Date Resolved This is the date that the status of the item was changed to Resolved. Resolution is determined by the user.

User ID The User ID identifies the user who is responsible for following up on the item. In an actual practice, users are assigned login names and passwords in the Security Setup area of the program.

ENTERING A TICKLER ITEM

A new tickler item is created by pressing the New button in the Collection List dialog box. This action opens the Tickler Item dialog box. The Tickler Item dialog box is displayed in Figure 10-11.

The Tickler Item dialog box contains two tabs for information: Tickler and Office Notes.

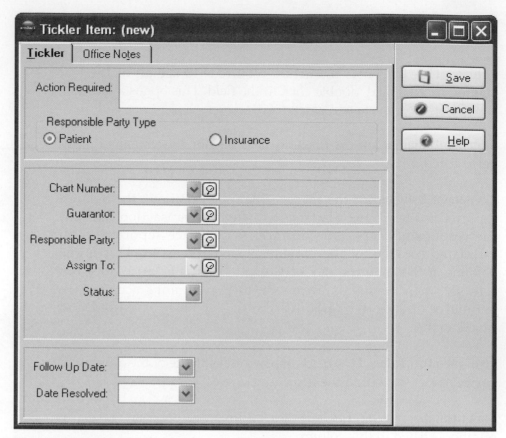

Figure 10-11 Tickler Item Dialog Box

Tickler Tab

The following information is entered in the Tickler tab:

Action Required   The Action Required field specifies the action that is to be taken to remedy the problem. Up to eighty characters of text can be entered.

Responsible Party Type   The button selected in this field indicates whether the patient or the insurance carrier is responsible for the account balance. This entry also controls the contents of the drop-down lists for the Responsible Party field below.

Chart Number   The patient's chart number is selected from the list.

Guarantor   The Guarantor field lists the account guarantor chart number for this tickler item.

Responsible Party   If the responsible party type is Patient, a chart number is selected from the drop-down list. If the responsible party type is Insurance, the code for an insurance carrier is selected.

Assign To   The Assign To box lists the name of the individual responsible for following up on the tickler item. These names are set up by selecting Security Setup on the File menu. *Note:* This feature is not demonstrated in this text/workbook, so the field is grayed out, and an entry cannot be made.

Status   The status of the tickler item is chosen from a drop-down list. The options are Open, Resolved, or Deleted.

Follow Up Date   This is the date the tickler will appear on the collection list if the Date range in the Collection List window is used. By default, Medisoft enters the current date—the Windows System Date—in this field.

Date Resolved   This field lists the date on which the status of the item was changed to Resolved. When the status is set to Resolved, the Date Resolved is set to the current date. Again, this is determined by the Windows System Date.

Office Notes Tab

The Office Notes tab consists of several buttons and a large area in which to enter notes. Notes that relate to the collection process of the selected tickler are entered in the large box.

When the right mouse button is clicked within the typing area, a shortcut menu is displayed (see Figure 10-12). Using this menu, notes can be edited, formatted, and printed from within the Office Notes tab.

Once a new tickler has been saved, the program automatically assigns a unique identifier code to the item.

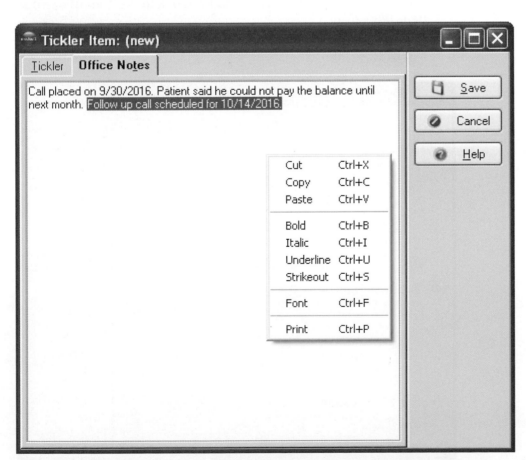

Figure 10-12   Office Notes Tab of the Tickler Item Dialog Box with Shortcut Menu Displayed

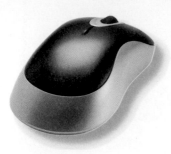

Using the information in Exercise 10-3, create a tickler item for the patient whose account is more than sixty days overdue.

Date: September 30, 2016

1. Change the Medisoft Program Date to September 30, 2016.
2. Select Collection List on the Activities menu.
3. Change the entries in the Date fields to **9/30/2016** and **9/30/2016**.
4. Click the New button to display the Tickler Item dialog box.
5. In the Action Required box, enter **Telephone call about overdue balance. See notes.**
6. Select Patient as the Responsible Party Type.
7. Select the patient's chart number in the Chart Number field.
8. Select the guarantor in the Guarantor field.
9. Complete the Responsible Party field.
10. Leave the Assign To field blank. (In a real practice setting, this field would contain the name of the staff member who was assigned to follow up on this collection list item.)
11. Set the Status of the item to Open.
12. Change the entry in the Follow Up Date box to the current exercise date, 9/30/2016.
13. Leave the Date Resolved field blank. Check your work against Figure 10-13.

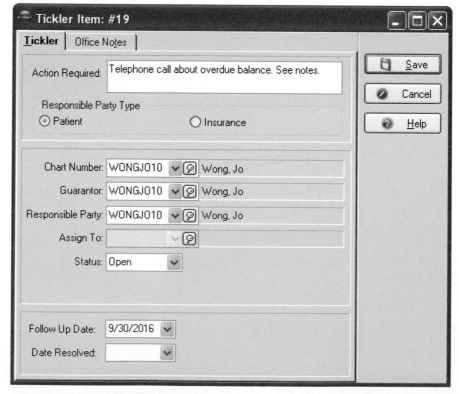

Figure 10-13   Completed Tickler Tab

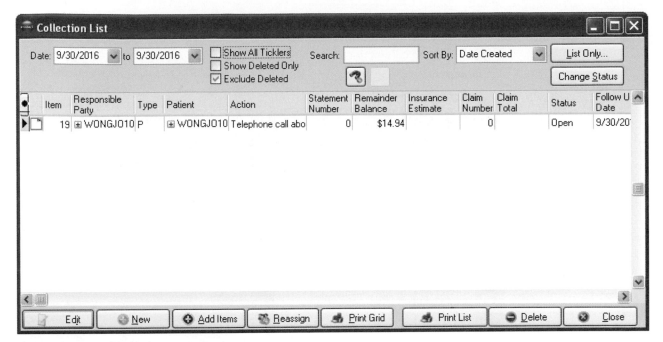

Figure 10-14   Tickler Added to Collection List

14. Click on the Office Notes tab, and enter the following text: **Patient said she could not pay the balance on the account until her Social Security check was deposited early next week.**

15. Click the Save button. The item is added to the collection list. Your screen should look like the window in Figure 10-14.

16. Click the Close button to close the Collection List dialog box. **CiMC**

 You have completed Exercise 10-4.

When an account is added to the collection list, the current balance for the tickler is determined. Once recorded in the tickler, it is not updated when new transactions are entered in the program.

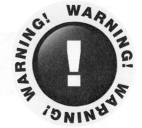

For patient-responsible ticklers, the balance is the balance shown in the Transaction Entry window. It could also include insurance balances. For insurance-responsible ticklers, the balance is the estimated amount due from the assigned insurance carrier.

10.8 CREATING COLLECTION LETTERS

A number of actions must be taken within Medisoft before collection letters can be sent. A patient-responsible tickler item for the patient's account must be entered in the collection list. Also, a collection letter report must be created. This report is generated when the Patient Collection Letters option is selected

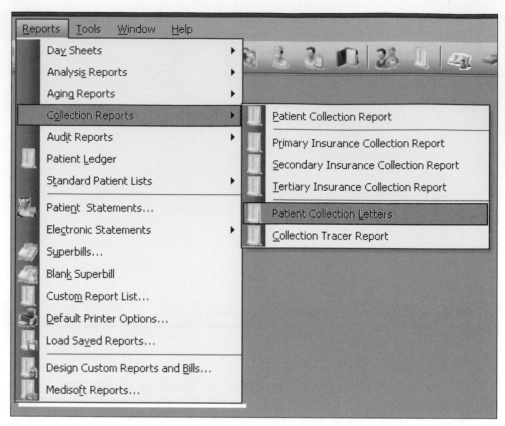

Figure 10-15   Patient Collection Letters Selected on the Collection Reports Submenu

Family Care Center
Collection Letter Report
10/31/2016

User ID:

Item	Status	Responsible Party	Patient Chart	Date Created	Date Resolved	Follow Up Date	Balance	# Days Old
21	Open	Kristin Zapata	ZAPATKR0	10/31/2016		10/31/2016	$247.50	0
20	Open	Elizabeth Jones	JONESEL0	10/31/2016		10/31/2016	$28.64	0

Figure 10-16   Collection Letter Report

on the Collection Reports submenu of the Reports menu (see Figure 10-15). The collection letter report lists patients with overdue accounts to whom statements have been mailed (see Figure 10-16).

After the patient collection report is printed (or the Preview window is closed), the program displays a Confirm window that asks whether to print collection letters (see Figure 10-17).

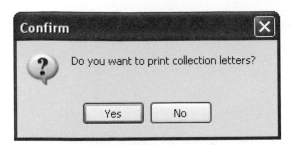

Figure 10-17   Confirm Dialog Box

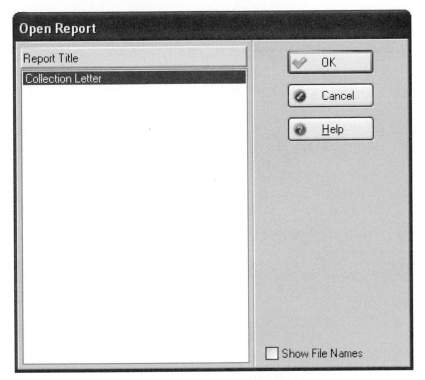

Figure 10-18   Open Report Window for Printing Collection Letters

If the Yes button is clicked, an Open Report dialog box appears (see Figure 10-18).

Once the OK button in the Open Report window is clicked, the program generates collection letters (see Figure 10-19).

After printing collection letters, an account alert appears in the Transaction Entry, Quick Ledger, and Appointment Entry windows and remains until the patient no longer has an open tickler in the collection list. There are three account alert abbreviations:

- RB   The patient has a remainder balance greater than the amount specified in the General tab in the Program Options window.

- DP   The patient is delinquent on his or her payment plan.

- IC   The patient account is in collections. (For this message to appear, a collection letter must have been printed.)

Family Care Center
285 Stephenson Boulevard
Stephenson, OH 60089
(614)555-0000

Kristin Zapata
109 East Milan Avenue
Stephenson, OH 60089

10/3/2016
Patient Account: Zapata, Kristin

Dear Kristin Zapata

Our records indicate that your account with us is overdue. The total unpaid amount is *$ 282.50

If you have already forwarded your payment, please disregard this letter; otherwise, please forward your payment immediately.

Please contact us at (614)555-0000 if you have any questions or concerns about your account.

Sincerely,

Katherine Yan

ZAPATKR0

*Balance does not reflect any outstanding insurance payments

Figure 10-19   Patient Collection Letter

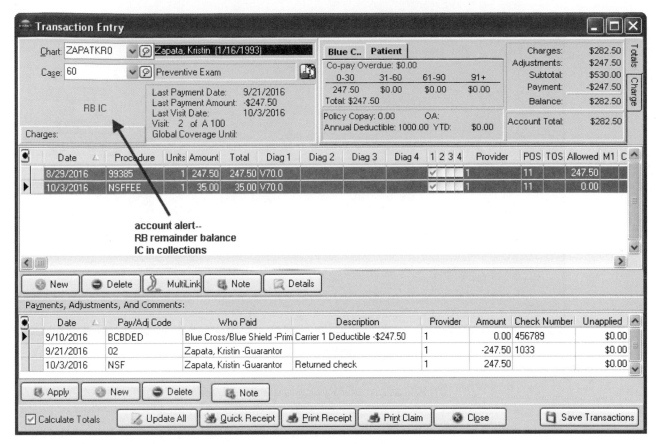

Figure 10-20   Transaction Entry Dialog Box with Account Alert Message Displayed

A sample account alert in the Transaction Entry window is displayed in Figure 10-20.

CREATING A COLLECTION LETTER	EXERCISE 10-5

Create a collection letter for the patient you added to the collection list in Exercise 10-4.

Date: September 30, 2016

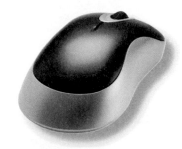

1. Select Collection Reports > Patient Collection Letters on the Reports menu. The Print Report Where? dialog box appears. Accept the default entry to preview the report on the screen, and click the Start button. The Data Selection Questions dialog box appears.

2. Leave the Responsible Party Range and the Patient Range boxes blank. Enter **9/30/2016** in both Follow Up Date Range boxes.

3. Leave the other boxes as they are, except for the check boxes at the bottom of the dialog box. Click the box Exclude items that follow Payment Plan.

4. Click the Generate Collection Letters box. The Add to Collection Tracer box will automatically be checked. Compare your screen to Figure 10-21.

5. Click the OK button. The collection letter report appears.

6. Click the Close button to exit the Preview window.

Collection Letter Report: Data Selection Questions

NOTE: A blank field indicates no limitation, all records will be included.

Responsible Party Range:	[▼ 🔍]	to	[▼ 🔍]
Patient Range:	[▼ 🔍]	to	[▼ 🔍]
Follow Up Date Range:	9/30/2016 ▼	to	9/30/2016 ▼
Date Created Range:	[▼]	to	[▼]
Item Number Range:	[ ]	to	[ ]
Balance Range:	0.01	to	99999
Status Match:	0 ▼		

☑ Exclude items that follow Payment Plan

☑ Generate Collection Letters

☑ Add To Collection Tracer

[✔ OK]
[⊘ Cancel]
[❓ Help]

Figure 10-21 Data Selection Questions Dialog Box Completed

7. A Confirm dialog box is displayed, asking if collection letters should be printed. Click the Yes button. The Open Report window appears.

8. Select Collection Letter if it is not already selected, and click OK.

9. The Print Report Where? dialog box appears. Select the option to send the report directly to the printer, and click the Start button. (*Note:* If the letter is not actually printed, the account alert message feature will not work in the next step.)

10. Open the Transaction Entry dialog box, and select Jo Wong in the Chart field. Notice that the letters *RB IC* appear in red in the upper-left section of the window. This is an account alert message, indicating that the account has a remainder balance and is in collections. Close the Transaction Entry dialog box.

Note: The date shown in the collection letter is the current date—the Windows System Date. In an actual office setting, this date would be the actual date the letter was created.

☑ **You have completed Exercise 10-5.**

10.9 CREATING A COLLECTION TRACER REPORT

collection tracer report a tool for keeping track of collection letters that were sent

A **collection tracer report** is used to keep track of collection letters that were sent. The report lists the tickler item number, the responsible party, the chart number, the account balance (as of the date the tickler was created), the date the collection letter was sent, and the reasons the account is in collections (see Figure 10-22).

Family Care Center

Collection Tracer Report

10/31/2016

Item #	Responsible Party	Patient Chart	Balance	Date Letter Sent	Reasons
Elizabeth Jones					
2	Elizabeth Jones	JONESEL0	28.64	10/31/2016	The outstanding balance is greater than 0.01.
					Total Letters Sent: 1
Kristin Zapata					
3	Kristin Zapata	ZAPATKR0	247.50	10/31/2016	The outstanding balance is greater than 0.01.
					Total Letters Sent: 1

Figure 10-22 Collection Tracer Report

CREATING A COLLECTION TRACER REPORT	EXERCISE 10-6

Create a collection tracer report.

Date: September 30, 2016

1. Select Collection Reports > Collection Tracer Report on the Reports menu.

2. In the Print Report Where? dialog box, click the Start button to preview the report on the screen.

3. In the Data Selection Questions dialog box, select Jo Wong in both Responsible Party Range boxes.

4. Leave the Date Letter Sent Range boxes blank to include all dates.

5. Click the OK button.

6. The report appears in the Preview window. When you are finished viewing the report, close the Preview window. **CiMC**

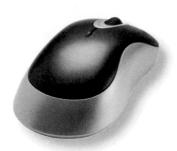

 You have completed Exercise 10-6.

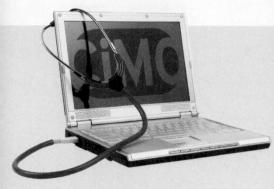

APPLYING YOUR SKILLS
9: PRINT A PATIENT AGING REPORT

December 30, 2016
Print a Date Accurate Patient Aging by Date of Service report for charges, payments, and adjustments on or before 12/30/2016. (This report is included in the new Medisoft Reports feature, in the Aging Power Pack folder.) Review the status of Lisa Wright's account.

APPLYING YOUR SKILLS
10: ADD A PATIENT TO THE COLLECTION LIST

December 30, 2016
Add an item to the collection list for patient Lisa Wright. Notice that her account has an overdue balance. Add a tickler to the collection list indicating that her account is overdue. Enter *12/30/2016* as the follow-up date.

APPLYING YOUR SKILLS
EXERCISE 11: CREATE A COLLECTION LETTER

December 30, 2016
Create a collection letter for Lisa Wright. When setting up the collection letter report, be sure to enter Lisa Wright's chart number in the Responsible Party Range boxes; check the Exclude items that follow Payment Plan box and the Generate Collection Letters box. The Add to Collection Tracer box will be checked automatically.

Remember to create a backup of your work before exiting Medisoft! To help you keep track of your work, name the backup file after the chapter you are working on, for example, StudentID-c10.mbk.

Name: _____ Date: _____

After completing all the exercises in the chapter, answer the following questions in the spaces provided.

1. *[LO 10.4]* In Exercise 10-1, what is the amount of the payment entered on 10/31/2016?

   _____

2. *[LO 10.5]* In Exercise 10-2, what is entered in the Pay/Adj Code box for the entry on 11/30/2016?

   _____

3. *[LO 10.6]* In Exercise 10-4, who is listed in the Responsible Party field of the Tickler Item dialog box?

   _____

4. *[LO 10.7]* In Exercise 10-4, what is listed in the Status column of the Collection List dialog box?

   _____

5. *[LO 10.6]* In the collection letter printed in Exercise 10-5, what is listed as the total unpaid amount?

   _____

6. *[LO 10.8]* After completing Exercise 10-5, what four letters are displayed under the Case field in the Transaction Entry dialog box for Jo Wong?

   _____

7. *[LO 10.9]* In the report created in Applying Your Skills Exercise 9, how many patients have accounts that are more than 121 days late?

   _____

8. *[LO 10.9]* What is listed in the Guarantor field in the Tickler Item dialog box in Applying Your Skills Exercise 10?

   _____

9. *[LO 10.9]* In Applying Your Skills Exercise 11, whose name appears after the closing "Sincerely,"?

   _____

10. *[LO 10.9]* In Applying Your Skills Exercise 11, what is listed as the total unpaid amount in the letter to Lisa Wright?

    _____

10.1 Explain the importance of prompt payment laws. Page 344	Prompt payment laws require insurance carriers to pay claims in a timely manner.
10.2 Summarize the importance of a financial policy in a medical office. Pages 344–347	A financial policy is used to communicate how a practice handles financial matters, such as past-due balances and payments for services not covered by insurance. When patients are aware of and understand a practice's financial policy, they are more likely to pay their accounts on time.
10.3 Identify the laws that regulate collections from patients. Pages 347–348	The Fair Debt Collection Practices Act of 1977 and the Telephone Consumer Protection Act of 1991 regulate debt collections.
10.4 Demonstrate how to post a payment from a collection agency. Pages 348–350	1. On the Activities menu, click Enter Transactions. 2. Select the patient in the Chart box. 3. Verify that the correct case is active in the Case box. 4. In the Payments, Adjustments, and Comments section of the dialog box, click the New button. 5. Verify the entry in the Date box. 6. Click in the Pay/Adj Code box, and select the payment code 04—Patient pymt via collections. 7. Verify that the guarantor is listed in the Who Paid box. 8. Enter *Collections payment* in the Description field. 9. Enter the amount of the payment in the Amount box. 10. Click the Apply button. 11. Enter the amount of the payment that is to be applied to each charge until the unapplied amount is zero. 12. Click the Close button. 13. Click the Save Transactions button.

10.5 Discuss the process of writing off uncollectible accounts. Pages 350–352	1. Open the Transaction Entry dialog box. 2. Select the patient in the Chart box. 3. Verify that the correct case is active in the Case box. 4. In the Payments, Adjustments, and Comments section of the dialog box, click the New button. 5. Verify the entry in the Date box. 6. Click in the Pay/Adj Code box, and select WRITEOFF—Write Off as the adjustment code. 7. Verify that the guarantor is listed in the Who Paid box. 8. Enter the amount to be written off in the Amount box. 9. Click the Apply button. 10. Locate the Balance column. In the This Adjust. Column, enter an amount equal to the amount in the Balance column for each outstanding charge. 11. When all the charges have been adjusted, click the Close button. 12. Click the Save Transactions button. 13. Close the Transaction Entry dialog box.
10.6 Explain how to use a patient aging report to identify past-due accounts. Pages 352–353	The aging report shows the status of each patient's account over time. For each account, an aging report shows the patient's chart number and name, and the amount of unpaid charges categorized by the number of days past due. Using this report, it is possible to identify patients who have the largest outstanding balance, as well as the most overdue balance.
10.7 Demonstrate how to add an account to the collection list. Pages 353–361	1. Select Collection List on the Activities menu. 2. Make appropriate entries in the Date fields. 3. Click the New button to display the Tickler Item dialog box. 4. Make an appropriate entry in the Action Required box. 5. Select Patient as the Responsible Party Type. 6. Select the patient's chart number in the Chart Number field. 7. Select the guarantor in the Guarantor field. 8. Complete the Responsible Party field. 9. Leave the Assign To field blank. (In a real practice setting, this field would contain the name of the staff member who was assigned to follow up on this collection list item.) 10. Set the Status of the item to Open. 11. Enter a value in the Follow Up Date field. 12. Leave the Date Resolved field blank. 13. Click the Office Notes tab, and enter any additional notes. 14. Click the Save button. 15. The account is added to the collection list. Close the Collection List dialog box.

10.8 Demonstrate how to create a collection letter. Pages 361–366	1. Select Collection Reports > Patient Collection Letters on the Reports menu.
	2. The Print Report Where? dialog box appears. Make an appropriate entry. The Data Selection Questions dialog box appears.
	3. If needed, make selections in the following boxes:
	Responsible Party Range
	Patient Range
	Follow Up Date Range
	Date Created Range
	Item Number Range
	Balance Range
	Status Match
	4. Click in the Exclude items that follow Payment Plan box.
	5. Click in the Generate Collection Letters box. The Add to Collection Tracer box will automatically be checked.
	6. Click the OK button. The collection letter report appears.
	7. Click the Close button to exit the Preview window.
	8. A Confirm dialog box is displayed, asking if collection letters should be printed. Click the Yes button. The Open Report window appears.
	9. Select Collection Letter if it is not already selected, and click OK.
	10. The Print Report Where? dialog box appears. Select the option to send the report directly to the printer, and click the Start button. (*Note:* If the letter is not actually printed, the account alert message feature will not work.)
10.9 Demonstrate how to create a collection tracer report. Pages 366–367	1. Select Collection Reports > Collection Tracer Report on the Reports menu.
	2. In the Print Report Where? dialog box, click the Start button to preview the report on the screen.
	3. In the Data Selection Questions dialog box, enter information as needed in the Responsible Party Range and Date Letter Sent Range boxes.
	4. Click the OK button.
	5. The report appears in the Preview window. When you are finished viewing the report, close the Preview window.

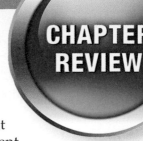

USING TERMINOLOGY

Match the terms on the left with the definitions on the right.

_____ **1.** *[LO 10.4]* collection agency

_____ **2.** *[LO 10.7]* collection list

_____ **3.** *[LO 10.9]* collection tracer report

_____ **4.** *[LO 10.3]* payment plan

_____ **5.** *[LO 10.1]* prompt payment laws

_____ **6.** *[LO 10.7]* tickler

_____ **7.** *[LO 10.5]* uncollectible account

_____ **8.** *[LO 10.5]* write-off

a. An agreement between a patient and a practice in which the patient agrees to make regular monthly payments over a specified period of time.

b. A reminder to follow up on an account.

c. An outside firm hired to collect on delinquent accounts.

d. An account that does not respond to collection efforts and is written off the practice's expected accounts receivable.

e. A balance that is removed from a patient's account.

f. Legislation that mandates a time period within which clean claims must be paid; if they are not, financial penalties are levied against the payer.

g. A tool for tracking activities that need to be completed as part of the collection process.

h. A tool for tracking collection letters that were sent.

CHECKING YOUR UNDERSTANDING

Write "T" or "F" in the blank to indicate whether you think the statement is true or false.

1. *[LO 10.2]* Accounts that are overdue are treated equally; accounts with small balances are just as likely to be sent for collections as accounts with large balances. _____

2. *[LO 10.3]* Collection activities regarding patient accounts are considered business collections and are not regulated by federal or state law. _____

3. *[LO 10.3]* By law, payment plans cannot include finance charges. _____

4. *[LO 10.6]* Aging reports are used to determine which accounts are overdue. _____

5. *[LO 10.6]* An account is considered current if it is paid within thirty days. _____

6. *[LO 10.7]* A tickler item entered on the collection list includes a follow-up date for action. _____

Choose the best answer.

1. *[LO 10.7]* In the Collection List dialog box, the entry in the Type field, which describes the responsible party, is either *P* for Patient or
   a. *G* for Guarantor
   b. *C* for Child
   c. *I* for Insurance

2. *[LO 10.3]* General guidelines for telephone collection practices recommend not calling before 8:00 A.M. or after
   a. 8:00 P.M.
   b. 9:00 P.M.
   c. 10:00 P.M.

3. *[LO 10.3]* An arrangement in which a patient agrees to make a regular monthly payment on an account for a specified period of time is known as a
   a. financial plan
   b. payment plan
   c. payment policy

4. *[LO 10.5]* An account that must be written off the practice's expected accounts receivable is
   a. an overdue account
   b. an uncollectible account
   c. a tickler account

APPLYING YOUR KNOWLEDGE

Answer the questions below in the space provided.

10.1. *[LO 10.2]* What is the purpose of a medical practice's financial policy?

_____

_____

10.2. *[LO 10.2]* What is the first step in the collection process?

_____

_____

10.3. *[LO 10.6]* How is an aging report used to identify accounts for collection?

_____

_____

10.4. *[LO 10.8]* What two steps need to occur before a collection letter can be printed in Medisoft?

_____

_____

THINKING ABOUT IT

Answer the questions below in the space provided.

10.1. *[LO 10. 2]* Why is it important for a medical practice to share its financial policy with patients?

_____

_____

10.2. *[LO 10.4]* What are the positive and negative factors in using an outside collection agency to pursue overdue patient accounts?

_____

_____

AT THE COMPUTER

Answer the following question at the computer.

10.1. *[LO 10.6]* Create a Date Accurate Patient Aging by Date of Service report for the period ending December 31, 2016. Which account has the largest total overdue balance (regardless of number of days past due)? Which patient has the smallest overdue balance?

_____

_____

chapter
11

Scheduling

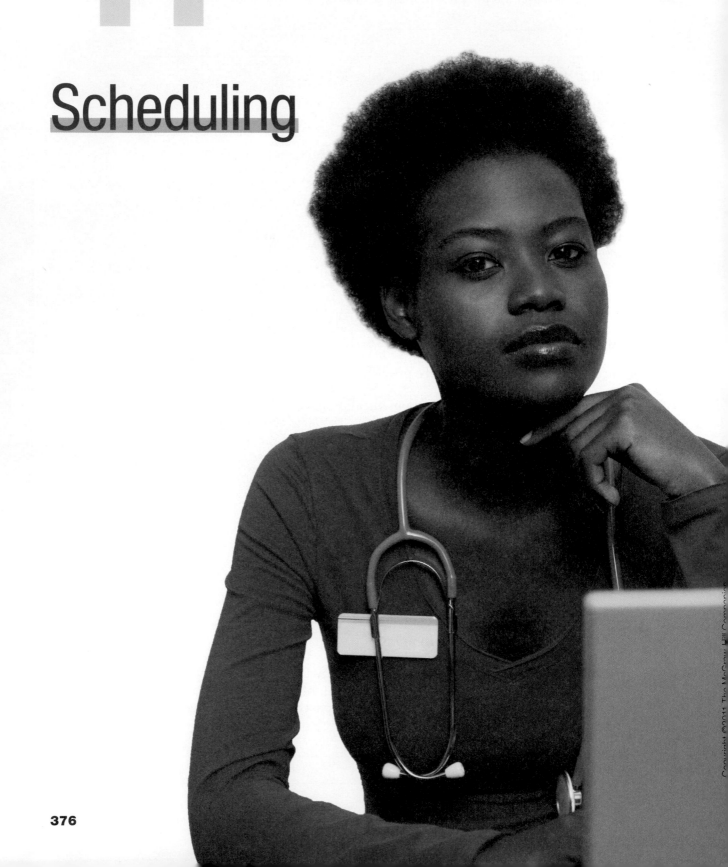

key terms

Office Hours break

Office Hours calendar

Office Hours patient
information

provider's daily schedule

provider selection box

learning outcomes

When you finish this chapter, you will be able to:

11.1 List the four main areas of the Office Hours window.

11.2 Demonstrate how to enter an appointment.

11.3 Demonstrate how to schedule a follow-up appointment.

11.4 Demonstrate how to search for an available time slot.

11.5 Demonstrate how to book an appointment for a new patient.

11.6 Demonstrate how to book repeating appointments.

11.7 Demonstrate how to reschedule an appointment.

11.8 Demonstrate how to create a recall list.

11.9 Demonstrate how to enter provider breaks in the schedule.

11.10 Demonstrate how to print a provider's schedule.

11.11 Demonstrate how to create an overdue balance report for upcoming appointments.

what you need to know

To use this chapter, you need to know how to:

- Start Medisoft, use menus, and enter and edit text.
- Work with chart numbers and codes.
- Locate patient information.

Appointment scheduling is one of the most important tasks in a medical office. Different medical procedures take different lengths of time, and each appointment must be the right length. On the one hand, a physician wants to be able to go from one appointment to another without unnecessary breaks. On the other hand, a patient should not be kept waiting more than a few minutes for a physician. Managing and juggling the schedule are usually the job of a medical office assistant working at the front desk. Medisoft® provides a special program called Office Hours to handle appointment scheduling.

11.1 THE OFFICE HOURS WINDOW

The Office Hours program has its own window (see Figure 11-1), including its own menu bar and toolbar. The Office Hours menu bar lists the menus available: File, Edit, View, Lists, Reports, Tools, and Help (see Figure 11-2). Under the menu bar is a toolbar with shortcut buttons. The functions of Office Hours are accessed by selecting a choice from one of the menus or by clicking a button on the toolbar.

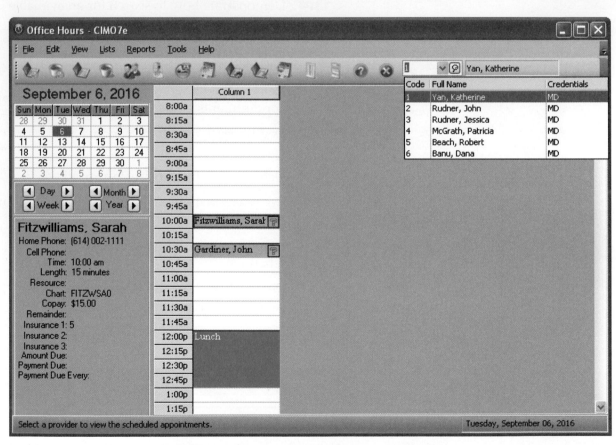

Figure 11-1   The Office Hours Window

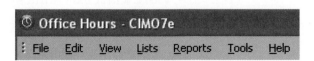

Figure 11-2   The Office Hours Menu Bar

Figure 11-3 The Office Hours Toolbar

Located just below the menu bar, the toolbar contains a series of buttons that represent the most common activities performed in Office Hours. These buttons are shortcuts for frequently used menu commands. The toolbar displays fifteen buttons (see Figure 11-3 and Table 11-1).

TABLE 11-1	Office Hours Toolbar Buttons		
Button	**Button Name**	**Associated Function**	**Activity**
	Appointment Entry	New Appointment Entry dialog box	Enter appointments
	Break Entry	New Break Entry dialog box	Enter breaks
	Appointment List	Appointment List dialog box	Display list of appointments
	Break List	Break List dialog box	Display list of breaks
	Patient List	Patient List dialog box	Display list of patients
	Provider List	Provider List dialog box	Display list of providers
	Resource List	Resource List dialog box	Display list of resources
	Go to a Date	Go to Date dialog box	Change calendar to a different date
	Search for Open Time Slot	Find Open Time dialog box	Locate first available time slot
	Search Again	Find Open Time dialog box	Locate next available time slot
	Go to Today		Return calendar to current date
	Print Appointment List		Print appointment list
	Edit Patient Notes in Final Draft	Final Draft word processor	Use Final Draft word processor
	Help	Office Hours Help	Display Office Hours Help contents
	Exit	Exit	Exit the Office Hours program

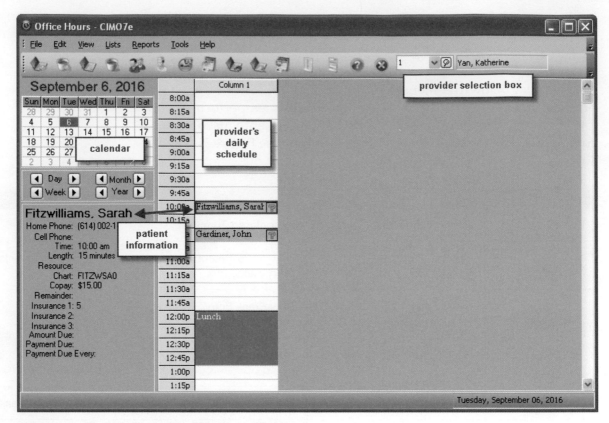

Figure 11-4 The Main Areas of the Office Hours Window

provider selection box
a selection box that determines which provider's schedule is displayed in the provider's daily schedule

provider's daily schedule
a listing of time slots for a particular day for a specific provider that corresponds to the date selected in the calendar

Office Hours calendar
an interactive calendar that is used to select or change dates in Office Hours

Office Hours patient information the area of the Office Hours window that displays information about the patient who is selected in the provider's daily schedule

In addition to the menu bar and toolbar, the Office Hours window contains four main areas (see Figure 11-4). The **provider selection box,** located at the far-right end of the toolbar, is where you select a provider. This selection determines which provider's schedule is displayed in the provider's daily schedule. The **provider's daily schedule,** shown in the right half of the screen, is a listing of time slots for a particular day for a specific provider. The schedule displayed corresponds to the date selected in the calendar, which is located on the left side of the window. The **Office Hours calendar** is used to select or change dates. The right and left arrows that surround Day, Week, Month, and Year are used to move back or ahead on the calendar. When a different date is clicked on the calendar, the calendar switches to the new date. Finally, the area just below the calendar contains **Office Hours patient information** about the patient who is selected in the provider's daily schedule.

PROGRAM OPTIONS

When Office Hours is installed in a medical practice, it is set up to reflect the needs of that particular practice. Most offices that use Medisoft already have Office Hours set up and running. However, if Medisoft is just being installed, the options to set up the Office Hours program can be found in the Program Options dialog box, which is accessed by clicking Program Options on the Office Hours File menu.

ENTERING AND EXITING OFFICE HOURS

Office Hours can be started from within Medisoft or directly from Windows. To access Office Hours from within Medisoft, Appointment Book is clicked on the Activities menu (see Figure 11-5). Office Hours can also be started by clicking the corresponding shortcut button on the toolbar (see Figure 11-6).

To start Office Hours without entering Medisoft first:

1. Click Start > All Programs.

2. Click Medisoft on the Programs submenu.

3. Click Office Hours on the Medisoft submenu.

The Office Hours program is closed by clicking Exit on the Office Hours File menu or by clicking the Exit button on its toolbar. If Office Hours was started from within Medisoft, exiting will return you to Medisoft. If Office Hours was started directly from Windows, clicking Exit will return you to the Windows desktop.

11.2 ENTERING APPOINTMENTS

Entering an appointment begins with selecting the provider for whom the appointment is being scheduled. The current provider is listed in the provider selection box at the upper-right of the screen (see Figure 11-7). Clicking the arrow button displays a drop-down list of providers in the system. To choose a different provider, click the name of the provider on the drop-down list.

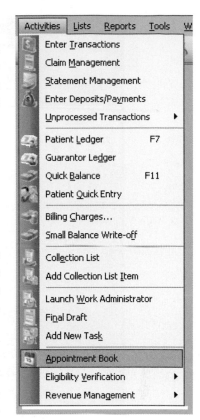

Figure 11-5 The Appointment Book Selection on the Activities Menu

Figure 11-6
The Office Hours Shortcut Button

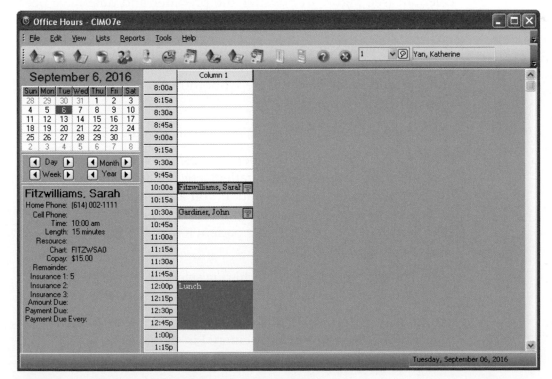

Figure 11-7 Office Hours Window with Provider Box Highlighted

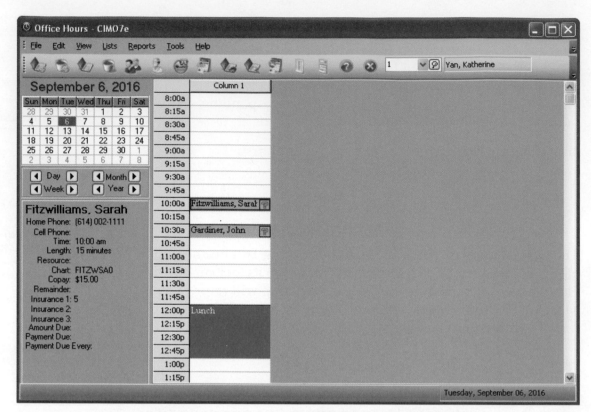

Figure 11-8 Office Hours Window with Day, Week, Month, and Year Arrow Buttons Highlighted

After the provider is selected, the date of the desired appointment must be chosen. Dates are changed by clicking the Day, Week, Month, and Year right and left arrow buttons located under the calendar (see Figure 11-8). After the provider and date have been selected, patient appointments can be entered.

Appointments are entered by clicking the Appointment Entry shortcut button or by double clicking in a time slot on the schedule. When either action is taken, the New Appointment Entry dialog box is displayed (see Figure 11-9).

The New Appointment Entry dialog box contains the following fields:

Chart A patient's chart number is chosen from the Chart dropdown list. To select the desired patient, click on the patient's name in the drop-down list and press Tab. If you are setting up an appointment for a new patient who has not been assigned a chart number, skip the Chart box, and key the patient's name in the blank box to the right of the Chart box.

Home Phone After a patient's chart is selected, that patient's home phone number is automatically entered in the Home Phone box.

Cell Phone After a patient's chart is selected, that patient's cell phone number is automatically entered in the Cell Phone box.

Resource This box is used if the practice assigns codes to resources, such as exam rooms or equipment.

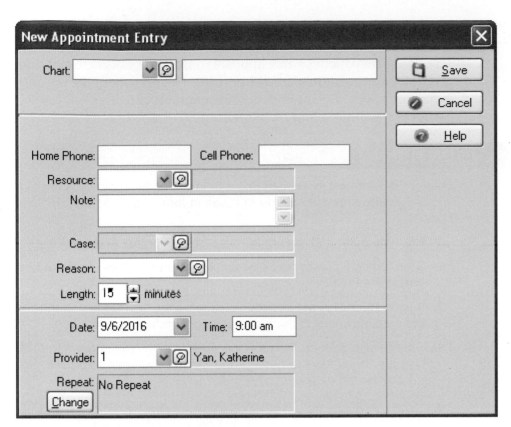

Figure 11-9   New Appointment Entry Dialog Box

Note   Any special information about an appointment is entered in the Note box.

Case   The case that pertains to the appointment is selected from the drop-down list of cases.

Reason   Reason codes can be set up in the program to reflect the reason for an appointment.

Length   The amount of time an appointment will take (in minutes) is entered in the Length box by keying the number of minutes or using the up and down arrows.

Date   The Date box displays the date that is currently displayed on the calendar. If this is not the desired date, it may be changed by keying in a different date or by clicking the arrow button and selecting a date from the pop-up calendar that appears.

Time   The Time box displays the appointment time that is currently selected on the schedule. If this is not the desired time, it may be changed by keying in a different time.

Provider   The provider who will be treating the patient during this appointment is selected from the drop-down list of providers.

Repeat   The Repeat box is used to enter appointments that recur on a regular basis.

After the boxes in the New Appointment Entry dialog box have been completed, clicking the Save button enters the information on the schedule. The patient's name appears in the time slot corresponding to the appointment time. In addition, information about the patient's insurance appears in the patient information section in the lower-left corner of the Office Hours window.

EXERCISE 11-1   ENTERING AN APPOINTMENT

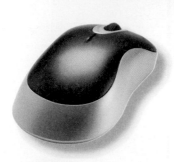

Enter an appointment for Herbert Bell at 3:00 P.M. on Monday, November 14, 2016. The appointment is sixty minutes in length and is with Dr. John Rudner.

1. Start Medisoft and restore the data from your last work session.

2. Start Office Hours by clicking the Appointment Book shortcut button on the toolbar.

3. If John Rudner is not already selected, click "2 - Rudner, John" on the drop-down list in the provider selection box to select him.

4. Change the date on the calendar to Monday, November 14, 2016. Use the arrow keys to change the month and year, and then click the day on the calendar.

5. Locate 3:00 P.M. in the schedule and click once to select it. (You may need to use the scroll bar to view 3:00 P.M.) Figure 11-10 shows the Office Hours window with John Rudner selected as provider, November 14, 2016, on the calendar, and the 3:00 P.M. time slot highlighted. Compare your screen to Figure 11-10.

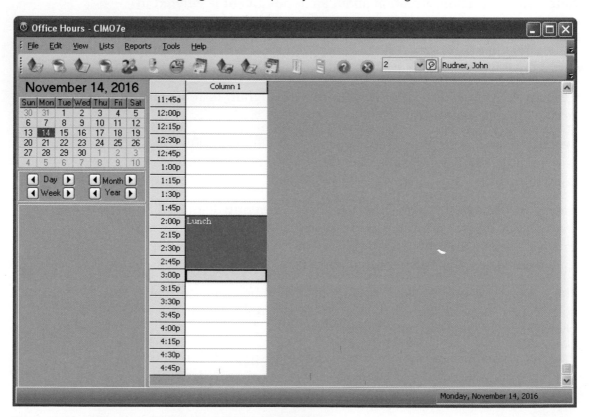

Figure 11-10   Office Hours Window with Selections Highlighted

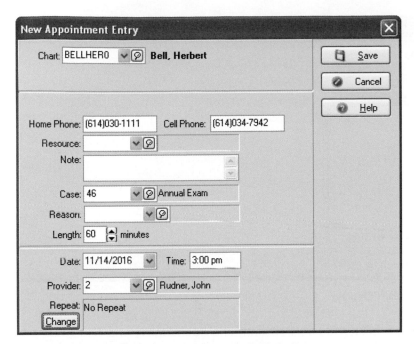

New Appointment Entry

Chart: BELLHERO ▾ 🔍 **Bell, Herbert**

Home Phone: (614)030-1111   Cell Phone: (614)034-7942

Resource: ▾ 🔍

Note:

Case: 46 ▾ 🔍 Annual Exam

Reason: ▾ 🔍

Length: 60 ⬍ minutes

Date: 11/14/2016 ▾   Time: 3:00 pm

Provider: 2 ▾ 🔍 Rudner, John

Repeat: No Repeat

[Change]

[💾 Save] [⊘ Cancel] [❓ Help]

Figure 11-11   Completed New Appointment Entry Dialog Box

6. In the schedule, double click the 3:00 P.M. time slot. The New Appointment Entry dialog box is displayed.

7. Click Herbert Bell from the list of names on the drop-down list in the Chart box, and press Tab. The system automatically fills in a number of boxes in the dialog box, such as the patient's name and home and cell phone numbers.

8. Accept the default entry in the Case box.

9. Notice that the Length box already contains an entry of fifteen minutes. This is the default appointment length set up in Medisoft. Since Herbert Bell's appointment is for an annual exam, this entry must be changed to sixty minutes. Key **60** in the Length box, or use the up arrow next to the Length box to change the appointment length to sixty minutes.

10. Check your entries against Figure 11-11, and then click the Save button. Medisoft saves the appointment and closes the dialog box. Herbert Bell's name is displayed in the 3:00 P.M. time slot on the schedule as well as in the patient information section on the left.

 You have completed Exercise 11-1.

LOOKING UP A PROVIDER AND ENTERING AN APPOINTMENT   **EXERCISE 11-2**

Enter a thirty-minute appointment on Thursday, November 10, 2016, at 9:00 A.M. for John Gardiner. You do not know his provider, so this information must be looked up before you enter the appointment.

1. Select Patient List on the Lists menu in Office Hours. The Patient List dialog box is displayed.

2. Enter **G** in the Search for box to select John Gardiner (see Figure 11-12).

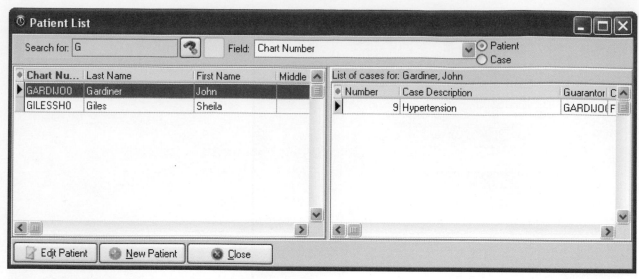

Figure 11-12 Patient List Dialog Box with John Gardiner Selected

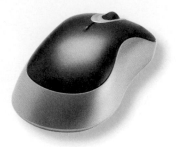

3. Double click the line that contains John Gardiner's chart number and name, or click the Edit Patient button. The Patient/Guarantor dialog box appears.

4. Click the Other Information tab, and locate the Assigned Provider field to determine the name of John Gardiner's provider.

5. To close the Patient/Guarantor dialog box, click the Cancel button.

6. Click the Close button to close the Patient List dialog box. You are back to the main Office Hours window.

7. Select John Gardiner's provider in the provider selection box on the toolbar, and enter the appointment. Remember to set the Office Hours calendar to the correct date. **CiMO**

 You have completed Exercise 11-2.

11.3 BOOKING FOLLOW-UP APPOINTMENTS

Often a patient will need a follow-up appointment at a certain time in the future. For example, suppose a physician would like a patient to return for a checkup in three weeks. The most efficient way to search for a future appointment in Office Hours is to use the Go to a Date shortcut button on the toolbar. (This feature can also be accessed on the Edit menu.)

Clicking the Go to a Date shortcut button displays the Go To Date dialog box (see Figure 11-13). Within the dialog box, five boxes offer options for choosing a future date.

Date From This box indicates the current date in the appointment search.

Figure 11-13 Go To Date Dialog Box

Go ___ Days This box is used to locate a date that is a specific number of days in the future. For example, if a patient needs an appointment ten days from the current day, *10* would be entered in this box.

Go ___ Weeks This box is used when a patient needs an appointment a specific number of weeks in the future, such as six weeks from the current day.

Go ___ Months This box is used when a patient needs an appointment a specific number of months in the future, such as three months from the current day.

Go ___ Years Similar to the weeks and months options, this box is used when an appointment is needed in one year or several years in the future.

After a future date option has been selected, clicking the Go button closes the dialog box and begins the search. The system locates the future date and displays the calendar schedule for that date.

BOOKING APPOINTMENTS, INCLUDING FOLLOW-UP — EXERCISE 11-3

Enter the following appointments with Dr. John Rudner.

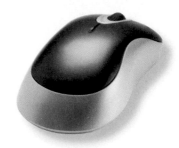

1. The first appointment is Monday, November 14, 2016, at 4:00 P.M. for John Fitzwilliams, thirty minutes in length. Select "2 Rudner, John" in the Provider box.

2. Change the date in the Office Hours calendar to Monday, November 14, 2016.

3. In the schedule, scroll down and double click the 4:00 P.M. time-slot box.

4. Select John Fitzwilliams on the Chart drop-down list.

5. Press the Tab key. The program automatically completes several boxes in the dialog box.

6. Press the Tab key until the entry in the Length box is highlighted.

7. Key *30* in the Length box, or click the up arrow once to change the length to thirty minutes.

8. Click the Save button. Verify that the appointment for John Fitzwilliams appears on the schedule for November 14, 2016, at 4:00 P.M. for a length of thirty minutes.

9. Enter an appointment on Monday, November 14, 2016, at 4:30 P.M. for Leila Patterson, fifteen minutes in length.

10. Enter an appointment on Tuesday, November 15, 2016, at 12:15 P.M. for James Smith, thirty minutes in length.

11. To schedule an appointment for James Smith two weeks after November 15, 2016, at 12:15 P.M., fifteen minutes in length, click the Go to a Date shortcut button.

12. Key **2** in the Go ___ Weeks box. Click the Go button. The program closes the Go To Date box and displays the appointment schedule for November 29, 2016, at 12:15 P.M.

13. Enter James Smith's appointment.

✓ **You have completed Exercise 11-3.**

| EXERCISE 11-4 | BOOKING FOLLOW-UP APPOINTMENTS |

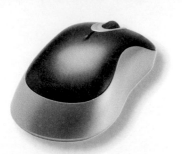

Enter these appointments with Dr. Jessica Rudner.

1. Click Dr. Jessica Rudner from the list of providers in the Provider drop-down list.

2. Enter a fifteen-minute appointment for Friday, November 18, 2016, at 3:00 P.M. for Janine Bell.

3. Use the Go to a Date feature to schedule an appointment three weeks from November 18, 2016, at 1:15 P.M. for Sarina Bell, thirty minutes in length.

4. Schedule a fifteen-minute appointment for Sarah Fitzwilliams one week from November 18, 2016, at 9:00 A.M.

✓ **You have completed Exercise 11-4.**

11.4 SEARCHING FOR AVAILABLE TIME SLOTS

Often it is necessary to search for available appointment space on a particular day of the week and at a specific time. For example, a patient needs a thirty-minute appointment and would like it to be during his lunch hour, which is from 12:00 P.M. to 1:00 P.M. He can get away from the office only on Mondays and Fridays. Office Hours makes it easy to locate an appointment slot that meets these requirements with the Search for Open Time Slot shortcut button.

| EXERCISE 11-5 | SEARCHING FOR OPEN TIME, RAMOS |

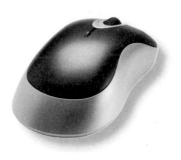

Maritza Ramos needs an appointment, but she has very limited times she can come in to the office. Search for the next available appointment slot with Dr. Yan on a Tuesday, 30 minutes in length, between 11:00 A.M. and 2:00 P.M., beginning November 10, 2016.

1. Select Dr. Katherine Yan in the Provider box on the toolbar, and change the calendar to November 10, 2016.

2. On the Edit menu, click Find Open Time, or click the Search for Open Time Slot shortcut button. The Find Open Time dialog box is displayed (see Figure 11-14).

3. Key **30** in the Length box. Press the Tab key.

4. Key **11** in the Start Time box. Press the Tab key.

5. Key **2** in the End Time box. Press the Tab key.

6. To search for an appointment on Tuesday, click the Tuesday box in the Day of Week area of the dialog box. The Find Open Time dialog box should look like Figure 11-15.

7. Click the Search button to begin looking for an appointment slot. The Find Open Time dialog box closes and locates the first available time slot that meets these specifications. The time slot is outlined on the schedule.

8. Double click the selected time slot. Click Maritza Ramos on the drop-down list in the Chart box.

9. Press the Tab key until the cursor is in the Length box.

10. Key **30**, and press the Tab key.

11. Click the Save button.

12. Verify that the appointment has been entered by looking at the schedule. **CIMC**

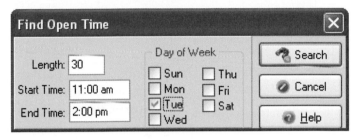

Figure 11-14   Find Open Time Dialog Box

Figure 11-15   Completed Find Open Time Dialog Box

☑ **You have completed Exercise 11-5.**

SEARCHING FOR OPEN TIME, KLEIN   EXERCISE 11-6

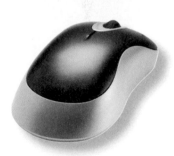

Schedule Randall Klein for a thirty-minute appointment with Dr. John Rudner sometime after November 14, 2016. Mr. Klein is available only on Mondays between 3:00 P.M. and 5:00 P.M.

1. Click the desired provider in the Provider box.

2. Change the calendar to November 14, 2016.

3. Click Find Open Time on the Edit menu to display the Find Open Time dialog box.

4. Key **30** in the Length box. Press the Tab key to move the cursor to the Start Time box.

5. Key **3** in the Start Time box. Click on "am" to highlight it, and then key **p** to change "am" to "pm." Press Tab to move to the End Time box.

6. Key **5** in the End Time box. Press Tab.

7. In the Day of Week boxes, select Monday. If necessary, deselect any other days that are selected.

8. Click the Search button. The first available slot that meets the requirements is outlined on the schedule.

9. Double click in the time slot to open the New Appointment Entry dialog box.

10. Click Randall Klein in the drop-down list in the Chart box. Press tab several times to move the cursor to the Length box.

11. Key *30* in the Length box, and press the Tab key.

12. Click the Save button. The dialog box closes, and Randall Klein's appointment appears on the schedule.

✓ **You have completed Exercise 11-6.**

11.5 ENTERING APPOINTMENTS FOR NEW PATIENTS

When a new patient phones the office for an appointment, the appointment can be scheduled in Office Hours before the patient information is entered in Medisoft. In these instances, it is possible to enter an appointment before a chart number has been assigned to the patient. However, while the prospective patient is still on the phone, most offices obtain basic data and enter it in the appropriate Medisoft dialog boxes (Patient/Guarantor and Case).

| EXERCISE 11-7 | ENTERING AN APPOINTMENT FOR A NEW PATIENT |

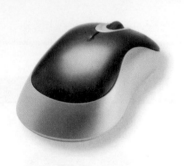

Schedule Lisa Green, a new patient, for a forty-five-minute appointment with Dr. John Rudner on November 14, 2016, at 1:15 P.M.

1. Verify that Dr. John Rudner is selected as the provider, and change the calendar to November 14, 2016.

2. Double click the 1:15 P.M. time slot.

3. Click in the blank box to the right of the Chart box, and key *Green, Lisa*. Press the Tab key to move the cursor to the Home Phone box.

4. Key *6145553604* in the Home Phone box, and press Tab to go to the Cell Phone box.

5. Enter *6145559671* in the Cell Phone box. Press Tab repeatedly to go to the Length box.

6. Key *45* in the Length box.

7. Click the Save button. The appointment is displayed on the November 14, 2016, schedule.

✓ **You have completed Exercise 11-7.**

11.6 BOOKING REPEATED APPOINTMENTS

Some patients require appointments on a repeated basis, such as every Thursday for eight weeks. Repeated appointments are also set up in the New Appointment Entry dialog box. The Repeat feature is located at the bottom of the dialog box (see Figure 11-16). When the Change button is clicked, the Repeat Change dialog box is displayed.

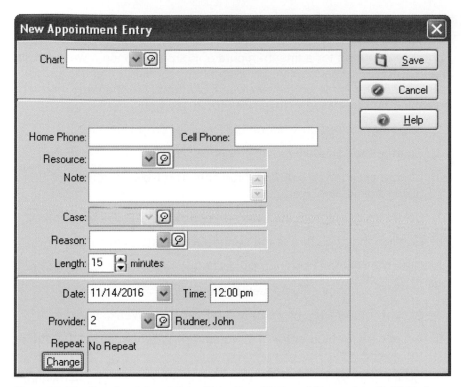

Figure 11-16   New Appointment Entry Dialog Box with Repeat Change Area Highlighted

The Repeat Change dialog box provides a number of choices for setting up repeating appointments (see Figure 11-17).

The left side of the dialog box contains information about the frequency of the appointments. The default is set to None. Other options include Daily, Weekly, Monthly, and Yearly. When an option other than None is selected, the center section of the dialog box changes and displays additional options for setting up the appointments (see Figure 11-18).

In the center section, an option is provided to indicate how often the appointments should be scheduled, such as once every week. Below that there is an option to indicate the day of the week on which the appointments should be scheduled. Finally, there is a box to indicate when the repeating appointments should stop. When all the information has been entered, clicking the OK button closes the Repeat Change dialog box, and the New Appointment Entry dialog box is once again visible. Clicking the Save button enters the repeating appointments on the schedule.

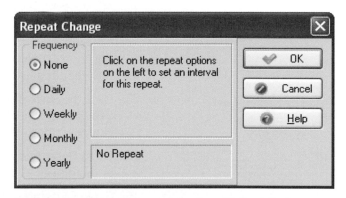

Figure 11-17   Repeat Change Dialog Box with the Default Settings (None Button Selected)

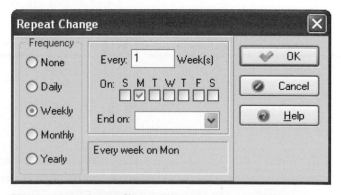

Figure 11-18   Repeat Change Dialog Box When an Option Other Than None Is Selected

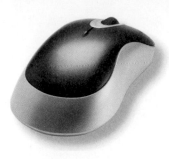

Schedule Jo Wong for a fifteen-minute appointment once a week for six weeks with Dr. Katherine Yan. Mr. Wong has requested that the appointments be at the same time every week, preferably in the early morning, beginning on Wednesday, November 16, 2016.

1. Click the desired provider on the Provider drop-down list.

2. Change the schedule to November 16, 2016.

3. Double click in the 8:00 A.M. time slot. The New Appointment Entry dialog box is displayed.

4. Select Jo Wong from the Chart drop-down list. Press the Tab key.

5. Confirm that the entry in the Length box is fifteen minutes.

6. Click the Change button to schedule the repeating appointments.

7. In the Frequency column, select Weekly.

8. Accept the default entry of 1 in the Every ____ Week(s) box.

9. Accept the default entry of W to accept Wednesday as the day of the week.

10. Click the arrow for the drop-down list in the End on box. A calendar box pops up. Locate November 16, 2016, in the calendar box.

11. Count six weeks from November 16, 2016. When you find the sixth Wednesday (counting November 16 as the first week), click in the calendar box for that day. The date 12/21/2016 appears in the End on box.

12. Click the OK button. Notice that "Every week on Wed" is displayed in the Repeat area of the New Appointment Entry dialog box.

13. Click the Save button to enter the appointments. Notice that "Occurs every week on Wed" appears in the lower-left corner of the Office Hours window, below the patient information.

14. Go to December 21, 2016, to verify that Mr. Wong is scheduled for an appointment at 8:00 A.M.

15. Go to December 28, 2016, and confirm that Mr. Wong is not scheduled. This is the seventh week, and his repeating appointments were scheduled for six weeks, so no appointment should appear on December 28, 2016. **CiMC**

 You have completed Exercise 11-8.

11.7 RESCHEDULING AND CANCELING APPOINTMENTS

It is often necessary to reschedule a patient's appointment. Changing an appointment is accomplished with the Cut and Paste commands on the Office Hours Edit menu. Similarly, an appointment can be canceled and not rescheduled simply by using the Cut command.

The following steps are used to reschedule an appointment:

1. Locate the appointment that needs to be changed. Make sure the appointment slot is visible on the schedule.

2. Click on the existing time-slot box. A black border surrounds the slot to indicate that it is selected.

3. Click Cut on the Edit menu. The appointment disappears from the schedule.

4. Click the date on the calendar when the appointment is to be rescheduled.

5. Click the desired time-slot box on the schedule. The slot becomes active.

6. Click Paste on the Edit menu. The patient's name appears in the new time-slot box.

The following steps are used to cancel an appointment without rescheduling:

1. Locate the appointment on the schedule.

2. Click the time-slot box to select the appointment.

3. Click Cut on the Edit menu. The appointment disappears from the schedule.

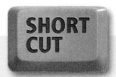

CUTTING AND PASTING

Instead of using the Cut and Paste commands to change or delete an appointment, select the appointment, and press the right mouse button. A shortcut menu appears with several options, including Cut, Copy, and Delete.

RESCHEDULING APPOINTMENTS	EXERCISE 11-9

Change Janine Bell's and John Gardiner's appointments.

1. Click Jessica Rudner on the Provider box drop-down list.

2. Go to Friday, November 18, 2016, on the calendar.

3. Locate Janine Bell's 3:00 P.M. appointment on the schedule. Click the 3:00 P.M. time-slot box.

4. Click Cut on the Edit menu. Janine Bell's appointment is removed from the 3:00 P.M. time-slot box. (You may also use the right-mouse-click shortcut.)

5. Click the 4:00 P.M. time-slot box.

6. Click Paste on the Edit menu. Janine Bell's name is displayed in the 4:00 P.M. time-slot box.

7. Click Katherine Yan on the Provider drop-down list.

8. Go to Thursday, November 10, 2016, on the calendar.

9. Locate John Gardiner's 9:00 A.M. appointment. Remove his appointment from the 9:00 A.M. time slot.

10. Go to Friday, November 18, 2016, on the calendar.

11. Enter John Gardiner's appointment in the 9:15 A.M. time slot.

12. Exit Office Hours.

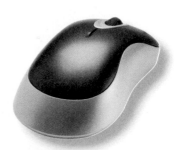

 You have completed Exercise 11-9.

11.8 CREATING A PATIENT RECALL LIST

Medical offices frequently must keep track of patients who need to return for future appointments. Some offices schedule future appointments when the patient is leaving the office. For example, if a patient has just seen a physician and needs to return for a follow-up appointment in six weeks, the appointment is usually made before the patient leaves the office. However, when the appointment is needed farther in the future, such as one year later, it is not always practical to set up the appointment. It is difficult for the patient and the physician to know their schedules a year in advance. For this reason, many offices keep lists of patients who need to be contacted for future appointments.

In Medisoft, a recall list can be created and maintained by clicking Patient Recall on the Lists menu. *Note:* The Patient Recall feature is in Medisoft, not Office Hours. Patients can also be added to the recall list by clicking the Patient Recall Entry shortcut button on the toolbar. When Patient Recall is selected from the Lists menu, the Patient Recall List dialog box is displayed (see Figure 11-19). This dialog box organizes the recall information in a column format. The scroll bar is used to display the last three columns on the right.

Date of Recall   Lists the date on which the recall is scheduled.

Name   Displays the patient's name.

Phone   Lists the patient's phone number, making it easy to call patients for appointments without having to look up phone numbers in another dialog box.

Extension   Lists the patient's phone extension.

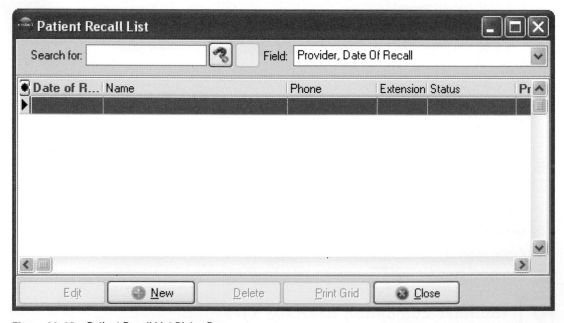

Figure 11-19   Patient Recall List Dialog Box

Status Indicates the patient's recall status: Call, Call Again, Appointment Set, or No Appointment.

Provider Displays the provider code for the patient's provider.

Message Displays the entry made in the Message box of the Patient Recall dialog box.

Chart Number Displays the patient's chart number.

Procedure Code Lists the procedure code for the procedure for which the patient is being recalled.

The Patient Recall List dialog box contains the following boxes:

Search For The Search For box is used to locate a specific patient on the recall list. Entering the first few letters or numbers in the Search For box displays the selection that is the closest match to the search criteria.

Field The choices in the Field box determine the order in which patients are listed in the dialog box. There are three sorting options:

1. Provider, Date of Recall
2. Chart Number, Date of Recall
3. Date of Recall, Provider, Chart Number

The Patient Recall List dialog box also contains these buttons: Edit, New, Delete, Print Grid, and Close.

Edit Clicking the Edit button displays the Patient Recall dialog box for the patient whose entry is highlighted. The information on the patient can then be edited by making different selections in the boxes.

New Clicking the New button displays an empty Patient Recall dialog box in which data on a new recall patient can be entered.

Delete Clicking the Delete button deletes data on the patient whose entry is highlighted from the patient recall list.

Print Grid Clicking the Print Grid button displays options to print the grid that is used in the Patient Recall dialog box.

Close The Close button is used to exit the Patient Recall List dialog box.

ADDING A PATIENT TO THE RECALL LIST

Patients are added to the recall list by clicking the New button in the Patient Recall List dialog box or by clicking the Patient Recall Entry shortcut button. When either of these actions is performed, the Patient Recall dialog box is displayed (see Figure 11-20).

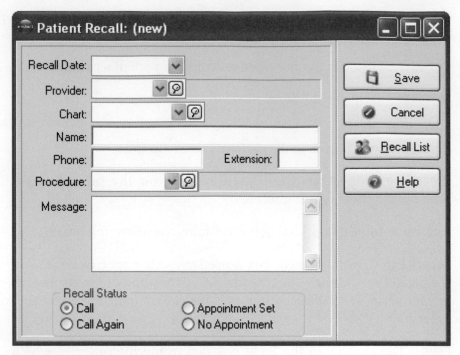

Figure 11-20   Patient Recall (new) Dialog Box

The Patient Recall dialog box contains the following boxes:

Recall Date   The date a patient needs to return to see a physician is entered in the Recall Date box.

Provider   A patient's provider is selected from the drop-down list.

Chart   A patient's chart number is selected from the drop-down list, or the first few letters of a patient's chart number are entered in the Chart box.

Name, Phone, Extension   After a chart number is entered, the system automatically completes the Name, Phone, and Extension boxes.

Procedure   If the procedure for which a patient is returning is known, it is entered in the Procedure box in one of two ways. The procedure code can be selected from the drop-down list, or the first few numbers can be entered so that the drop-down list will display the entry that most closely matches the entered numbers. This is especially valuable in practices that use hundreds of procedure codes because it eliminates the need to scroll through the codes to locate the desired one.

Message   The Message box is used to record any special notes, reminders, or instructions about a patient and his or her appointment.

Recall Status   The choices in the Recall Status box are used to indicate the action that needs to be taken. They include:

- *Call*   The Call button is used when a patient needs to be telephoned about a future appointment.

- *Call Again*   The Call Again button is used when a patient has been called once, but contact was not made and an additional call is necessary.

- *Appointment Set*   The Appointment Set button is used when a patient has an appointment already scheduled.

- *No Appointment*   The No Appointment button is used when a patient has been contacted for an appointment but has declined for some reason.

After the information has been entered in the dialog box, clicking the Save button saves the data and adds the patient to the recall list. In addition to the Save button, the Patient Recall dialog box contains Cancel, Recall List, and Help buttons. The Cancel button exits the dialog box without saving the data entered. The Recall List button in the Patient Recall dialog box is used to display the Patient Recall List dialog box. The Help button displays Medisoft's online help for the Patient Recall dialog box.

ADDING A PATIENT TO THE RECALL LIST	EXERCISE 11-10

John Fitzwilliams needs to receive a phone call one year from November 14, 2016, to set up an appointment for an annual physical. Add John Fitzwilliams to the recall list.

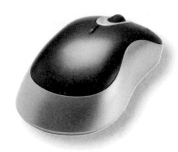

1. Click the Patient Recall Entry shortcut button. The Patient Recall dialog box is displayed. *Note:* The shortcut button is in Medisoft, not Office Hours.

2. In the Recall Date box, enter November 14, 2017. Press Tab.

3. Determine which physician is John Fitzwilliams's provider. (Look in the Patient/Guarantor dialog box for this information.)

4. Click John Fitzwilliams's provider on the drop-down list in the Provider box. Press Tab.

5. Enter John Fitzwilliams's chart number in the Chart box by keying the first few letters of his last name and pressing Tab. Notice that the system automatically completes the Name and Phone boxes. (The Extension box would also be completed if there were an extension.)

6. Enter the procedure code in the Procedure box by keying **99396** (Preventive est., 40–64 years) and pressing Tab.

7. Verify that the Call radio button in the Recall Status box is selected.

8. Click the Save button to save the entry.

9. Click Patient Recall on the Lists menu.

10. Verify that the entry for John Fitzwilliams has been added to the recall list.

11. Close the Patient Recall List dialog box.   **ciMC**

 You have completed Exercise 11-10.

11.9 CREATING PROVIDER BREAKS

Office Hours break a block of time when a physician is unavailable for appointments with patients

Office Hours provides features for inserting standard breaks in providers' schedules. The **Office Hours break** is a block of time when a physician is unavailable for appointments with patients. Some examples of breaks include Lunch, Meeting, Personal, Emergency, Break, Vacation, Seminar, Holiday, Trip, and Surgery. In Office Hours, breaks can be created one at a time or on a recurring basis for all providers. One-time breaks, such as those for vacations, are set up for individual providers. Other breaks, such as staff meetings, can be entered once for multiple providers.

Often breaks need to be inserted into a provider's schedule when he or she is not available for appointments with patients. For example, if a physician will be in surgery on Thursday from 9 A.M. until 12:00 P.M., that time period must be marked as unavailable on his or her schedule.

To set up a break for a current provider (that is, the provider listed in the Office Hours Provider box), click the Break Entry shortcut button. This action causes the New Break Entry dialog box to appear (see Figure 11-21).

The dialog box contains the following options:

Name   The Name field is used to store a name or description of the break.

Date   The Date field displays the current date on the Office Hours calendar. If this is not the correct date for the break entry, a different date can be entered.

Time   The starting time of the break is entered in this box.

Length   This box indicates the length of the break in minutes (from 0 to 720).

Resource   The drop-down list entries in the Resource box display the different types of breaks already set up in Office Hours.

Change   The Change button next to the Repeat box is used to enter breaks that recur at a regular interval.

Color   By selecting a different color from the drop-down list, the color of the break time slot in the schedule can be changed.

Figure 11-21   New Break Entry Dialog Box

All Columns   If the All Columns box is checked, the break will appear across all columns of the schedule (if a practice uses multiple columns in Office Hours).

Provider(s)   The Provider(s) buttons are used to indicate whether a break is to be set for the current provider (the provider selected in the Provider box in Office Hours), some providers, or all providers. If Some is selected, a Provider Selection dialog box will be displayed when the Save button is clicked. The appropriate providers can then be selected.

When all the information has been entered, clicking the Save button closes the dialog box and enters the break(s) in Medisoft.

ENTERING A PROVIDER BREAK	EXERCISE 11-11

Dr. Jessica Rudner will be attending a seminar from 10:00 A.M. to 12:00 P.M. on Monday, Tuesday, and Wednesday, December 12–14, 2016. Enter this as a break on her schedule.

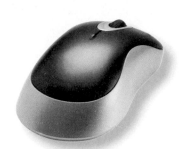

1. Open Office Hours and select Jessica Rudner from the Provider drop-down list.

2. Change the date on the calendar to December 12, 2016.

3. Click once in the 10:00 A.M. time slot (do not double click).

4. Click the Break Entry shortcut button. The New Break Entry dialog box appears.

5. Enter **HITECH Update Seminar** in the Name box.

6. Confirm that the date and time are correct.

7. Enter **120** in the Length box to change the length of time to 120 minutes.

8. Select Seminar Break in the Resource box.

9. Press the Change button (to repeat the break for two additional days). The Repeat Change dialog box is displayed.

10. If it is not already selected, click the Daily button in the Frequency column.

11. Accept the default entry of 1 in the Every ___ Day(s) box, since the break occurs every day for a period of three days.

12. Key **12/14/2016** in the End on box.

13. Click the OK button. You are returned to the New Break Entry dialog box.

14. Click the Save button to enter the break in Office Hours. Notice that the time slot from 10:00 A.M. to 12:00 P.M. on December 12, 2016, has been filled in on the calendar.

15. Change the calendar to December 13 and 14, 2016, to verify that the break has been entered correctly. **CiMO**

 You have completed Exercise 11-11.

11.10 PRINTING SCHEDULES

In most medical offices, providers' schedules are printed on a daily basis. To view a list of all appointments for a provider for a given day, the Appointment List option on the Office Hours Reports menu is used. A single provider and date are specified in the Data Selection dialog box for the report. (If the Provider boxes are left blank, schedules are created for all providers.) The schedule created is based on the provider and date specified in the Data Selection dialog box rather than the provider and date selected in the Office Hours window.

The report can be previewed on the screen or sent directly to the printer. If the preview option is selected, the appointment list is displayed in a preview window (see Figure 11-22). Various buttons are used to view the schedule at different sizes, to move from page to page, to print the schedule, and to save the schedule as a file. Clicking the Close button closes the preview window.

The schedule can also be printed without using the Appointment List option on the Office Hours Reports menu by clicking the Print Appointment List shortcut button. If this option is chosen, Office Hours prints the schedule for the date selected in the calendar and for the provider who is listed in the Provider box. To print the schedule for a different date or provider, change the date on the calendar and the entry in the Provider box before printing the schedule.

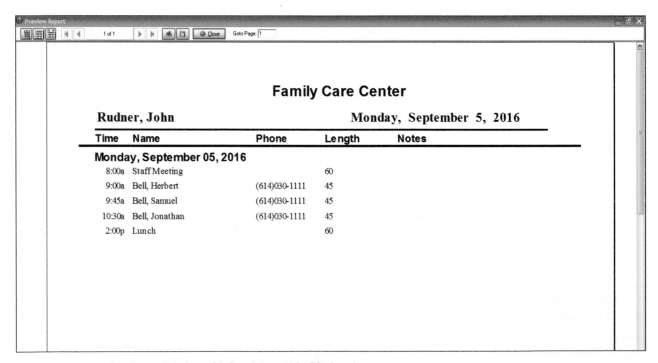

Figure 11-22 Preview Report Window with Appointment List Displayed

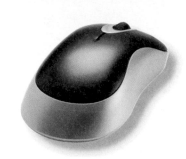

Print Dr. John Rudner's schedule for November 14, 2016, using the Appointment List option on the Office Hours Reports menu.

1. Click Appointment List on the Office Hours Reports menu. The Report Setup dialog box appears.

2. Under Print Selection, click the button that sends the report directly to the printer.

3. Click the Start button. The Data Selection dialog box is displayed.

4. Enter *11/14/2016* in both Dates boxes.

5. Select John Rudner in both Providers boxes.

6. Click the OK button. The Print dialog box appears.

7. Click OK to print the report. **CiMC**

✓ **You have completed Exercise 11-12.**

11.11 CREATING AN OVERDUE BALANCE REPORT FOR PATIENTS WITH APPOINTMENTS

Medical practices have discovered that it is much easier to collect on overdue accounts when the patient is in the office, rather than by phone or mail. As a result, it is useful to have account balance information available at the front desk when patients check in. In Medisoft, the Appointment List with Remainder Balance report provides this information.

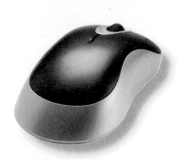

The practice has a new policy and would like a list of patients with appointments scheduled in the current month who have overdue balances.

1. Minimize the Office Hours window by clicking the minimize button.

2. In Medisoft, select Medisoft Reports on the Reports menu.

3. In the left-hand column titled All Folders, double click on the Plus Pack folder. The contents of the Plus Pack folder appear in the pane on the right.

4. Double click on the report titled Appointment List with Remainder Balance (Patient). The Search box appears.

5. Enter *11/1/2016* in the first Date box and *11/30/2016* in the second Date box.

6. Leave the other fields blank and click the OK button.

7. The report is displayed. Notice that the report has more than one page. Each page lists patients for a different provider.

8. Close the Print Preview window. Close the Medisoft Reports window. Click the Office Hours button on the status bar to display it on the screen again.

☑ **You have completed Exercise 11-13.**

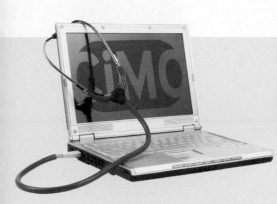

APPLYING YOUR SKILLS

12: ENTER AN APPOINTMENT

December 5, 2016
Book a fifteen-minute appointment for Lisa Wright as soon as possible. She is still complaining of a cough, especially at night. The appointment will need to be at 3:00 P.M. or later.

APPLYING YOUR SKILLS

13: RESCHEDULE AN APPOINTMENT

November 21, 2016
James Smith calls to say that he will be out of town and cannot make his appointment on November 29. He is available after 12:00 P.M. beginning on December 5. Reschedule his appointment.

APPLYING YOUR SKILLS

14: PRINT A PHYSICIAN'S SCHEDULE

December 5, 2016
Print today's appointment list for Dr. Jessica Rudner.

Remember to create a backup of your work before exiting Medisoft! To help you keep track of your work, name the backup file after the chapter you are working on, for example, StudentID-c11.mbk.

ELECTRONIC HEALTH RECORD EXCHANGE

Transferring Appointment Information

The first time Medisoft exchanges information with an electronic health record, all appointments and patient demographics are transferred. After that first transmission, only new or edited appointments and demographics are transmitted. The figure below shows the settings required to exchange appointment information with an electronic health record such as Medisoft Clinical.

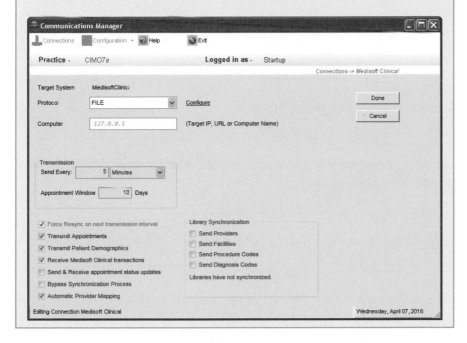

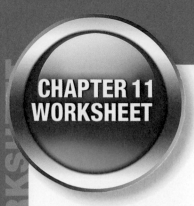
Name: _____ Date: _____

After completing all the exercises in the chapter, answer the following questions in the spaces provided.

1. *[LO 11.2]* In Exercise 11-1, what is listed on the appointment schedule immediately before Herbert Bell's appointment?

   _____

2. *[LO 11.2]* In Exercise 11-2, who is John Gardiner's provider?

   _____

3. *[LO 11.2]* In Exercise 11-3, what is listed on the appointment schedule immediately after John Fitzwilliams's appointment on November 14, 2016?

   _____

4. *[LO 11.2]* In Exercise 11-3, how long is James Smith's appointment on November 15, 2016?

   _____

5. *[LO 11.10]* In Exercise 11-4, are there any other patient appointments with Dr. Jessica Rudner on the day of Janine Bell's appointment?

   _____

6. *[LO 11.4]* In Exercise 11-5, what is the date and time of the next available slot for Maritza Ramos to see Dr. Yan?

   _____

7. *[LO 11.2]* In Exercise 11-6, what is the date and time of Randall Klein's appointment?

   _____

8. *[LO 11.10]* In Exercise 11-8, what is the date of Jo Wong's last fifteen-minute appointment with Dr. Yan?

   _____

9. *[LO 11.2]* In Exercise 11-11, what is listed in the 10:00 A.M. time slot for Dr. Jessica Rudner on December 14, 2016?

   _____

10. *[LO 11.10]* In Exercise 11-12, who has the last appointment with Dr. John Rudner on November 14, 2016?

    _____

11.1 List the four main areas of the Office Hours window. Pages 378–381	1. Provider selection box 2. Provider's daily schedule 3. Office Hours calendar 4. Office Hours patient information
11.2 Demonstrate how to enter an appointment. Pages 381–386	1. Start Office Hours. 2. Select the appropriate provider in the Provider box. 3. Change the date on the calendar to the desired date. 4. Locate the desired time slot in the schedule. 5. Double click in the time slot. 6. Select the patient in the Chart box. 7. Complete the other fields as required, being sure to enter the appointment length in the Length box. 8. When you are finished entering information, click the Save button.
11.3 Demonstrate how to schedule a follow-up appointment. Pages 386–388	1. Verify that the correct provider is selected in the Provider box. 2. Click the Go to a Date shortcut button. 3. Confirm the entry in the Date From box. 4. Make an entry in the Go ___ Days, Weeks, Months, or Years boxes. 5. Click the Go button. 6. The calendar changes to the specified date. 7. Double click in the time slot. 8. Select the patient in the Chart box. 9. Complete the other fields as required, being sure to enter the appointment length in the Length box. 10. When you are finished entering information, click the Save button.
11.4 Demonstrate how to search for an available time slot. Pages 388–390	1. Verify that the correct provider is selected in the Provider box. 2. Click the Search Open Time Slot button. 3. Make appropriate entries in the Length, Start Time, End Time, and Day of Week boxes. 4. Click the Search button. 5. The calendar displays the first available time slot that matches the specifications. 6. Double click in the time slot. 7. Select the patient in the Chart box. 8. Complete the other fields as required, being sure to enter the appointment length in the Length box. 9. When you are finished entering information, click the Save button.

11.5 Demonstrate how to book an appointment for a new patient. Page 390	1. Verify that the correct provider is selected in the Provider box. 2. Locate the desired date and time for the appointment. 3. Double click in the desired time slot. 4. Click in the blank box to the right of the Chart box, and enter the patient's name (last name, first name). Press the Tab key to move the cursor to the Home Phone box. 5. Enter the patient's home phone. Press Tab to go to the Cell Phone box. 6. Finish entering information in the boxes, as appropriate. 7. Click the Save button.
11.6 Demonstrate how to book repeating appointments. Pages 390–392	1. Click the desired provider on the Provider drop-down list. 2. Change the calendar to the appropriate date. 3. Double click in the desired time slot. The New Appointment Entry dialog box is displayed. 4. Select the patient in the Chart box. 5. Finish completing the boxes in the dialog box. 6. Click the Change button to schedule the repeating appointments. The Repeat Change dialog box appears. 7. Make a selection in the Frequency column. 8. Make entries in the additional boxes that appear. (These will vary depending on whether you selected Daily, Weekly, Monthly, or Yearly in the Frequency column.) 9. Click the arrow for the drop-down list in the End on box. A calendar pops up. Set the calendar to the date when the repeating appointment should stop. 10. Click the OK button. 11. Check the calendar to be sure the repeating appointments are correct.
11.7 Demonstrate how to reschedule an appointment. Pages 392–393	1. Locate the appointment that needs to be changed. Make sure the appointment slot is visible on the provider's daily schedule. 2. Click on the existing time-slot box. A black border surrounds the slot to indicate that it is selected. 3. Click Cut on the Edit menu. The appointment disappears from the schedule. 4. Click the date on the calendar when the appointment is to be rescheduled. 5. Click the desired time-slot box on the schedule. The slot becomes active. 6. Click Paste on the Edit menu. The patient's name appears in the new time-slot box.

11.8 Demonstrate how to create a recall list. Pages 394–397	1. In Medisoft, click the Patient Recall Entry shortcut button. The Patient Recall dialog box is displayed. 2. In the Recall Date box, enter the date the patient needs to have a follow-up appointment. Press Tab. 3. Select the patient's provider from the drop-down list in the Provider box. Press Tab. 4. Select the patient in the Chart box. 5. Enter the procedure code that corresponds to the appointment, if known. 6. Verify that the appropriate radio button is selected in the Recall Status box. 7. Click the Save button to save the entry.
11.9 Demonstrate how to enter provider breaks in the schedule. Pages 398–399	1. Select the provider from the Provider drop-down list. 2. Change the date on the calendar to the date of the break. 3. Click once in the appropriate time slot (do not double click). 4. Click the Break Entry shortcut button. The New Break Entry dialog box appears. 5. Enter a description of the break in the Name box. 6. Confirm that the date and time are correct. 7. Make the appropriate selection in the Length box. 8. Make a selection in the Resource box. 9. If the break is for more than one day, press the Change button. The Repeat Change dialog box is displayed. 10. Complete the Repeat Change box if necessary and click OK. 11. Click the Save button to enter the break in Office Hours. 12. Verify that the break has been entered correctly.
11.10 Demonstrate how to print a provider's schedule. Pages 400–401	1. Click Appointment List on the Office Hours Reports menu. The Report Setup dialog box appears. 2. Under Print Selection, click the button that sends the report directly to the printer. 3. Click the Start button. The Data Selection box is displayed. 4. Enter the desired date in both Dates boxes. 5. Select the appropriate provider in both Providers boxes. 6. Click the OK button. The Print dialog box appears. 7. Click OK to print the report.

11.11 Demonstrate how to create an overdue balance report for upcoming appointments. Pages 401–402	1. In Medisoft, select Medisoft Reports on the Reports menu. 2. In the left column titled All Folders, double click on the Plus Pack folder. The contents of the Plus Pack folder appear in the pane on the right. 3. Double click on the report titled Appointment List with Remainder Balance (Patient). The Search box appears. 4. Enter the desired dates in both Date boxes. 5. Complete the other fields if appropriate. 6. Click the OK button. 7. The report is displayed. Notice that the report has more than one page. Each page lists patients for a different provider.

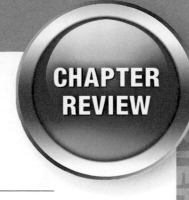

USING TERMINOLOGY

Define the terms below as they apply to Office Hours.

1. *[LO 11.9]* Office Hours break

_____

_____

2. *[LO 11.1]* Office Hours calendar

_____

_____

3. *[LO 11.1]* Office Hours patient information

_____

_____

4. *[LO 11.1]* provider's daily schedule

_____

_____

5. *[LO 11.1]* provider selection box

_____

_____

CHECKING YOUR UNDERSTANDING

Answer the questions below in the space provided.

1. *[LO 11.1]* What are the different ways of starting Office Hours?

_____

_____

2. *[LO 11.2]* How do you display the schedule for a specific date?

_____

_____

3. *[LO 11.2]* If the Office Hours calendar shows October 6, how do you move to November 6?

_____

_____

4. *[LO 11.2]* How do you display the schedule for a specific provider?

_____

_____

5. *[LO 11.2]* How do you schedule a new appointment in Office Hours?

_____

_____

6. *[LO 11.8]* How is a patient added to the Recall List?

_____

_____

7. *[LO 11.7]* How is an appointment rescheduled?

_____

_____

8. *[LO 11.2]* Suppose your office has set up Office Hours so that the default appointment length is fifteen minutes. If you need to make a one-hour appointment for a patient, in what box do you change fifteen to sixty?

_____

_____

APPLYING YOUR KNOWLEDGE

Answer the questions below in the space provided.

11.1. *[LO 11.9]* After you entered a personal break for Dr. Katherine Yan for February 24, she tells you that she gave you the wrong date. The break should be February 25. How do you correct the schedule?

_____

_____

11.2. *[LO 11.2]* A patient calls to request an appointment on a specific day next week. You determine that the appointment is for a routine checkup, not an emergency. What steps should you follow to schedule the appointment?

_____

_____

THINKING ABOUT IT

Answer the questions below in the space provided.

11.1. *[LO 11.2]* Why would an office switch from a paper-based system to a computer-based scheduling system? What are some advantages of a computerized scheduling system?

_____

_____

11.2. *[LO 11.11]* How does efficient scheduling contribute to the financial success of the practice?

_____

_____

AT THE COMPUTER

Answer the following questions at the computer.

11.1. *[LO 11.2]* Today is Friday, September 2, 2016. Dr. Katherine Yan asks you to find out when Sarah Fitzwilliams is coming in for her next two appointments. Locate the appointments in Office Hours. *Hint:* Use the Appointment List option on the Office Hours Lists menu, or click the Appointment List button on the Office Hours toolbar.

_____

_____

11.2. *[LO 11.4]* Today is November 14, 2016. Samuel Bell needs to be scheduled with Dr. John Rudner as soon as possible for a thirty-minute appointment between 10:00 A.M. and 12:00 P.M. When is the next available time slot that meets these requirements? How did you locate the open slot?

_____

_____

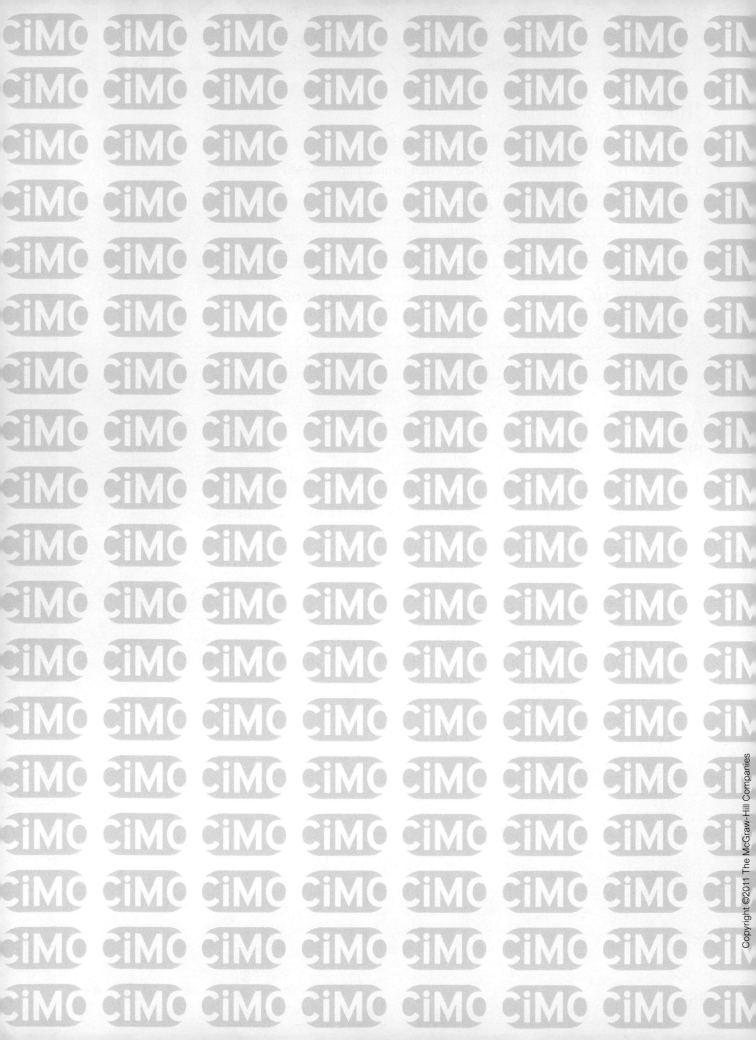

part 3

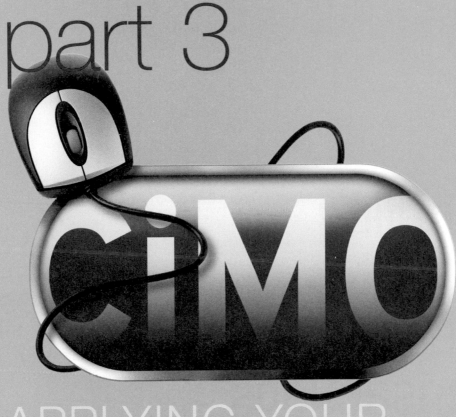

APPLYING YOUR SKILLS

chapter
12

Handling Patient Records and Transactions

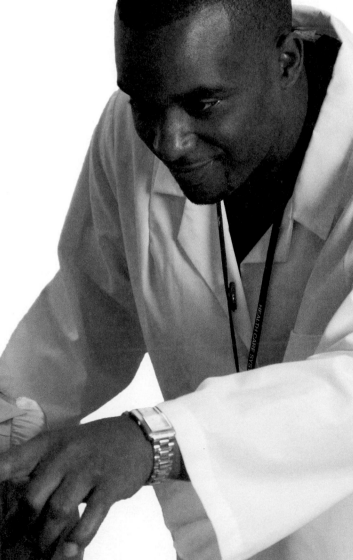

an overview of chapters 12–15

Chapters 12–15 provide you with an opportunity to practice what you learned in Chapters 1–11. These last chapters differ from the others in several ways:

- The purpose of these chapters is to see how well you have mastered the Medisoft® skills taught in earlier chapters, rather than to cover new topics.

- Convenient cross-references are provided to pages in the earlier chapters that teach each Medisoft skill, in case you need to review a procedure or refresh your skills. These references are listed at the beginning of each chapter, under the heading What You Need to Know, for each Medisoft function.

- Minimal instructions are provided for the exercises in Chapters 12, 13, and 14. In Chapter 15, you are on your own—no Medisoft steps are provided.

- There are no objectives, key terms, or end-of-chapter exercises.

what you need to know

To complete the exercises in this chapter, you need to know how to:

- Locate patient information. (Chapter 4, pages 121–126)

- Change the Medisoft Program Date. (Chapter 3, pages 76–80)

- Assign a new chart number and enter information on a new patient. (Chapter 4, pages 109–121)

- Create a new case for a patient. (Chapter 5, pages 136–141)

- Change information on an established patient. (Chapter 4, pages 126–127)

- Enter procedures, charges, and diagnoses. (Chapter 6, pages 177–188)

- Record payments from patients and insurance carriers. (Chapter 6, pages 188–197 and Chapter 8, pages 253–260)

- Print walkout receipts. (Chapter 6, pages 197–200)

All office personnel at the Family Care Center (FCC) know how to input patient information in the Patient/Guarantor dialog box and in the Case dialog box. Whenever possible, information for both dialog boxes is entered into the computer as soon as patients complete the handwritten information sheet and return it to the receptionist. On busy days, however, or when the office is understaffed because one of the medical assistants is sick or on vacation, input operations may be delayed.

EXERCISE 12-1 INPUTTING PATIENT INFORMATION

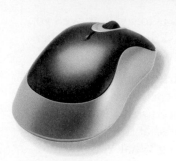

For this exercise, you need Source Documents 13–19.

It is Monday, November 14, 2016. You are a records/billing clerk at the Family Care Center. On your desk is a small pile of information sheets and encounter forms from Friday afternoon, November 11. You decide to input all patient information first, and then go back to record the transactions. First, you arrange the papers alphabetically:

> Battistuta
>
> Brooks
>
> Hsu
>
> Syzmanski

Then you begin. (Remember to change the Medisoft Program Date to November 11, 2016.)

PATIENT 1: ANTHONY BATTISTUTA

Record the address change that is written on Mr. Battistuta's encounter form (Source Document 13).

1. Start Medisoft, and restore the data from your last work session.
2. Click Patients/Guarantors and Cases on the Lists menu. The Patient List dialog box is displayed.
3. Select Anthony Battistuta from the list of patients.
4. Click the Edit Patient button. The Patient/Guarantor dialog box is displayed, with the Name, Address tab active.
5. Enter the new address.
6. Click the Save button.

PATIENT 2: LAWANA BROOKS

You can see from the encounter form (Source Document 14) that Ms. Brooks is an established patient. There are no changes to be made in the Patient/Guarantor dialog box. The work you need to do must take place in the Case dialog box. Ms. Brooks has had an accident at work, so a new case must be created.

1. After saving the changes for Mr. Battistuta in the Patient/Guarantor dialog box, the Patient List dialog box is redisplayed.
2. In the list of patients, click the listing for Brooks to select her as the patient. In the list of cases, click the ankle sprain case. You will not enter new information in the ankle sprain case; instead, you will copy information from the ankle sprain case to create a new case.

3. Click the Copy Case button to copy the information from the existing case into a new case. A duplicate case is displayed.

4. Using Source Documents 14 and 15, edit the information in the case to reflect the information relevant to the new case by changing the information in the Medisoft boxes listed below. If a box is not listed, either the information in that box does not need to be changed or the box is to remain blank.

Personal Tab

Description

Diagnosis Tab

Principal Diagnosis

Default Diagnosis 2

Default Diagnosis 3

Condition Tab

Injury/Illness/LMP Date

Illness Indicator

First Consultation Date (when a message about the date entry appears, click the No button)

Employment Related

Emergency

Accident
   Related to
   Nature of

5. Save your work.

TIP When entering information on different tabs within a dialog box, it is not necessary to click the Save button after completing work on each tab. However, the Save button must be clicked once all the tabs are complete and before exiting the dialog box.

PATIENT 3: EDWIN HSU

The information you need to make the necessary changes for Edwin Hsu is on Source Documents 16 and 17. Changes need to be made in Edwin Hsu's Patient/Guarantor and Case dialog boxes.

1. If the Patient List dialog box is not still displayed, open it now. Select Edwin Hsu from the list of patients, and click the Edit Patient button.

2. Move to the Street box, and enter the new address.

3. Move to the Home Phone box, and enter the new phone number.

4. Save the information you just entered.

5. Create a new case for Edwin Hsu by copying his existing case.

6. Using Source Documents 16 and 17, edit the information in the copied case to reflect the information relevant to the new case. Change information in the following boxes:

Personal Tab

Description

Diagnosis Tab

Principal Diagnosis

7. Click the Save button to save the new case.

PATIENT 4: HANNAH SYZMANSKI

Use Source Documents 18 and 19 to enter information on a new patient, Hannah Syzmanski. Hannah is the daughter of Michael and Debra Syzmanski, who are Dr. Dana Banu's patients. Hannah's pediatrician, Dr. Harold Gearhart, has referred her to the Family Care Center. This is noted on Source Document 19.

1. Go to the Patient List dialog box, click the Patient radio button to make the Patient section of the dialog box active, and then click the New Patient button.

2. Key **SYZMAHAØ** in the Chart Number box.

3. Complete the boxes for name, address, phone, birth date, sex, and Social Security number.

4. Complete the following boxes in the Other Information tab:

    Type

    Assigned Provider

    Flag (East Ohio PPO)

    Signature on File

    Signature Date

5. Save your work. (If a message about the signature date appears, click the No button, click OK, and then save your work.)

6. Click the Case radio button to make the Case portion of the Patient List dialog box active.

7. Click the New Case button to open a new Case dialog box.

8. Complete the following tabs in the Case dialog box:

Personal Tab

Description

Guarantor

Marital Status

Student Status

Account Tab

Referring Provider

Price Code (accept the default value of A)

Diagnosis Tab

Principal Diagnosis

Allergies and Notes

Policy 1 Tab

When you attempt to complete the Policy 1 tab, you notice that Hannah has not filled in her insurance information. Since she is covered under her father's policy, it is easy to locate the information required to complete the Policy 1 tab.

First save your work on Hannah's case. As before, open the Case dialog box for the acne case for Michael Syzmanski. This time go to the Policy 1 tab. Use the information on that tab to fill in the missing insurance data for Hannah Syzmanski.

When completing the Policy 1 tab for Hannah, remember to list Michael Syzmanski in the Policy Holder 1 box and to click Child in the Relationship to Insured field. Also be sure that all of the Insurance Coverage Percents by Service Classification boxes at the bottom are set to 100.

9. Save your work.

 You have completed Exercise 12-1.

ENTERING AN EMERGENCY VISIT	EXERCISE 12-2

You will need Source Document 20 for this exercise.

It is still Monday morning, November 14, 2016. Carlos Lopez has just seen Dr. McGrath on an emergency basis. Mr. Lopez was experiencing chest tightness. Dr. McGrath has determined that he was suffering from heart palpitations. You need to enter the procedure charges, accept Mr. Lopez's payment, and print a walkout receipt. Make sure all transaction information is properly recorded in the database.

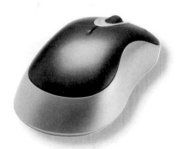

1. Change the Medisoft Program Date to November 14, 2016.

2. From the Patient List dialog box, create a new case for Carlos Lopez by copying the information in the case that already exists.

3. Using Source Document 20, complete the following boxes:

Personal Tab

Description

Diagnosis Tab

Default Diagnosis 1

Condition Tab

Injury/Illness/LMP Date

Illness Indicator

First Consultation Date

Emergency

4. Save your work. Close the Patient List dialog box.

5. Click Enter Transactions on the Activities menu.

6. Select Mr. Lopez in the Chart box.

7. Select Heart Palpitations in the Case box. (You may have given the case a slightly different name—this is okay.)

8. Click the New button in the Charges section to create a new transaction.

9. Verify that the entry in the Date box is 11/14/2016.

10. Enter the procedures marked on the encounter form.

11. Enter Lopez's payment. Remember to enter a check number in the Check Number box. Then click the Apply button, and apply the payment.

12. Click the Save Transactions button to save your work. When the Date of Service Validation boxes appear, click Yes to save the transactions.

13. Click the Quick Receipt button to print a walkout statement.

14. Close the Transaction Entry dialog box.

✓ **You have completed Exercise 12-2.**

EXERCISE 12-3 INPUTTING TRANSACTION DATA

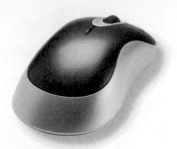

For this exercise, you need Source Documents 13, 14, 16, and 19.

You are now ready to record the transactions from Friday's four encounter forms. Before you begin, set the Medisoft Program Date to November 11, 2016.

ANTHONY BATTISTUTA

1. Click Enter Transactions on the Activities menu.

2. Select Anthony Battistuta in the Chart box.

3. Verify that Diabetes is displayed to the right of the Case box.

4. Record the procedures, one at a time.

5. Save your work.

LAWANA BROOKS

Follow essentially the same procedures to enter the transaction data. Remember to save your work.

EDWIN HSU

Follow essentially the same procedures to enter the transaction data. Then enter Hsu's payment, apply the payment to the charges, and save your work.

HANNAH SYZMANSKI

Follow essentially the same procedures to enter the transaction data. You need to record the date and procedure and Syzmanski's payment. Apply the payment to the charges, and save your work.

✓ **You have completed Exercise 12-3.**

ENTERING A NEW PATIENT AND TRANSACTIONS | EXERCISE 12-4

For this exercise, you need Source Documents 21 and 22.

The date is November 11, 2016. Enter patient information and all transactions for Christopher Palmer, a new patient of Dr. Beach. (*Note:* When completing the Policy 1 tab in the Case dialog box, enter 100 in all of the Insurance Coverage by Service Classification boxes.)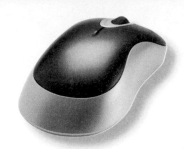

 You have completed Exercise 12-4.

ENTERING AND APPLYING AN INSURANCE CARRIER PAYMENT | EXERCISE 12-5

For this exercise, you need Source Document 23.

The date is November 11, 2016. A remittance advice and electronic funds transfer (EFT) have just been received from East Ohio PPO. Enter the deposit in Medisoft, and apply the payment to the appropriate patient accounts.

1. Open the Deposit List dialog box.

2. If necessary, change the date in the Deposit Date box to November 11, 2016.

3. Enter the deposit.

4. Apply the payment to the patient charges. Be sure to click the Save Payments/Adjustments button after each patient. Notice that as you enter and save payments, the amount listed in the Unapplied box decreases.

5. When you are finished, click the Detail button in the Deposit List dialog box to verify that the amount in the Unapplied column for each patient is 0.00.

6. Payments entered in the Deposit List dialog box are automatically linked to data in the Transaction Entry dialog box. Open the Transaction Entry dialog box, and confirm that the insurance company payments and adjustments appear in the transaction list at the bottom of the window for each patient in this exercise. Close the Transaction Entry dialog box.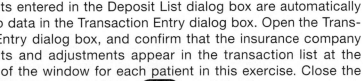

 You have completed Exercise 12-5.

Remember to create a backup of your work before exiting Medisoft! To help you keep track of your work, name the backup file after the chapter you are working on, for example, StudentID-c12.mbk.

chapter
13

Setting Up Appointments

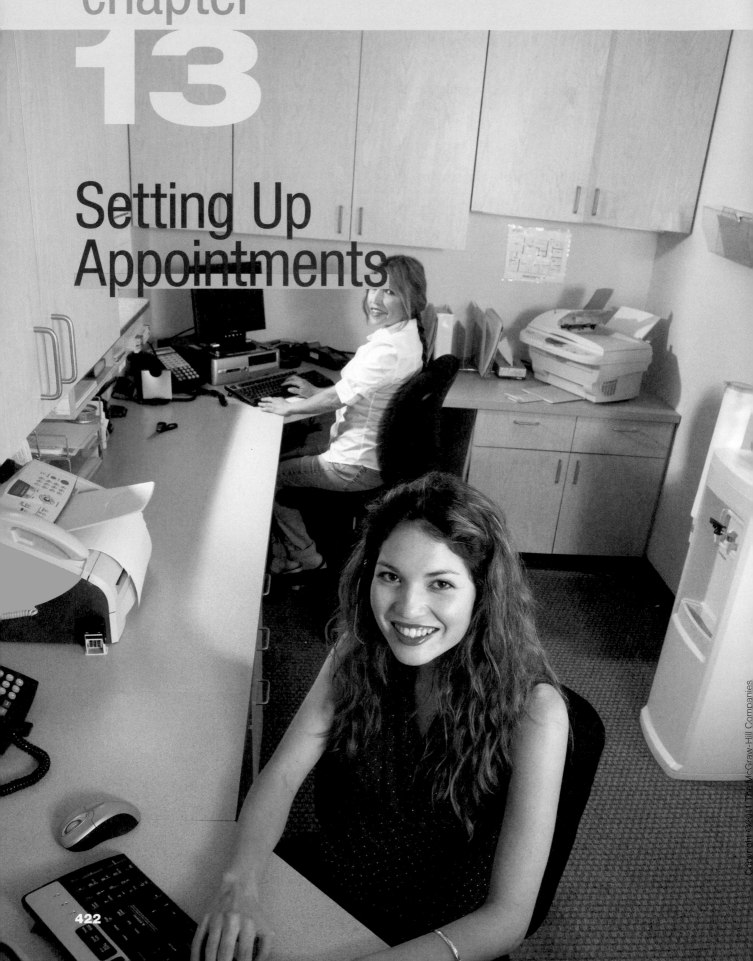

what you need to know

To complete the exercises in this chapter, you need to know how to:

- Start Office Hours. (Chapter 11, page 381)
- Move around in the schedule. (Chapter 11, pages 381–386)
- Enter appointments. (Chapter 11, pages 381–386)
- Change appointment information. (Chapter 11, pages 392–393)
- Move or copy an appointment. (Chapter 11, pages 392–393)
- Schedule a recall appointment. (Chapter 11, pages 394–397)
- Create a new case record for a patient. (Chapter 4, pages 136–141)
- Change a transaction record. (Chapter 6, pages 184–185)

The Family Care Center uses Office Hours as the primary tool for recording appointments. For the simulations in this chapter, assume that you are the front-desk receptionist and are responsible for most of the center's scheduling tasks. Remember, you can access Office Hours at any time, no matter what you are working on. For example, suppose you are typing a letter for one of the doctors and a patient calls to make an appointment. All you have to do is click the Start button on the task bar, select Programs—Medisoft and then Office Hours, enter the appointment, exit Office Hours, and return to your word-processing program. Office Hours can also be accessed from within Medisoft®, either by clicking the shortcut button or by clicking Appointment Book on the Activities menu.

EXERCISE 13-1 — SCHEDULING APPOINTMENTS

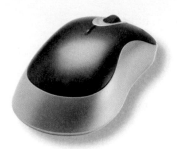

It is Monday, November 14, 2016. In Office Hours, schedule the following patient appointments on December 9, 2016:

Patient	Provider	Time	Length
Nancy Stern	P. McGrath	9:30	30 minutes
Sheila Giles	R. Beach	10:00	45 minutes
Raji Patel	D. Banu	2:45	30 minutes

1. Start Medisoft, and restore the data from your last work session.

2. Set the Medisoft Program Date to November 14, 2016.

3. Open Office Hours.

4. Go to December 9, 2016, on the Office Hours calendar.

5. Select each patient's provider from the Provider drop-down list, and enter the appointments.

✓ **You have completed Exercise 13-1.**

EXERCISE 13-2 — MAKING AN APPOINTMENT CHANGE

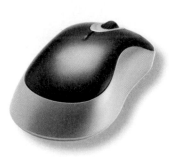

Carlos Lopez has just called to say that he lost his appointment card and cannot remember the time of his November 30 appointment. He thinks he may have a scheduling conflict. If the appointment is in the morning, he wants it changed to 2:00 the same day. If the 2:00 slot is not available, he needs to make the appointment for the next day at the earliest possible time.

1. In Office Hours, go to November 30, 2016.

2. Find out who Lopez's doctor is by calling up the Patient/Guarantor dialog box in Medisoft. Select the Other Information tab, and check the Assigned Provider box. Then select Lopez's provider from the Provider drop-down list in Office Hours.

TIP You may use the Patients/Guarantors and Cases option on the Medisoft Lists menu or the Patient List option on the Office Hours Lists menu to access the Patient/Guarantor dialog box.

3. Locate Mr. Lopez's appointment.

4. Check to see whether 2:00 P.M., the time he wants the appointment changed to, is available.

5. Since 2:00 is not available, move to December 1 on the calendar, and see if 8:00 A.M. is available.

6. Go back to November 30. Move Mr. Lopez's appointment from November 30 to December 1. (If you do not remember how to move an appointment, see Chapter 11.)

 You have completed Exercise 13-2.

JUGGLING SCHEDULES	EXERCISE 13-3

Mrs. Jackson's sister is on the phone. She will be taking care of the Jackson twins, Darnell and Tyrone, on Saturday, December 10, 2016, and she needs to make appointments for both of them for physicals and tetanus shots sometime after 9:00 A.M. That is the only day they can come in, so she hopes you can accommodate her. She does not remember the name of their doctor.

1. Find out who the boys' doctor is by looking up the information in Medisoft.

2. Go into Office Hours, and check the provider's schedule for December 10. The doctor is booked solid from 8:00 A.M. until she leaves at 1:00 P.M.

3. Check the schedules of Dr. McGrath and Dr. Beach. Since Dr. McGrath is unavailable, book Darnell in the 10:30 A.M. time slot and Tyrone in the 10:45 A.M. slot with Dr. Beach.

 You have completed Exercise 13-3.

ADDING PATIENTS TO THE RECALL LIST	EXERCISE 13-4

Darnell and Tyrone Jackson need to be called back for follow-up appointments in six months. Add both names to the recall list for six months from December 10, 2016.

1. Click Patient Recall on the Lists menu in Medisoft. The Patient Recall List dialog box is displayed.

2. Click the New button.

3. Enter June 10, 2017, in the Recall Date box.

4. Select Dr. Dana Banu in the Provider box.

5. Select Darnell Jackson's chart number from the drop-down list in the Chart box. Press the Tab key.

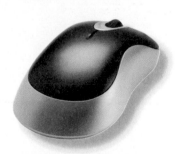

6. In the Message box, key *Six month follow-up appointment needed.*

7. Verify that the Call radio button in the Recall Status box is selected.

8. Click the Save button to save the entry.

9. Repeat the steps to add Tyrone Jackson to the patient recall list.

10. Close the Patient Recall List dialog box.

✅ **You have completed Exercise 13-4.**

EXERCISE 13-5 — DIANE HSU AND MICHAEL SYZMANSKI

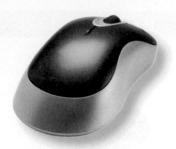

For this exercise, you will need Source Documents 24 and 25.

It is Monday, November 14, 2016. Diane Hsu and Michael Syzmanski are leaving the office after their appointments. Use the information on Source Documents 24 and 25 to perform the following tasks.

1. Create new cases for both patients by copying existing cases.

For Hsu, complete the boxes listed below in the Personal and Diagnosis tabs:

Personal Tab
Description

Diagnosis Tab
Principal Diagnosis

For Syzmanski, complete the following boxes in the Personal and Diagnosis tabs:

Personal Tab
Description

Diagnosis Tab
Principal Diagnosis

2. Record the charges in the Transaction Entry dialog box.

3. Record the payments, and apply the payments to the charges.

4. Make the appointment indicated on Mrs. Hsu's encounter form using Office Hours.

✅ **You have completed Exercise 13-5.**

Just as you finish making Mrs. Hsu's appointment, Dr. Robert Beach comes to the desk to say that he thinks he forgot to add the strep test he performed on Christopher Palmer on November 11, 2016, to the encounter form. He asks you to check and to add the charge if necessary.

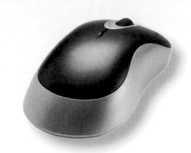

1. Go to the Transaction Entry dialog box. Check through the entries to find out whether the charge was entered. (It was not.)

2. Enter the new charge. (*Hint:* Remember to change the default date entry in the Date box to November 11, 2016.)

☑ You have completed Exercise 13-6.

Remember to create a backup of your work before exiting Medisoft! To help you keep track of your work, name the backup file after the chapter you are working on, for example, StudentID-c13.mbk.

Printing Lists and Reports

what you need to know

To complete the exercises in this chapter, you need to know how to:

- Create a day sheet report. (Chapter 9, pages 307–313)

- Understand what aging means in an accounting sense. (Chapter 9, page 326)

- Create a patient aging report. (Chapter 9, page 326)

- Create a practice analysis report. (Chapter 9, pages 313–317)

- Enter a new patient (Chapter 4, pages 109–121)

- Create a new case (Chapter 5, pages 136–144)

- Enter transactions. (Chapter 6, pages 177–188)

- Print an appointment list. (Chapter 11, pages 400–401)

- Add an item to the collection list. (Chapter 10, pages 353–361)

Because Medisoft® is an accounting package, its most powerful features involve computerized manipulation of account data for patients. Medisoft uses information in the system to produce reports on any facet of patients' or insurers' accounts and to generate bills for patients and for insurance companies. For example, as long as the office personnel in the Family Care Center have entered transactions correctly and have performed basic accounting procedures, Medisoft can be used to print current reports on the center's finances. You can print a report showing details of a day's transactions for any one of the center's physicians or for all physicians. You can print a report of late accounts for a particular patient or for all patients, for one insurance company or for all insurance companies.

Before starting the exercises in this chapter, you should understand some basic aspects of medical office accounting procedures.

Every medical office must keep a daily record of charges for and payments made for and by every patient of every doctor. For charges, the record usually includes the name of the patient, the type of service provided, and the amount of the charge. For payments, the record usually includes the name of the patient whose account is being credited and the payment amount.

EXERCISE 14-1 FINDING A PATIENT'S BALANCE

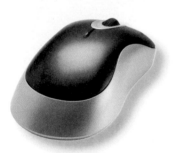

It is still Monday, November 14, 2016. Anthony Battistuta calls. He would like to know the amount of the charges from November 11 that he is responsible for, assuming that Medicare pays its portion (80 percent) of the total charges. How can you find the amount he is responsible for?

1. Start Medisoft, set the Program Date to November 14, 2016, and restore the data from your last work session.

2. On the Activities menu, click Enter Transactions.

3. In the Chart box, select Anthony Battistuta's chart number.

4. Verify that the Diabetes case is active in the Case box.

5. Look at the Allowed column in the Charges section for the three procedures on 11/11/2016. Add up the amounts in the Allowed column to determine how much Medicare is likely to pay. Since Medicare pays 80 percent of the allowed amount and the patient is responsible for the remaining 20 percent, calculate how much the patient is likely to owe for the November 11th visit. **CiMC**

 You have completed Exercise 14-1.

Print the appointment schedule for Dr. Dana Banu for Saturday, December 10, 2016.

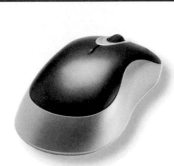

1. Open Office Hours.

2. Click Appointment List on the Office Hours Reports menu.

3. Select the option to print the report on the printer.

4. Click the Start button. The Data Selection dialog box appears.

5. Enter **12/10/2016** in both Dates boxes.

6. Enter **6** in both Providers boxes.

7. Click the OK button.

8. When the Print dialog box is displayed, click the OK button.

9. Exit Office Hours. **CiMC**

✓ **You have completed Exercise 14-2.**

PRINTING DAY SHEET REPORTS   EXERCISE 14-3

Patient day sheets and procedure day sheets can be viewed and/or printed using options on the Reports menu.

MEDISOFT PROGRAM DATE: NOVEMBER 11, 2016

CREATING A PATIENT DAY SHEET REPORT

1. On the Reports menu, click Day Sheets and then Patient Day Sheet.

2. Select the option to preview the report, then click the Start button.

3. In the Search dialog box, click in the Show all values of the Date Created field box to select it.

4. Change the entries in both Date From field boxes to November 11, 2016.

5. Accept the default entries in the other boxes.

6. Click the OK button.

7. The patient day sheet report is displayed on the screen.

8. Print the report, and then close the Preview Report window.

CREATING A PROCEDURE DAY SHEET REPORT

1. On the Reports menu, click Day Sheets and then Procedure Day Sheet.

2. Select the option to send the report directly to the printer, then click the Start button.

3. Confirm that the Show all values of the Procedure Code field box is checked.

4. Click in the Show all values of the Date Created field box to select it.

5. Change the entries in both Date From field boxes to November 11, 2016.

6. Confirm that the Show all values of the Attending Provider field box is checked.

7. Print the report.

✓ **You have completed Exercise 14-3.**

CREATING A PATIENT AGING REPORT

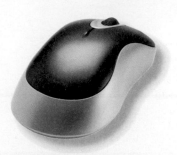

Create a Date Accurate Patient Aging by Date of Service report. The report shows which accounts are overdue and how long they have been overdue.

MEDISOFT PROGRAM DATE: NOVEMBER 30, 2016

1. On the Reports menu, click Medisoft Reports.

2. Double click the Aging Power Pack folder.

3. Double click the Date Accurate Patient Aging by Date of Service report.

4. Leave the Chart Number fields blank.

5. Enter 11/30/2016 in the Charges/Payment/Adj is on or before field.

6. Leave the Attending Provider boxes blank.

7. Click the OK button.

8. The Patient Aging Applied Payment report is displayed on the screen.

9. Print the report.

✓ **You have completed Exercise 14-4.**

ADDING ITEMS TO THE COLLECTION LIST

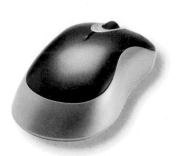

Study the Patient Aging Applied Payment report created in Exercise 14-4. Determine which patients have outstanding balances of greater than $5.00 that are more than ninety days past due.

Add these patient accounts to the collection list. (*Note:* Do not include Jo Wong's account, since you added it to the list in Chapter 10.)

MEDISOFT PROGRAM DATE: NOVEMBER 30, 2016

1. Select Collection List on the Activities menu.

2. Click the New button.

3. Change the entries in both Date fields to November 30, 2016.

4. Complete the following fields in the Tickler tab:

   Action Required

   Responsible Party Type

   Chart Number

   Guarantor

   Responsible Party

   Status

   Follow Up Date

5. Click the Save button.

6. Close the Collection List dialog box.

 You have completed Exercise 14-5.

Print a practice analysis report for the month of November 2016.

MEDISOFT PROGRAM DATE: NOVEMBER 30, 2016

1. On the Reports menu, click Analysis Reports and then Practice Analysis.

2. Select the option to preview the report.

3. Confirm that the Show all values of the Code 1 field box is checked.

4. Confirm that the Show all values of the Date Created field box is checked.

5. Change the entry in the first Date From field box to November 1, 2016, and change the entry in the second box to November 30, 2016.

6. Accept the default selections to show all values of the Attending Provider and Place of Service field boxes.

7. Click the OK button. The practice analysis report is displayed on the screen.

8. Print the report, and then close the Preview Report window.

 You have completed Exercise 14-6.

You need Source Documents 26 and 27 for this exercise, which has two parts.

PART ONE: DECEMBER 9, 2016

A new patient of Dr. Beach, Stewart Robertson, has stopped by to schedule an appointment and to fill out a patient information form. He wants an appointment for a routine physical in December, specifically for the third Saturday of the month, as early as possible.

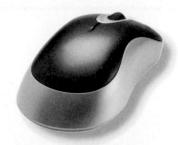

MEDISOFT PROGRAM DATE: DECEMBER 9, 2016

1. Using Source Document 26, enter the patient information for Mr. Robertson. Complete the Patient/Guarantor dialog box and the Case dialog box. You need to create a new case. Since Stewart's insurance is a capitated plan, remember to check the Capitated Plan box in the Policy 1 tab of the Case folder. Also enter 100 in all of the Insurance Coverage Percents by Service Classification boxes.

2. In Office Hours, schedule Robertson for his appointment (sixty minutes).

PART TWO: DECEMBER 17, 2016

Stewart Robinson completes his office visit with Dr. Beach.

MEDISOFT PROGRAM DATE: DECEMBER 17, 2016

1. Using Source Document 27, enter Robertson's diagnosis in Medisoft.

2. Enter the charges and payments for Stewart Robertson's visit.

✓ **You have completed Exercise 14-7.**

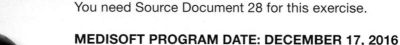

| EXERCISE 14-8 | MICHAEL SYZMANSKI |

You need Source Document 28 for this exercise.

MEDISOFT PROGRAM DATE: DECEMBER 17, 2016

Read the following account of Michael Syzmanski's visit to the Family Care Center on December 17, 2016:

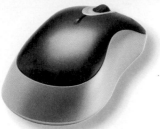

1. While driving to his daughter Hannah's soccer game, Syzmanski had a minor automobile accident in Jefferson and has a cut on his eyelid. He has come in to see Dr. Banu on an emergency basis. Dr. Banu is unavailable, so he is treated by Dr. McGrath. She determines that there has been no serious damage. After an examination using a local anesthetic, Dr. McGrath stitches the cut and tells Syzmanski to come back in a week. The procedure is simple suture.

2. In Medisoft, enter all the information pertaining to this visit using Source Document 28. *Hint:* Remember to change the default entry in the Provider column in the Transaction Entry dialog box.

3. Close the Transaction Entry dialog box.

✓ **You have completed Exercise 14-8.**

Remember to create a backup of your work before exiting Medisoft! To help you keep track of your work, name the backup file after the chapter you are working on, for example, StudentID-c14.mbk.

Putting It All Together

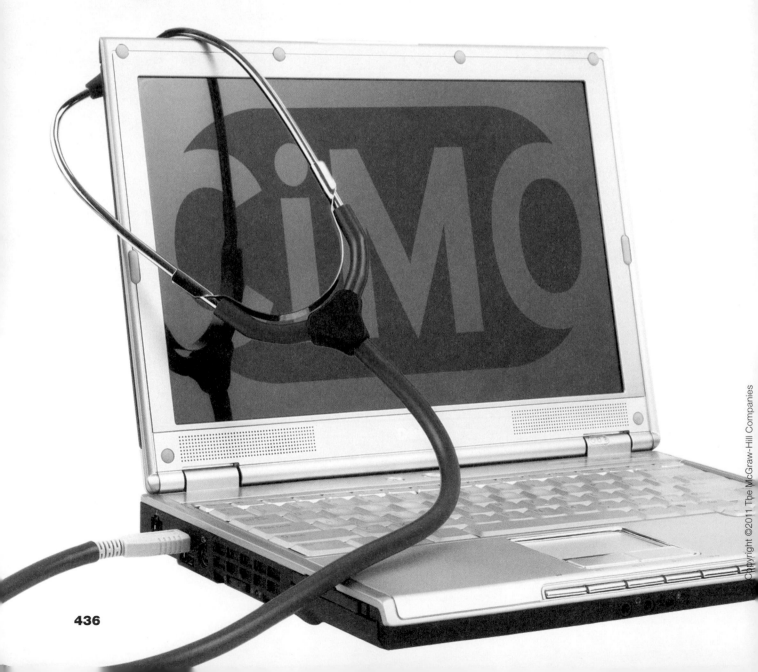

what you need to know

To complete the exercises in this chapter, you need to know how to:

- Schedule appointments. (Chapter 11, pages 381–385)
- Create cases. (Chapter 5, pages 141–163)
- Enter charges for procedures. (Chapter 6, pages 177–188)
- Enter copayments from patients. (Chapter 6, pages 188–197)
- Create claims. (Chapter 7, pages 221–223)
- Enter payments from insurance carriers. (Chapter 8, pages 253–260)
- Create patient statements. (Chapter 8, pages 278–282)
- Print reports. (Chapter 9, pages 300–329)
- Add items to the collection list. (Chapter 10, pages 353–361)
- Create collection letters. (Chapter 10, pages 361–366)

In this chapter, you need to use almost all the skills you have practiced throughout the exercises in the book. If you have any problems, refer back to the chapters in the book that cover the material.

EXERCISE 15-1 SCHEDULING APPOINTMENTS

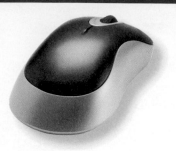

1. Start Medisoft, and restore the data from your last work session.

2. Schedule appointments for January 4, 2017, for the following patients. Make sure they are scheduled for the right doctors.

Jackson, Luther	30 minutes	9:00 A.M.
Hsu, Edwin	15 minutes	9:15 A.M.
Simmons, Jill	15 minutes	10:15 A.M.
Stern, Nancy	1 hour	9:30 A.M.
Syzmanski, Debra	30 minutes	9:30 A.M.
Giles, Sheila	15 minutes	9:00 A.M.
Battistuta, Pauline	30 minutes	10:30 A.M.

3. Switch the appointment times for Giles and Simmons.

4. Cancel the appointment for Edwin Hsu.

5. Print the appointment lists for January 4, 2017, for Dr. Banu, Dr. Beach, and Dr. McGrath.

 You have completed Exercise 15-1.

EXERCISE 15-2 CREATING CASES

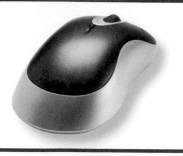

Create new cases for all patients with appointments on January 4, 2017, using the information found on Source Documents 29–34.

✓ **You have completed Exercise 15-2.**

EXERCISE 15-3 ENTERING TRANSACTIONS

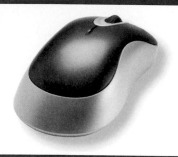

Using Source Documents 29–34, record the charge and payment transactions for all of the patients who had appointments. CiMC

✓ **You have completed Exercise 15-3.**

CREATING CLAIMS — EXERCISE 15-4

Create insurance claims for all transactions that have not already been placed on claims. (*Hint:* Leave the Transaction Dates boxes blank in the Create Claims dialog box.) Change the status of the newly created claims from Ready to Send to Sent. **CiMO**

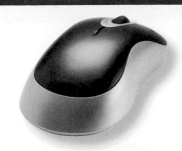

 You have completed Exercise 15-4.

ENTERING INSURANCE PAYMENTS — EXERCISE 15-5

Change the Medisoft Program Date to December 30, 2016. Enter the insurance payments listed on Source Documents 35–39, and apply the payments to patient charges. For capitated payments, remember to identify patients covered by this plan who had visited the practice during the month of November 2016, using the List Only . . . button in the Claim Management window, then enter a zero insurance deposit to adjust capitated patient accounts to a zero balance. **CiMO**

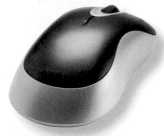

 You have completed Exercise 15-5.

CREATING PATIENT STATEMENTS — EXERCISE 15-6

Create remainder statements as of December 30, 2016 for patients whose last names begin with the letters *J* through *Z*. Print any statements that were created. **CiMO**

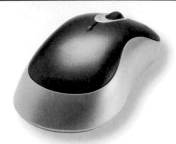

 You have completed Exercise 15-6.

PRINTING REPORTS — EXERCISE 15-7

Print a patient day sheet for January 4, 2017.

Print a practice analysis report for the period of January 1, 2016 to December 31, 2016. **CiMO**

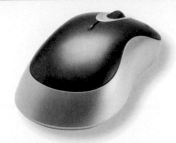

 You have completed Exercise 15-7.

EXERCISE 15-8	ENTERING PATIENT PAYMENTS AND REVIEWING OVERDUE ACCOUNTS

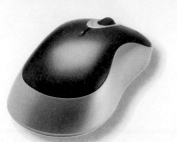

Date: December 30, 2016

Collection Agency Payment

A notice of an electronic payment from a collection agency has come in for Kristin Zapata's account. The agency collected the full amount owed to the practice, $282.50. The payment to the practice is the full amount minus the 25 percent fee charged by the agency. Calculate the net amount of the payment and enter it in Medisoft. Write off the remaining balance.

Patient Payment

A check has been received from Lisa Wright in the amount of $46.40. Enter the payment. The check number is 4629.

Aging Report

Print a Date Accurate Patient Aging by Date of Service report for transactions through December 30, 2016.

✓ **You have completed Exercise 15-8.**

EXERCISE 15-9	ADDING PATIENTS TO THE COLLECTION LIST AND CREATING COLLECTION LETTERS

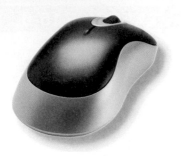

Date: December 30, 2016

Collection List

Study the patient aging report you created in Exercise 15-8. Determine which patients have account balances of greater than $5.00 whose accounts are more than sixty days late. These patients must be added to the collection list and sent collection letters. *Note:* If a patient is already on the collection list, they do not need to be added. *Hint:* To view all items on the collection list, be sure to check the box Show All Ticklers in the Collection List dialog box.

When completing the Tickler Item dialog box, enter *Call about overdue account* in the Action Required box and *12/30/2016* in the Follow Up Date box. Complete the other fields as appropriate.

Collection Letters

Create collection letters for the patients you just added to the collection list. *Hint:* In the Collection Letter Report dialog box, enter *12/30/2016* in both Follow Up Date Range boxes. Don't forget to check the Exclude Items that follow Payment Plan box and the Generate Collection Letters box.

✓ **You have completed Exercise 15-9.**

Remember to create a backup of your work before exiting Medisoft! To help you keep track of your work, name the backup file after the chapter you are working on, for example, StudentID-c15.mbk.

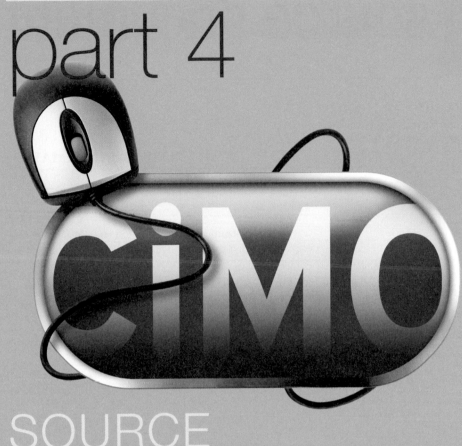

part 4

SOURCE DOCUMENTS

FAMILY CARE CENTER
285 Stephenson Boulevard
Stephenson, OH 60089-4000
614-555-0000

PATIENT INFORMATION FORM

Patient

Last Name	First Name	MI	Sex	Date of Birth
Tanaka	Hiro		__ M X F	2 / 20 / 1981

Address	City	State	Zip
80 Cedar Lane	Stephenson	OH	60089

Home Ph # (614) 555-7373	Cell Ph # (614) 555-0162	Marital Status Single	Student Status

SS# 812-73-6000	Email htanaka@abc.com	Allergies: penicillin

Employment Status Full-time	Employer Name McCray Manufacturing Inc.	Work Ph # (614) 555-1001	Primary Insurance ID# 812736000 Group HJ31

Employer Address 1311 Kings Highway	City Stephenson	State OH	Zip 60089

Referred By Dr. Bertram Brown	Ph # of Referral (614) 567-7896

Responsible Party (Complete this section if the person responsible for the bill is not the patient)

Last Name	First Name	MI	Sex __ M __ F	Date of Birth / /

Address	City	State	Zip	SS#

Relation to Patient __ Spouse __ Parent __ Other	Employer Name	Work Phone # ( )

Spouse, or Parent (if minor):	Home Phone # ( )

Insurance (If you have multiple coverage, supply information from both carriers)

Primary Carrier Name OhioCare HMO	Secondary Carrier Name
Name of the Insured (Name on ID Card) Hiro Tanaka	Name of the Insured (Name on ID Card)
Patient's relationship to the insured X Self __ Spouse __ Child	Patient's relationship to the insured __ Self __ Spouse __ Child
Insured ID # 812736000	Insured ID #
Group # or Company Name Group HJ31	Group # or Company Name
Insurance Address 147 Central Ave., Haleville, OH 60890	Insurance Address

Phone # 614-555-0101	Copay $ 20	Phone #	Copay $
	Deductible $		Deductible $

Other Information

Is patient's condition related to: __ Employment X Auto Accident (if yes, state in which accident occurred: OH) __ Other Accident	Reason for visit: Accident - back pain

Date of Accident: 9/25/2016   Date of First Symptom of Illness: 9/25/2016

Financial Agreement and Authorization for Treatment

I authorize treatment and agree to pay all fees and charges for the person named above. I agree to pay all charges shown by statements, promptly upon their presentation, unless credit arrangements are agreed upon in writing.

I authorize payment directly to FAMILY CARE CENTER of insurance benefits otherwise payable to me. I hereby authorize the release of any medical information necessary in order to process a claim for payment in my behalf.

Signed: Hiro Tanaka

Date: 10/3/2016

FAMILY CARE CENTER
285 Stephenson Boulevard
Stephenson, OH 60089-4000
614-555-0000

PATIENT INFORMATION FORM

Patient				
Last Name Wright	First Name Lisa	MI	Sex __ M __X_ F	Date of Birth 3 / 15/ 1976
Address 39 Woodlake Rd.	City Stephenson		State OH	Zip 60089
Home Ph # (614) 555-7059 Cell Ph # (614) 505-1397		Marital Status Divorced		Student Status
SS# 333-46-7904	Email lwright@abc.com		Allergies: none	
Employment Status Full-time	Employer Name Wheeler, Sampson, & Hull	Work Ph # (614) 086-9000	Primary Insurance ID# 0032697 Group A4	
Employer Address 100 Central Ave.	City Stephenson		State OH	Zip 60089
Referred By Dr. Marion Davis	Ph # of Referral (614) 444-3200			

Responsible Party (Complete this section if the person responsible for the bill is not the patient)

Last Name	First Name	MI	Sex __ M __ F	Date of Birth / /
Address	City	State Zip	SS#	

Relation to Patient __ Spouse __ Parent __ Other	Employer Name	Work Phone # ( )
Spouse, or Parent (if minor):		Home Phone # ( )

Insurance (If you have multiple coverage, supply information from both carriers)

Primary Carrier Name Blue Cross Blue Shield	Secondary Carrier Name
Name of the Insured (Name on ID Card) Lisa Wright	Name of the Insured (Name on ID Card)
Patient's relationship to the insured _X_ Self __ Spouse __ Child	Patient's relationship to the insured __ Self __ Spouse __ Child
Insured ID # 0032697	Insured ID #
Group # or Company Name Group A4	Group # or Company Name
Insurance Address 340 Boulevard, Columbus, OH 60220	Insurance Address
Phone # 614-024-9000 Copay $ Deductible $ $500 (met)	Phone # Copay $ Deductible $

Other Information

Is patient's condition related to: Reason for visit: cough
__ Employment __ Auto Accident (if yes, state in which accident occurred: ___) __ Other Accident
Date of Accident: /   /   Date of First Symptom of Illness: /   /

Financial Agreement and Authorization for Treatment

I authorize treatment and agree to pay all fees and charges for the person named above. I agree to pay all charges shown by statements, promptly upon their presentation, unless credit arrangements are agreed upon in writing.

I authorize payment directly to FAMILY CARE CENTER of insurance benefits otherwise payable to me. I hereby authorize the release of any medical information necessary in order to process a claim for payment in my behalf.

Signed: Lisa Wright   Date: 10/3/2016

ENCOUNTER FORM

10/3/2016	3:00 pm
DATE	TIME
Hiro Tanaka	**TANAKHI0**
PATIENT NAME	CHART #

OFFICE VISITS - SYMPTOMATIC		
NEW		
99201	OF--New Patient Minimal	
99202	OF--New Patient Low	X
99203	OF--New Patient Detailed	
99204	OF--New Patient Moderate	
99205	OF--New Patient High	
ESTABLISHED		
99211	OF--Established Patient Minimal	
99212	OF--Established Patient Low	
99213	OF--Established Patient Detailed	
99214	OF--Established Patient Moderate	
99215	OF--Established Patient High	
PREVENTIVE VISITS		
NEW		
99381	Under 1 Year	
99382	1 - 4 Years	
99383	5 - 11 Years	
99384	12 - 17 Years	
99385	18 - 39 Years	
99386	40 - 64 Years	
99387	65 Years & Up	
ESTABLISHED		
99391	Under 1 Year	
99392	1 - 4 Years	
99393	5 - 11 Years	
99394	12 - 17 Years	
99395	18 - 39 Years	
99396	40 - 64 Years	
99397	65 Years & Up	
PROCEDURES		
12011	Simple suture--face--local anes.	
29125	App. of short arm splint; static	
29540	Strapping, ankle	
50390	Aspiration of renal cyst by needle	
71010	Chest x-ray, single view, frontal	

PROCEDURES		
71020	Chest x-ray, two views, frontal & lateral	
71030	Chest x-ray, complete, four views	
73070	Elbow x-ray, AP & lateral views	
73090	Forearm x-ray, AP & lateral views	
73100	Wrist x-ray, AP & lateral views	
73510	Hip x-ray, complete, two views	
73600	Ankle x-ray, AP & lateral views	
LABORATORY		
80019	19 clinical chemistry tests	
80048	Basic metabolic panel	
80061	Lipid panel	
82270	Blood screening, occult; feces	
82947	Glucose screening--quantitative	
82951	Glucose tolerance test, three specimens	
83718	HDL cholesterol	
84478	Triglycerides test	
85007	Manual differential WBC	
85018	Hemoglobin	
85651	Erythrocyte sedimentation rate--non-auto	
86580	TB Mantoux test	
87072	Culture by commercial kit, nonurine...	
87076	Culture, anerobic isolate	
87077	Bacterial culture, aerobic isolate	
87086	Urine culture and colony count	
87430	Strep test	
87880	Direct streptococcus screen	
INJECTIONS		
90471	Immunization administration	
90703	Tetanus injection	
96372	Injection	
92516	Facial nerve function studies	
93000	Electrocardiogram--ECG with interpretation	
93015	Treadmill stress test, with physician...	
96900	Ultraviolet light treatment	
99070	Supplies and materials provided	

FAMILY CARE CENTER
285 Stephenson Blvd.
Stephenson, OH 60089
614-555-0000

☐ DANA BANU, M.D.
☐ ROBERT BEACH, M.D.
☐ PATRICIA MCGRATH, M.D.

☐ JESSICA RUDNER, M.D.
☐ JOHN RUDNER, M.D.
☒ KATHERINE YAN, M.D.

NOTES

REFERRING PHYSICIAN	NPI	AUTHORIZATION #
Bertram Brown, MD	**1234567890**	

DIAGNOSIS
724.2

PAYMENT AMOUNT
$20, check #123

FAMILY CARE CENTER
285 Stephenson Boulevard
Stephenson, OH 60089
614-555-0000

KATHERINE YAN, M.D.
PHYSICIAN'S NOTES

PATIENT NAME	Hiro Tanaka
CHART NUMBER	TANAKHI0
DATE	10/3/2016
CASE	Accident - Back Pain

NOTES

Condition related to auto accident in Stephenson, Ohio that occurred on 9/25/16.

Patient was hospitalized from 9/25/16 to 9/26/16.

Patient was totally disabled from 9/25/16 to 9/26/16.

Patient was partially disabled from 9/27/16 to 10/3/16.

Patient was unable to work from 9/25/16 to 10/3/16.

ENCOUNTER FORM

10/3/2016	**9:45 am**
DATE	TIME
Elizabeth Jones	**JONESEL0**
PATIENT NAME	CHART #

OFFICE VISITS - SYMPTOMATIC

NEW

99201	OF--New Patient Minimal	
99202	OF--New Patient Low	
99203	OF--New Patient Detailed	
99204	OF--New Patient Moderate	
99205	OF--New Patient High	

ESTABLISHED

99211	OF--Established Patient Minimal	
99212	OF--Established Patient Low	
99213	OF--Established Patient Detailed	X
99214	OF--Established Patient Moderate	
99215	OF--Established Patient High	

PREVENTIVE VISITS

NEW

99381	Under 1 Year	
99382	1 - 4 Years	
99383	5 - 11 Years	
99384	12 - 17 Years	
99385	18 - 39 Years	
99386	40 - 64 Years	
99387	65 Years & Up	

ESTABLISHED

99391	Under 1 Year	
99392	1 - 4 Years	
99393	5 - 11 Years	
99394	12 - 17 Years	
99395	18 - 39 Years	
99396	40 - 64 Years	
99397	65 Years & Up	

PROCEDURES

12011	Simple suture--face--local anes.	
29125	App. of short arm splint; static	
29540	Strapping, ankle	
50390	Aspiration of renal cyst by needle	
71010	Chest x-ray, single view, frontal	

PROCEDURES

71020	Chest x-ray, two views, frontal & lateral	
71030	Chest x-ray, complete, four views	
73070	Elbow x-ray, AP & lateral views	
73090	Forearm x-ray, AP & lateral views	
73100	Wrist x-ray, AP & lateral views	
73510	Hip x-ray, complete, two views	
73600	Ankle x-ray, AP & lateral views	

LABORATORY

80019	19 clinical chemistry tests	
80048	Basic metabolic panel	
80061	Lipid panel	
82270	Blood screening, occult; feces	
82947	Glucose screening--quantitative	
82951	Glucose tolerance test, three specimens	
83718	HDL cholesterol	
84478	Triglycerides test	
85007	Manual differential WBC	
85018	Hemoglobin	
85651	Erythrocyte sedimentation rate--non-auto	
86580	TB Mantoux test	
87072	Culture by commercial kit, nonurine...	
87076	Culture, anerobic isolate	
87077	Bacterial culture, aerobic isolate	
87086	Urine culture and colony count	
87430	Strep test	
87880	Direct streptococcus screen	

INJECTIONS

90471	Immunization administration	
90703	Tetanus injection	
96372	Injection	
92516	Facial nerve function studies	
93000	Electrocardiogram--ECG with interpretation	
93015	Treadmill stress test, with physician...	
96900	Ultraviolet light treatment	
99070	Supplies and materials provided	

FAMILY CARE CENTER
285 Stephenson Blvd.
Stephenson, OH 60089
614-555-0000

☐ DANA BANU, M.D.	☐ JESSICA RUDNER, M.D.
☐ ROBERT BEACH, M.D.	☐ JOHN RUDNER, M.D.
☐ PATRICIA MCGRATH, M.D.	☒ KATHERINE YAN, M.D.

NOTES

REFERRING PHYSICIAN	NPI	AUTHORIZATION #

DIAGNOSIS
250.00
PAYMENT AMOUNT

ENCOUNTER FORM

10/3/2016
DATE

11:00 am
TIME

John Fitzwilliams
PATIENT NAME

FITZWJO0
CHART #

OFFICE VISITS - SYMPTOMATIC		
NEW		
99201	OF--New Patient Minimal	
99202	OF--New Patient Low	
99203	OF--New Patient Detailed	
99204	OF--New Patient Moderate	
99205	OF--New Patient High	
ESTABLISHED		
99211	OF--Established Patient Minimal	
99212	OF--Established Patient Low	X
99213	OF--Established Patient Detailed	
99214	OF--Established Patient Moderate	
99215	OF--Established Patient High	
PREVENTIVE VISITS		
NEW		
99381	Under 1 Year	
99382	1 - 4 Years	
99383	5 - 11 Years	
99384	12 - 17 Years	
99385	18 - 39 Years	
99386	40 - 64 Years	
99387	65 Years & Up	
ESTABLISHED		
99391	Under 1 Year	
99392	1 - 4 Years	
99393	5 - 11 Years	
99394	12 - 17 Years	
99395	18 - 39 Years	
99396	40 - 64 Years	
99397	65 Years & Up	
PROCEDURES		
12011	Simple suture--face--local anes.	
29125	App. of short arm splint; static	
29540	Strapping, ankle	
50390	Aspiration of renal cyst by needle	
71010	Chest x-ray, single view, frontal	

PROCEDURES		
71020	Chest x-ray, two views, frontal & lateral	
71030	Chest x-ray, complete, four views	
73070	Elbow x-ray, AP & lateral views	
73090	Forearm x-ray, AP & lateral views	
73100	Wrist x-ray, AP & lateral views	
73510	Hip x-ray, complete, two views	
73600	Ankle x-ray, AP & lateral views	
LABORATORY		
80019	19 clinical chemistry tests	
80048	Basic metabolic panel	
80061	Lipid panel	
82270	Blood screening, occult; feces	X
82947	Glucose screening--quantitative	
82951	Glucose tolerance test, three specimens	
83718	HDL cholesterol	
84478	Triglycerides test	
85007	Manual differential WBC	
85018	Hemoglobin	
85651	Erythrocyte sedimentation rate--non-auto	
86580	TB Mantoux test	
87072	Culture by commercial kit, nonurine...	
87076	Culture, anaerobic isolate	
87077	Bacterial culture, aerobic isolate	
87086	Urine culture and colony count	
87430	Strep test	
87880	Direct streptococcus screen	
INJECTIONS		
90471	Immunization administration	
90703	Tetanus injection	
96372	Injection	
92516	Facial nerve function studies	
93000	Electrocardiogram--ECG with interpretation	
93015	Treadmill stress test, with physician...	
96900	Ultraviolet light treatment	
99070	Supplies and materials provided	

FAMILY CARE CENTER
285 Stephenson Blvd.
Stephenson, OH 60089
614-555-0000

☐ DANA BANU, M.D.
☐ ROBERT BEACH, M.D.
☐ PATRICIA MCGRATH, M.D.

☐ JESSICA RUDNER, M.D.
☒ JOHN RUDNER, M.D.
☐ KATHERINE YAN, M.D.

NOTES

REFERRING PHYSICIAN

NPI

AUTHORIZATION #

DIAGNOSIS
531.30

PAYMENT AMOUNT
$15 copay, check #456

ENCOUNTER FORM

10/3/2016	1:00 pm
DATE	TIME
Lisa Wright	**WRIGHLI0**
PATIENT NAME	CHART #

OFFICE VISITS - SYMPTOMATIC

NEW

99201	OF--New Patient Minimal	
99202	OF--New Patient Low	
99203	OF--New Patient Detailed	X
99204	OF--New Patient Moderate	
99205	OF--New Patient High	

ESTABLISHED

99211	OF--Established Patient Minimal	
99212	OF--Established Patient Low	
99213	OF--Established Patient Detailed	
99214	OF--Established Patient Moderate	
99215	OF--Established Patient High	

PREVENTIVE VISITS

NEW

99381	Under 1 Year	
99382	1 - 4 Years	
99383	5 - 11 Years	
99384	12 - 17 Years	
99385	18 - 39 Years	
99386	40 - 64 Years	
99387	65 Years & Up	

ESTABLISHED

99391	Under 1 Year	
99392	1 - 4 Years	
99393	5 - 11 Years	
99394	12 - 17 Years	
99395	18 - 39 Years	
99396	40 - 64 Years	
99397	65 Years & Up	

PROCEDURES

12011	Simple suture--face--local anes.	
29125	App. of short arm splint; static	
29540	Strapping, ankle	
50390	Aspiration of renal cyst by needle	
71010	Chest x-ray, single view, frontal	

PROCEDURES

71020	Chest x-ray, two views, frontal & lateral	X
71030	Chest x-ray, complete, four views	
73070	Elbow x-ray, AP & lateral views	
73090	Forearm x-ray, AP & lateral views	
73100	Wrist x-ray, AP & lateral views	
73510	Hip x-ray, complete, two views	
73600	Ankle x-ray, AP & lateral views	

LABORATORY

80019	19 clinical chemistry tests	
80048	Basic metabolic panel	
80061	Lipid panel	
82270	Blood screening, occult; feces	
82947	Glucose screening--quantitative	
82951	Glucose tolerance test, three specimens	
83718	HDL cholesterol	
84478	Triglycerides test	
85007	Manual differential WBC	
85018	Hemoglobin	
85651	Erythrocyte sedimentation rate--non-auto	
86580	TB Mantoux test	
87072	Culture by commercial kit, nonurine...	
87076	Culture, anerobic isolate	
87077	Bacterial culture, aerobic isolate	
87086	Urine culture and colony count	
87430	Strep test	
87880	Direct streptococcus screen	

INJECTIONS

90471	Immunization administration	
90703	Tetanus injection	
96372	Injection	
92516	Facial nerve function studies	
93000	Electrocardiogram--ECG with interpretation	
93015	Treadmill stress test, with physician...	
96900	Ultraviolet light treatment	
99070	Supplies and materials provided	

FAMILY CARE CENTER
285 Stephenson Blvd.
Stephenson, OH 60089
614-555-0000

☐ DANA BANU, M.D.	☒ JESSICA RUDNER, M.D.
☐ ROBERT BEACH, M.D.	☐ JOHN RUDNER, M.D.
☐ PATRICIA MCGRATH, M.D.	☐ KATHERINE YAN, M.D.

NOTES

REFERRING PHYSICIAN	NPI	AUTHORIZATION #

DIAGNOSIS
490

PAYMENT AMOUNT

CHAMPVA
240 CENTER ST.
COLUMBUS, OH 60220

PROVIDER REMITTANCE
THIS IS NOT A BILL
A PAYMENT SUMMARY AND AN EXPLANATION OF
CODES ARE AT THE END OF THIS STATEMENT

FAMILY CARE CENTER
285 STEPHENSON BLVD.
STEPHENSON, OH 60089-4000

PAGE:	1 OF 1
DATE:	10/03/2016
ID NUMBER:	214778924

PROVIDER: JOHN RUDNER, M.D.

PATIENT: FITZWILLIAMS JOHN   CLAIM: 123456789

FROM DATE	THRU DATE	PROC CODE	UNITS	AMOUNT BILLED	AMOUNT ALLOWED	DEDUCT	COPAY/ COINS	PROV PAID	REASON CODE
09/06/16	09/06/16	99211	1	36.00	20.68	.00	15.00	5.68	
09/06/16	09/06/16	84478	1	29.00	8.04	.00	.00	8.04	
	CLAIM TOTALS			64.00	28.72	.00	15.00	13.72	

PROVIDER: KATHERINE YAN, M.D.

PATIENT: FITZWILLIAMS SARAH   CLAIM: 234567891

FROM DATE	THRU DATE	PROC CODE	UNITS	AMOUNT BILLED	AMOUNT ALLOWED	DEDUCT	COPAY/ COINS	PROV PAID	REASON CODE
09/06/16	09/06/16	90471	1	15.00	15.00	.00	15.00	.00	
09/06/16	09/06/16	90703	1	29.00	14.30	.00	.00	14.30	
	CLAIM TOTALS			44.00	29.30	.00	15.00	14.30	

****************** CHECK #214778924 IN THE AMOUNT OF $28.02 IS ATTACHED ******************

PAYMENT SUMMARY			TOTAL ALL CLAIMS	
TOTAL AMOUNT PAID	28.02		AMOUNT CHARGED	108.00
PRIOR CREDIT BALANCE	.00		AMOUNT ALLOWED	58.02
CURRENT CREDIT DEFERRED	.00		DEDUCTIBLE	.00
PRIOR CREDIT APPLIED	.00		COPAY	30.00
NEW CREDIT BALANCE	.00		OTHER REDUCTION	.00
NET DISBURSED	28.02			

STATUS CODES:
A - APPROVED   AJ - ADJUSTMENT   IP - IN PROCESS   R - REJECTED   V - VOID

EAST OHIO PPO
10 CENTRAL AVENUE
HALEVILLE, OH 60890

PROVIDER REMITTANCE
THIS IS NOT A BILL
A PAYMENT SUMMARY AND AN EXPLANATION OF
CODES ARE AT THE END OF THIS STATEMENT

FAMILY CARE CENTER
285 STEPHENSON BLVD.
STEPHENSON, OH 60089-4000

PAGE: 1 OF 2
DATE: 10/03/2016
ID NUMBER: 00146972

PROVIDER: ROBERT BEACH, M.D.

PATIENT: ARLEN SUSAN   CLAIM: 123456789

FROM DATE	THRU DATE	PROC CODE	UNITS	AMOUNT BILLED	AMOUNT ALLOWED	DEDUCT	COPAY/ COINS	PROV PAID	REASON CODE
09/05/16	09/05/16	99212	1	54.00	48.60	.00	20.00	28.60	
	CLAIM TOTALS			54.00	48.60	.00	20.00	28.60	

PROVIDER: JOHN RUDNER, M.D.

PATIENT: BELL HERBERT   CLAIM: 234567891

FROM DATE	THRU DATE	PROC CODE	UNITS	AMOUNT BILLED	AMOUNT ALLOWED	DEDUCT	COPAY/ COINS	PROV PAID	REASON CODE
09/05/16	09/05/16	99211	1	36.00	32.40	.00	20.00	12.40	
	CLAIM TOTALS			36.00	32.40	.00	20.00	12.40	

PATIENT: BELL SAMUEL   CLAIM: 34567891

FROM DATE	THRU DATE	PROC CODE	UNITS	AMOUNT BILLED	AMOUNT ALLOWED	DEDUCT	COPAY/ COINS	PROV PAID	REASON CODE
09/05/16	09/05/16	99212	1	54.00	48.60	.00	20.00	28.60	
	CLAIM TOTALS			54.00	48.60	.00	20.00	28.60	

PROVIDER: KATHERINE YAN, M.D.

PATIENT: BELL JANINE   CLAIM: 45678912

FROM DATE	THRU DATE	PROC CODE	UNITS	AMOUNT BILLED	AMOUNT ALLOWED	DEDUCT	COPAY/ COINS	PROV PAID	REASON CODE
09/05/16	09/05/16	99213	1	72.00	64.80	.00	20.00	44.80	
09/05/16	09/05/16	73510	1	124.00	111.60	.00	.00	111.60	
	CLAIM TOTALS			196.00	176.40	.00	20.00	156.40	

PATIENT: BELL JONATHAN   CLAIM: 56789123

FROM DATE	THRU DATE	PROC CODE	UNITS	AMOUNT BILLED	AMOUNT ALLOWED	DEDUCT	COPAY/ COINS	PROV PAID	REASON CODE
09/05/16	09/05/16	99394	1	222.00	199.80	.00	20.00	179.80	
	CLAIM TOTALS			222.00	199.80	.00	20.00	179.80	

STATUS CODES:
A - APPROVED   AJ - ADJUSTMENT   IP - IN PROCESS   R - REJECTED   V - VOID

source document 9

EAST OHIO PPO
10 CENTRAL AVENUE
HALEVILLE, OH 60890

PROVIDER REMITTANCE
THIS IS NOT A BILL
A PAYMENT SUMMARY AND AN EXPLANATION OF
CODES ARE AT THE END OF THIS STATEMENT

FAMILY CARE CENTER
285 STEPHENSON BLVD
STEPHENSON, OH 60089-4000

PAGE:	2 OF 2
DATE:	10/03/2016
ID NUMBER:	00146972

PROVIDER: KATHERINE YAN, M.D.

PATIENT: BELL SARINA   CLAIM: 56789123

FROM DATE	THRU DATE	PROC CODE	UNITS	AMOUNT BILLED	AMOUNT ALLOWED	DEDUCT	COPAY/ COINS	PROV PAID	REASON CODE
09/05/16	09/05/16	99213	1	72.00	64.80	.00	20.00	44.80	
	CLAIM TOTALS			72.00	64.80	.00	20.00	44.80	

PAYMENT SUMMARY		TOTAL ALL CLAIMS		EFT INFORMATION	
TOTAL AMOUNT PAID	450.60	AMOUNT CHARGED	634.00	NUMBER	00146972
PRIOR CREDIT BALANCE	.00	AMOUNT ALLOWED	570.60	DATE	10/03/16
CURRENT CREDIT DEFERRED	.00	DEDUCTIBLE	.00	AMOUNT	450.60
PRIOR CREDIT APPLIED	.00	COPAY	120.00		
NEW CREDIT BALANCE	.00	OTHER REDUCTION	.00		
NET DISBURSED	450.60	AMOUNT APPROVED	450.60		

STATUS CODES:
A - APPROVED   AJ - ADJUSTMENT   IP - IN PROCESS   R - REJECTED   V - VOID

BLUE CROSS/BLUE SHIELD
340 BOULEVARD
COLUMBUS, OH 60220

PROVIDER REMITTANCE
THIS IS NOT A BILL
A PAYMENT SUMMARY AND AN EXPLANATION OF
CODES ARE AT THE END OF THIS STATEMENT

FAMILY CARE CENTER
285 STEPHENSON BLVD.
STEPHENSON, OH 60089-4000

PAGE: 1 OF 1
DATE: 11/03/2016
ID NUMBER: 001234

PROVIDER: ROBERT BEACH, M.D.

PATIENT: GILES SHEILA   CLAIM: 123456789

FROM DATE	THRU DATE	PROC CODE	UNITS	AMOUNT BILLED	AMOUNT ALLOWED	DEDUCT	COPAY/ COINS	PROV PAID	REASON CODE
10/28/16	10/28/16	99213	1	72.00	72.00	.00	.00	57.60	
10/28/16	10/28/16	71010	1	91.00	91.00	.00	.00	72.80	
10/28/16	10/28/16	87430	1	29.00	.00	.00	.00	.00	R
	CLAIM TOTALS			192.00	163.00	.00	.00	130.40	

R* OUTSIDE LAB WORK NOT BILLABLE BY PROVIDER

PATIENT: SIMMONS JILL   CLAIM: 234567891

FROM DATE	THRU DATE	PROC CODE	UNITS	AMOUNT BILLED	AMOUNT ALLOWED	DEDUCT	COPAY/ COINS	PROV PAID	REASON CODE
10/28/16	10/28/16	99212	1	54.00	54.00	.00	.00	43.20	
10/28/16	10/28/16	87086	1	51.00	51.00	.00	.00	40.80	
	CLAIM TOTALS			105.00	105.00	.00	.00	84.00	

PAYMENT SUMMARY		TOTAL ALL CLAIMS		EFT INFORMATION	
TOTAL AMOUNT PAID	214.40	AMOUNT CHARGED	297.00	NUMBER	001234
PRIOR CREDIT BALANCE	.00	AMOUNT ALLOWED	268.00	DATE	11/03/16
CURRENT CREDIT DEFERRED	.00	DEDUCTIBLE	.00	AMOUNT	214.40
PRIOR CREDIT APPLIED	.00	COINSURANCE	.00		
NEW CREDIT BALANCE	.00	OTHER REDUCTION	.00		
NET DISBURSED	214.40	AMOUNT APPROVED	214.40		

STATUS CODES:
A - APPROVED   AJ - ADJUSTMENT   IP - IN PROCESS   R - REJECTED   V - VOID

OHIOCARE HMO
147 CENTRAL AVENUE
HALEVILLE, OH 60890

FAMILY CARE CENTER
285 STEPHENSON BLVD.
STEPHENSON, OH 60089-4000

PAGE:	1 OF 1
DATE:	10/30/2016
ID NUMBER:	001006003

OHIOCARE HMO CAPITATION STATEMENT
MONTH OF OCTOBER 2016

PROVIDERS
BANU DANA
BEACH ROBERT
MCGRATH PATRICIA
RUDNER JESSICA
RUDNER JOHN
YAN KATHERINE

MEMBER NUMBER	MEMBER NAME	CONTRACT NUMBER	CONTRACT STATUS
0003602149	FAMILY CARE CENTER	YG34906	APPROVED

AMOUNT OF PAYMENT $2,500.00
EFT STATUS: SENT 10/30/16 8:46AM
TRANSACTION #343434

BLUE CROSS/BLUE SHIELD
340 BOULEVARD
COLUMBUS, OH 60220

PROVIDER REMITTANCE
THIS IS NOT A BILL
A PAYMENT SUMMARY AND AN EXPLANATION OF
CODES ARE AT THE END OF THIS STATEMENT

FAMILY CARE CENTER
285 STEPHENSON BLVD.
STEPHENSON, OH 60089-4000

PAGE: 1 OF 1
DATE: 10/28/2016
ID NUMBER: 2000000

PROVIDER: JESSICA RUDNER, M.D.

PATIENT: WRIGHT LISA   CLAIM: 345678901

FROM DATE	THRU DATE	PROC CODE	UNITS	AMOUNT BILLED	AMOUNT ALLOWED	DEDUCT	COPAY/ COINS	PROV PAID	REASON CODE
10/03/16	10/03/16	99203	1	120.00	120.00	.00	.00	96.00	
10/03/16	10/03/16	71020	1	112.00	112.00	.00	.00	89.60	
	CLAIM TOTALS			232.00	232.00	.00	.00	185.60	

PAYMENT SUMMARY		TOTAL ALL CLAIMS		EFT INFORMATION	
TOTAL AMOUNT PAID	185.60	AMOUNT CHARGED	232.00	NUMBER	2000000
PRIOR CREDIT BALANCE	.00	AMOUNT ALLOWED	232.00	DATE	10/28/16
CURRENT CREDIT DEFERRED	.00	DEDUCTIBLE	.00	AMOUNT	185.60
PRIOR CREDIT APPLIED	.00	COINSURANCE	.00		
NEW CREDIT BALANCE	.00	OTHER REDUCTION	.00		
NET DISBURSED	185.60	AMOUNT APPROVED	185.60		

STATUS CODES:
A - APPROVED   AJ - ADJUSTMENT   IP - IN PROCESS   R - REJECTED   V - VOID

ENCOUNTER FORM

11/11/2016
DATE

9:00 am
TIME

Anthony Battistuta
PATIENT NAME

BATTIAN0
CHART #

OFFICE VISITS - SYMPTOMATIC		
NEW		
99201	OF--New Patient Minimal	
99202	OF--New Patient Low	
99203	OF--New Patient Detailed	
99204	OF--New Patient Moderate	
99205	OF--New Patient High	
ESTABLISHED		
99211	OF--Established Patient Minimal	
99212	OF--Established Patient Low	X
99213	OF--Established Patient Detailed	
99214	OF--Established Patient Moderate	
99215	OF--Established Patient High	
PREVENTIVE VISITS		
NEW		
99381	Under 1 Year	
99382	1 - 4 Years	
99383	5 - 11 Years	
99384	12 - 17 Years	
99385	18 - 39 Years	
99386	40 - 64 Years	
99387	65 Years & Up	
ESTABLISHED		
99391	Under 1 Year	
99392	1 - 4 Years	
99393	5 - 11 Years	
99394	12 - 17 Years	
99395	18 - 39 Years	
99396	40 - 64 Years	
99397	65 Years & Up	
PROCEDURES		
12011	Simple suture--face--local anes.	
29125	App. of short arm splint; static	
29540	Strapping, ankle	
50390	Aspiration of renal cyst by needle	
71010	Chest x-ray, single view, frontal	

PROCEDURES		
71020	Chest x-ray, two views, frontal & lateral	
71030	Chest x-ray, complete, four views	
73070	Elbow x-ray, AP & lateral views	
73090	Forearm x-ray, AP & lateral views	
73100	Wrist x-ray, AP & lateral views	
73510	Hip x-ray, complete, two views	
73600	Ankle x-ray, AP & lateral views	
LABORATORY		
80019	19 clinical chemistry tests	
80048	Basic metabolic panel	
80061	Lipid panel	
82270	Blood screening, occult; feces	
82947	Glucose screening--quantitative	
82951	Glucose tolerance test, three specimens	X
83718	HDL cholesterol	
84478	Triglycerides test	
85007	Manual differential WBC	
85018	Hemoglobin	
85651	Erythrocyte sedimentation rate--non-auto	
86580	TB Mantoux test	
87072	Culture by commercial kit, nonurine...	
87076	Culture, anaerobic isolate	
87077	Bacterial culture, aerobic isolate	
87086	Urine culture and colony count	X
87430	Strep test	
87880	Direct streptococcus screen	
INJECTIONS		
90471	Immunization administration	
90703	Tetanus injection	
96372	Injection	
92516	Facial nerve function studies	
93000	Electrocardiogram--ECG with interpretation	
93015	Treadmill stress test, with physician...	
96900	Ultraviolet light treatment	
99070	Supplies and materials provided	

FAMILY CARE CENTER
285 Stephenson Blvd.
Stephenson, OH 60089
614-555-0000

☐ DANA BANU, M.D.
☐ ROBERT BEACH, M.D.
☒ PATRICIA MCGRATH, M.D.

☐ JESSICA RUDNER, M.D.
☐ JOHN RUDNER, M.D.
☐ KATHERINE YAN, M.D.

NOTES

**New address:
36 Grant Blvd.
Grandville, OH
60092**

REFERRING PHYSICIAN

NPI

AUTHORIZATION #

DIAGNOSIS
Diabetes mellitus, type II
PAYMENT AMOUNT

ENCOUNTER FORM

11/11/2016	**10:00 am**
DATE	TIME
Lawana Brooks	**BROOKLA0**
PATIENT NAME	CHART #

OFFICE VISITS - SYMPTOMATIC

NEW

99201	OF--New Patient Minimal	
99202	OF--New Patient Low	
99203	OF--New Patient Detailed	
99204	OF--New Patient Moderate	
99205	OF--New Patient High	

ESTABLISHED

99211	OF--Established Patient Minimal	
99212	OF--Established Patient Low	X
99213	OF--Established Patient Detailed	
99214	OF--Established Patient Moderate	
99215	OF--Established Patient High	

PREVENTIVE VISITS

NEW

99381	Under 1 Year	
99382	1 - 4 Years	
99383	5 - 11 Years	
99384	12 - 17 Years	
99385	18 - 39 Years	
99386	40 - 64 Years	
99387	65 Years & Up	

ESTABLISHED

99391	Under 1 Year	
99392	1 - 4 Years	
99393	5 - 11 Years	
99394	12 - 17 Years	
99395	18 - 39 Years	
99396	40 - 64 Years	
99397	65 Years & Up	

PROCEDURES

12011	Simple suture--face--local anes.	
29125	App. of short arm splint; static	X
29540	Strapping, ankle	
50390	Aspiration of renal cyst by needle	
71010	Chest x-ray, single view, frontal	

PROCEDURES

71020	Chest x-ray, two views, frontal & lateral	
71030	Chest x-ray, complete, four views	
73070	Elbow x-ray, AP & lateral views	
73090	Forearm x-ray, AP & lateral views	X
73100	Wrist x-ray, AP & lateral views	
73510	Hip x-ray, complete, two views	
73600	Ankle x-ray, AP & lateral views	

LABORATORY

80019	19 clinical chemistry tests	
80048	Basic metabolic panel	
80061	Lipid panel	
82270	Blood screening, occult; feces	
82947	Glucose screening--quantitative	
82951	Glucose tolerance test, three specimens	
83718	HDL cholesterol	
84478	Triglycerides test	
85007	Manual differential WBC	
85018	Hemoglobin	
85651	Erythrocyte sedimentation rate--non-auto	
86580	TB Mantoux test	
87072	Culture by commercial kit, nonurine...	
87076	Culture, anerobic isolate	
87077	Bacterial culture, aerobic isolate	
87086	Urine culture and colony count	
87430	Strep test	
87880	Direct streptococcus screen	

INJECTIONS

90471	Immunization administration	
90703	Tetanus injection	
96372	Injection	
92516	Facial nerve function studies	
93000	Electrocardiogram--ECG with interpretation	
93015	Treadmill stress test, with physician...	
96900	Ultraviolet light treatment	
99070	Supplies and materials provided	

FAMILY CARE CENTER
285 Stephenson Blvd.
Stephenson, OH 60089
614-555-0000

☐ DANA BANU, M.D.	☐ JESSICA RUDNER, M.D.
☐ ROBERT BEACH, M.D.	☐ JOHN RUDNER, M.D.
☒ PATRICIA MCGRATH, M.D.	☐ KATHERINE YAN, M.D.

NOTES

Accidental fall at work

Workers' comp, no copayment collected from patient

REFERRING PHYSICIAN	NPI	AUTHORIZATION #

DIAGNOSIS
841.0   E885.9   E849.3

PAYMENT AMOUNT

FAMILY CARE CENTER
285 Stephenson Boulevard
Stephenson, OH 60089
614-555-0000

CASE NOTES

PATIENT NAME	Lawana Brooks
CHART NUMBER	BROOKLA0
DATE	11/11/16
CASE	Fall at work - Workers' Compensation

NOTES

Emergency visit for injuries sustained due to a fall at work on 11/11/16.

This is classified as a work injury - non-collision.

ENCOUNTER FORM

11/11/2016	**11:15 am**
DATE	TIME
Edwin Hsu	**HSUEDWI0**
PATIENT NAME	CHART #

OFFICE VISITS - SYMPTOMATIC

NEW

99201	OF--New Patient Minimal	
99202	OF--New Patient Low	
99203	OF--New Patient Detailed	
99204	OF--New Patient Moderate	
99205	OF--New Patient High	

ESTABLISHED

99211	OF--Established Patient Minimal	X
99212	OF--Established Patient Low	
99213	OF--Established Patient Detailed	
99214	OF--Established Patient Moderate	
99215	OF--Established Patient High	

PREVENTIVE VISITS

NEW

99381	Under 1 Year	
99382	1 - 4 Years	
99383	5 - 11 Years	
99384	12 - 17 Years	
99385	18 - 39 Years	
99386	40 - 64 Years	
99387	65 Years & Up	

ESTABLISHED

99391	Under 1 Year	
99392	1 - 4 Years	
99393	5 - 11 Years	
99394	12 - 17 Years	
99395	18 - 39 Years	
99396	40 - 64 Years	
99397	65 Years & Up	

PROCEDURES

12011	Simple suture--face--local anes.	
29125	App. of short arm splint; static	
29540	Strapping, ankle	
50390	Aspiration of renal cyst by needle	
71010	Chest x-ray, single view, frontal	

PROCEDURES

71020	Chest x-ray, two views, frontal & lateral	
71030	Chest x-ray, complete, four views	
73070	Elbow x-ray, AP & lateral views	
73090	Forearm x-ray, AP & lateral views	
73100	Wrist x-ray, AP & lateral views	
73510	Hip x-ray, complete, two views	
73600	Ankle x-ray, AP & lateral views	

LABORATORY

80019	19 clinical chemistry tests	
80048	Basic metabolic panel	
80061	Lipid panel	
82270	Blood screening, occult; feces	
82947	Glucose screening--quantitative	
82951	Glucose tolerance test, three specimens	
83718	HDL cholesterol	
84478	Triglycerides test	
85007	Manual differential WBC	
85018	Hemoglobin	
85651	Erythrocyte sedimentation rate--non-auto	
86580	TB Mantoux test	
87072	Culture by commercial kit, nonurine...	
87076	Culture, anerobic isolate	
87077	Bacterial culture, aerobic isolate	
87086	Urine culture and colony count	
87430	Strep test	
87880	Direct streptococcus screen	

INJECTIONS

90471	Immunization administration	
90703	Tetanus injection	
96372	Injection	
92516	Facial nerve function studies	
93000	Electrocardiogram--ECG with interpretation	
93015	Treadmill stress test, with physician...	
96900	Ultraviolet light treatment	
99070	Supplies and materials provided	

FAMILY CARE CENTER
285 Stephenson Blvd.
Stephenson, OH 60089
614-555-0000

☐ DANA BANU, M.D.	☐ JESSICA RUDNER, M.D.
☐ ROBERT BEACH, M.D.	☐ JOHN RUDNER, M.D.
☒ PATRICIA MCGRATH, M.D.	☐ KATHERINE YAN, M.D.

NOTES

REFERRING PHYSICIAN	NPI	AUTHORIZATION #

DIAGNOSIS
461.9 Acute sinusitis

PAYMENT AMOUNT
$20 copay, check #1066

FAMILY CARE CENTER
285 Stephenson Boulevard
Stephenson, OH 60089
614-555-0000

CASE NOTES
PAGE 1 OF 1

PATIENT NAME	Edwin Hsu
CHART NUMBER	HSUEDWI0
DATE	11/11/2016
CASE	Acute sinusitis

NOTES

Patient has moved--new address is:
56 Reynolds St.
Stephenson, OH 60089

Telephone: 614-034-6729

FAMILY CARE CENTER
285 Stephenson Boulevard
Stephenson, OH 60089-4000
614-555-0000

PATIENT INFORMATION FORM

Patient

Last Name	First Name	MI	Sex	Date of Birth
Syzmanski	Hannah		__ M X F	2 / 26 / 2006

Address	City	State	Zip
3 Broadbrook Lane	Stephenson	OH	60089

Home Ph # (614) 086-4444   Cell Ph # (   )   Marital Status Single   Student Status Full-time

SS# Email	Allergies
907-66-0003	Bee stings

Employment Status	Employer Name	Work Ph # ( )	Primary Insurance ID#

Employer Address	City	State	Zip

Referred By   Ph # of Referral (   )

Responsible Party (Complete this section if the person responsible for the bill is not the patient)

Last Name	First Name	MI	Sex	Date of Birth
Syzmanski	Michael		X M __ F	6 / 5 / 1976

Address	City	State	Zip	SS#
3 Broadbrook Lane	Stephenson	OH	60089	022-45-6789

Relation to Patient __ Spouse X Parent __ Other	Employer Name Nichol's Hardware	Work Phone # ( )

Spouse, or Parent (if minor):   Home Phone # (614) 086-4444

Insurance (If you have multiple coverage, supply information from both carriers)

Primary Carrier Name	Secondary Carrier Name
Name of the Insured (Name on ID Card)	Name of the Insured (Name on ID Card)
Patient's relationship to the insured __ Self __ Spouse __ Child	Patient's relationship to the insured __ Self __ Spouse __ Child
Insured ID #	Insured ID #
Group # or Company Name	Group # or Company Name
Insurance Address	Insurance Address
Phone # Copay $ Deductible $	Phone # Copay $ Deductible $

Other Information

Is patient's condition related to:	Reason for visit: general check up

__ Employment   __ Auto Accident (if yes, state in which accident occurred: ___)   __ Other Accident

Date of Accident: /   /   Date of First Symptom of Illness: /   /

Financial Agreement and Authorization for Treatment

I authorize treatment and agree to pay all fees and charges for the person named above. I agree to pay all charges shown by statements, promptly upon their presentation, unless credit arrangements are agreed upon in writing.

I authorize payment directly to FAMILY CARE CENTER of insurance benefits otherwise payable to me. I hereby authorize the release of any medical information necessary in order to process a claim for payment in my behalf.

Signed: Michael Syzmanski   Date: 11/11/2016

ENCOUNTER FORM

11/11/2016
DATE

10:00 am
TIME

Hannah Syzmanski
PATIENT NAME

SYZMAHA0
CHART #

OFFICE VISITS - SYMPTOMATIC		
NEW		
99201	OF--New Patient Minimal	
99202	OF--New Patient Low	
99203	OF--New Patient Detailed	
99204	OF--New Patient Moderate	
99205	OF--New Patient High	
ESTABLISHED		
99211	OF--Established Patient Minimal	
99212	OF--Established Patient Low	
99213	OF--Established Patient Detailed	
99214	OF--Established Patient Moderate	
99215	OF--Established Patient High	
PREVENTIVE VISITS		
NEW		
99381	Under 1 Year	
99382	1 - 4 Years	
99383	5 - 11 Years	X
99384	12 - 17 Years	
99385	18 - 39 Years	
99386	40 - 64 Years	
99387	65 Years & Up	
ESTABLISHED		
99391	Under 1 Year	
99392	1 - 4 Years	
99393	5 - 11 Years	
99394	12 - 17 Years	
99395	18 - 39 Years	
99396	40 - 64 Years	
99397	65 Years & Up	
PROCEDURES		
12011	Simple suture--face--local anes.	
29125	App. of short arm splint; static	
29540	Strapping, ankle	
50390	Aspiration of renal cyst by needle	
71010	Chest x-ray, single view, frontal	

PROCEDURES		
71020	Chest x-ray, two views, frontal & lateral	
71030	Chest x-ray, complete, four views	
73070	Elbow x-ray, AP & lateral views	
73090	Forearm x-ray, AP & lateral views	
73100	Wrist x-ray, AP & lateral views	
73510	Hip x-ray, complete, two views	
73600	Ankle x-ray, AP & lateral views	
LABORATORY		
80019	19 clinical chemistry tests	
80048	Basic metabolic panel	
80061	Lipid panel	
82270	Blood screening, occult; feces	
82947	Glucose screening--quantitative	
82951	Glucose tolerance test, three specimens	
83718	HDL cholesterol	
84478	Triglycerides test	
85007	Manual differential WBC	
85018	Hemoglobin	
85651	Erythrocyte sedimentation rate--non-auto	
86580	TB Mantoux test	
87072	Culture by commercial kit, nonurine...	
87076	Culture, anerobic isolate	
87077	Bacterial culture, aerobic isolate	
87086	Urine culture and colony count	
87430	Strep test	
87880	Direct streptococcus screen	
INJECTIONS		
90471	Immunization administration	
90703	Tetanus injection	
96372	Injection	
92516	Facial nerve function studies	
93000	Electrocardiogram--ECG with interpretation	
93015	Treadmill stress test, with physician...	
96900	Ultraviolet light treatment	
99070	Supplies and materials provided	

FAMILY CARE CENTER
285 Stephenson Blvd.
Stephenson, OH 60089
614-555-0000

☒ DANA BANU, M.D.
☐ ROBERT BEACH, M.D.
☐ PATRICIA MCGRATH, M.D.

☐ JESSICA RUDNER, M.D.
☐ JOHN RUDNER, M.D.
☐ KATHERINE YAN, M.D.

NOTES

REFERRING PHYSICIAN
Harold Gearhart, M.D.

NPI

AUTHORIZATION #

DIAGNOSIS
v20.2

PAYMENT AMOUNT
$20 copay, check #3019

ENCOUNTER FORM

11/14/2016	**9:00 am**
DATE	TIME
Carlos Lopez	**LOPEZCA0**
PATIENT NAME	CHART #

OFFICE VISITS - SYMPTOMATIC			
NEW			
99201	OF--New Patient Minimal		
99202	OF--New Patient Low		
99203	OF--New Patient Detailed		
99204	OF--New Patient Moderate		
99205	OF--New Patient High		
ESTABLISHED			
99211	OF--Established Patient Minimal		
99212	OF--Established Patient Low	X	
99213	OF--Established Patient Detailed		
99214	OF--Established Patient Moderate		
99215	OF--Established Patient High		
PREVENTIVE VISITS			
NEW			
99381	Under 1 Year		
99382	1 - 4 Years		
99383	5 - 11 Years		
99384	12 - 17 Years		
99385	18 - 39 Years		
99386	40 - 64 Years		
99387	65 Years & Up		
ESTABLISHED			
99391	Under 1 Year		
99392	1 - 4 Years		
99393	5 - 11 Years		
99394	12 - 17 Years		
99395	18 - 39 Years		
99396	40 - 64 Years		
99397	65 Years & Up		
PROCEDURES			
12011	Simple suture--face--local anes.		
29125	App. of short arm splint; static		
29540	Strapping, ankle		
50390	Aspiration of renal cyst by needle		
71010	Chest x-ray, single view, frontal		

PROCEDURES		
71020	Chest x-ray, two views, frontal & lateral	
71030	Chest x-ray, complete, four views	
73070	Elbow x-ray, AP & lateral views	
73090	Forearm x-ray, AP & lateral views	
73100	Wrist x-ray, AP & lateral views	
73510	Hip x-ray, complete, two views	
73600	Ankle x-ray, AP & lateral views	
LABORATORY		
80019	19 clinical chemistry tests	
80048	Basic metabolic panel	
80061	Lipid panel	
82270	Blood screening, occult; feces	
82947	Glucose screening--quantitative	
82951	Glucose tolerance test, three specimens	
83718	HDL cholesterol	
84478	Triglycerides test	
85007	Manual differential WBC	
85018	Hemoglobin	
85651	Erythrocyte sedimentation rate--non-auto	
86580	TB Mantoux test	
87072	Culture by commercial kit, nonurine...	
87076	Culture, anaerobic isolate	
87077	Bacterial culture, aerobic isolate	
87086	Urine culture and colony count	
87430	Strep test	
87880	Direct streptococcus screen	
INJECTIONS		
90471	Immunization administration	
90703	Tetanus injection	
96372	Injection	
92516	Facial nerve function studies	
93000	Electrocardiogram--ECG with interpretation	
93015	Treadmill stress test, with physician...	
96900	Ultraviolet light treatment	
99070	Supplies and materials provided	

FAMILY CARE CENTER
285 Stephenson Blvd.
Stephenson, OH 60089
614-555-0000

☐ DANA BANU, M.D.
☐ ROBERT BEACH, M.D.
☒ PATRICIA MCGRATH, M.D.
☐ JESSICA RUDNER, M.D.
☐ JOHN RUDNER, M.D.
☐ KATHERINE YAN, M.D.

NOTES

REFERRING PHYSICIAN	NPI	AUTHORIZATION #

DIAGNOSIS
v65.5

PAYMENT AMOUNT
$20 copay, check #1001

FAMILY CARE CENTER
285 Stephenson Boulevard
Stephenson, OH 60089-4000
614-555-0000

PATIENT INFORMATION FORM

Patient

Last Name	First Name	MI	Sex	Date of Birth
Palmer	Christopher		X M __ F	1 / 5 / 1960

Address	City	State	Zip
17 Red Oak Lane	Jefferson	OH	60093

Home Ph # (614) 077-2249 Cell Ph # (614) 077-2250	Marital Status Single	Student Status

SS# 607-50-7620	Email cpalmer@abc.com	Allergies

Employment Status Not employed	Employer Name	Work Ph # ( )	Primary Insurance ID# 607507620

Employer Address	City	State	Zip

Referred By Dr. Marion Davis	Ph # of Referral (614) 444-3200

Responsible Party (Complete this section if the person responsible for the bill is not the patient)

Last Name	First Name	MI	Sex __ M __ F	Date of Birth / /

Address	City	State	Zip	SS#

Relation to Patient __ Spouse __ Parent __ Other	Employer Name	Work Phone # ( )

Spouse, or Parent (if minor):	Home Phone # ( )

Insurance (If you have multiple coverage, supply information from both carriers)

Primary Carrier Name Medicaid	Secondary Carrier Name
Name of the Insured (Name on ID Card) Christopher Palmer	Name of the Insured (Name on ID Card)
Patient's relationship to the insured X Self __ Spouse __ Child	Patient's relationship to the insured __ Self __ Spouse __ Child
Insured ID # 607507620	Insured ID #
Group # or Company Name	Group # or Company Name
Insurance Address 248 West Main St., Cleveland, OH 60120	Insurance Address
Phone # 614-599-6000	Copay $ 10	Phone #	Copay $
	Deductible $		Deductible $

Other Information

Is patient's condition related to:	Reason for visit: **difficulty breathing**
__ Employment __ Auto Accident (if yes, state in which accident occurred: ___) __ Other Accident	
Date of Accident: / / Date of First Symptom of Illness: / /	

Financial Agreement and Authorization for Treatment

I authorize treatment and agree to pay all fees and charges for the person named above. I agree to pay all charges shown by statements, promptly upon their presentation, unless credit arrangements are agreed upon in writing.

I authorize payment directly to FAMILY CARE CENTER of insurance benefits otherwise payable to me. I hereby authorize the release of any medical information necessary in order to process a claim for payment in my behalf.

Signed: Christopher Palmer   Date: 11/11/2016

ENCOUNTER FORM

11/11/2016
DATE

10:00 am
TIME

Christopher Palmer
PATIENT NAME

PALMECH0
CHART #

OFFICE VISITS - SYMPTOMATIC

NEW

99201	OF--New Patient Minimal	X
99202	OF--New Patient Low	
99203	OF--New Patient Detailed	
99204	OF--New Patient Moderate	
99205	OF--New Patient High	

ESTABLISHED

99211	OF--Established Patient Minimal	
99212	OF--Established Patient Low	
99213	OF--Established Patient Detailed	
99214	OF--Established Patient Moderate	
99215	OF--Established Patient High	

PREVENTIVE VISITS

NEW

99381	Under 1 Year	
99382	1 - 4 Years	
99383	5 - 11 Years	
99384	12 - 17 Years	
99385	18 - 39 Years	
99386	40 - 64 Years	
99387	65 Years & Up	

ESTABLISHED

99391	Under 1 Year	
99392	1 - 4 Years	
99393	5 - 11 Years	
99394	12 - 17 Years	
99395	18 - 39 Years	
99396	40 - 64 Years	
99397	65 Years & Up	

PROCEDURES

12011	Simple suture--face--local anes.	
29125	App. of short arm splint; static	
29540	Strapping, ankle	
50390	Aspiration of renal cyst by needle	
71010	Chest x-ray, single view, frontal	

PROCEDURES

71020	Chest x-ray, two views, frontal & lateral	
71030	Chest x-ray, complete, four views	
73070	Elbow x-ray, AP & lateral views	
73090	Forearm x-ray, AP & lateral views	
73100	Wrist x-ray, AP & lateral views	
73510	Hip x-ray, complete, two views	
73600	Ankle x-ray, AP & lateral views	

LABORATORY

80019	19 clinical chemistry tests	
80048	Basic metabolic panel	
80061	Lipid panel	
82270	Blood screening, occult; feces	
82947	Glucose screening--quantitative	
82951	Glucose tolerance test, three specimens	
83718	HDL cholesterol	
84478	Triglycerides test	
85007	Manual differential WBC	
85018	Hemoglobin	
85651	Erythrocyte sedimentation rate--non-auto	
86580	TB Mantoux test	
87072	Culture by commercial kit, nonurine...	
87076	Culture, anaerobic isolate	
87077	Bacterial culture, aerobic isolate	
87086	Urine culture and colony count	
87430	Strep test	
87880	Direct streptococcus screen	

INJECTIONS

90471	Immunization administration	
90703	Tetanus injection	
96372	Injection	
92516	Facial nerve function studies	
93000	Electrocardiogram--ECG with interpretation	
93015	Treadmill stress test, with physician...	
96900	Ultraviolet light treatment	
99070	Supplies and materials provided	

FAMILY CARE CENTER
285 Stephenson Blvd.
Stephenson, OH 60089
614-555-0000

- ☐ DANA BANU, M.D.
- ☒ ROBERT BEACH, M.D.
- ☐ PATRICIA MCGRATH, M.D.
- ☐ JESSICA RUDNER, M.D.
- ☐ JOHN RUDNER, M.D.
- ☐ KATHERINE YAN, M.D.

NOTES

REFERRING PHYSICIAN
Dr. Marion Davis

NPI

AUTHORIZATION #

DIAGNOSIS
485 Bronchopneumonia

PAYMENT AMOUNT
$10 copay, cash

EAST OHIO PPO
10 CENTRAL AVENUE
HALEVILLE, OH 60890

PROVIDER REMITTANCE

FAMILY CARE CENTER
285 STEPHENSON BLVD.
STEPHENSON, OH 60089

PAGE:	1 OF 1
DATE:	11/11/2016
ID NUMBER:	4679323

PROVIDER: PATRICIA MCGRATH, M.D.

PATIENT: BROOKS LAWANA   CLAIM: 234567000

FROM DATE	THRU DATE	PROC CODE	UNITS	AMOUNT BILLED	AMOUNT ALLOWED	DEDUCT	COPAY/ COINS	PROV PAID	REASON CODE
10/28/16	10/28/16	99212	1	54.00	48.60	.00	20.00	28.60	
10/28/16	10/28/16	73600	1	96.00	86.40	.00	.00	86.40	
	CLAIM TOTALS			150.00	135.00	.00	20.00	115.00	

PATIENT: HSU DIANE   CLAIM: 345678901

FROM DATE	THRU DATE	PROC CODE	UNITS	AMOUNT BILLED	AMOUNT ALLOWED	DEDUCT	COPAY/ COINS	PROV PAID	REASON CODE
10/28/16	10/28/16	99213	1	72.00	64.80	.00	20.00	44.80	
10/28/16	10/28/16	80048	1	50.00	45.00	.00	.00	45.00	
	CLAIM TOTALS			122.00	109.80	.00	20.00	89.80	

PROVIDER: DANA BANU, M.D.

PATIENT: PATEL RAJI   CLAIM: 567890123

FROM DATE	THRU DATE	PROC CODE	UNITS	AMOUNT BILLED	AMOUNT ALLOWED	DEDUCT	COPAY/ COINS	PROV PAID	REASON CODE
10/28/16	10/28/16	99212	1	54.00	48.60	.00	20.00	28.60	
	CLAIM TOTALS			54.00	48.60	.00	20.00	28.60	

PATIENT: SYZMANSKI MICHAEL   CLAIM: 678901234

FROM DATE	THRU DATE	PROC CODE	UNITS	AMOUNT BILLED	AMOUNT ALLOWED	DEDUCT	COPAY/ COINS	PROV PAID	REASON CODE
10/28/16	10/28/16	99212	1	54.00	48.60	.00	20.00	28.60	
	CLAIM TOTALS			54.00	48.60	.00	20.00	28.60	

PAYMENT SUMMARY		TOTAL ALL CLAIMS		EFT INFORMATION	
TOTAL AMOUNT PAID	262.00	AMOUNT CHARGED	380.00	NUMBER	4679323
PRIOR CREDIT BALANCE	.00	AMOUNT ALLOWED	342.00	DATE	11/11/2016
CURRENT CREDIT DEFERRED	.00	DEDUCTIBLE	.00	AMOUNT	262.00
PRIOR CREDIT APPLIED	.00	COPAY	.00		
NEW CREDIT BALANCE	.00	COINSURANCE	80.00		
NET DISBURSED	262.00				

STATUS CODES:
A - APPROVED   AJ - ADJUSTMENT   IP - IN PROCESS   R - REJECTED   V - VOID

ENCOUNTER FORM

11/14/2016	11:30 am
DATE	TIME
Diane Hsu	**HSUDIAN0**
PATIENT NAME	CHART #

OFFICE VISITS - SYMPTOMATIC

NEW

99201	OF--New Patient Minimal	
99202	OF--New Patient Low	
99203	OF--New Patient Detailed	
99204	OF--New Patient Moderate	
99205	OF--New Patient High	

ESTABLISHED

99211	OF--Established Patient Minimal	
99212	OF--Established Patient Low	X
99213	OF--Established Patient Detailed	
99214	OF--Established Patient Moderate	
99215	OF--Established Patient High	

PREVENTIVE VISITS

NEW

99381	Under 1 Year	
99382	1 - 4 Years	
99383	5 - 11 Years	
99384	12 - 17 Years	
99385	18 - 39 Years	
99386	40 - 64 Years	
99387	65 Years & Up	

ESTABLISHED

99391	Under 1 Year	
99392	1 - 4 Years	
99393	5 - 11 Years	
99394	12 - 17 Years	
99395	18 - 39 Years	
99396	40 - 64 Years	
99397	65 Years & Up	

PROCEDURES

12011	Simple suture--face--local anes.	
29125	App. of short arm splint; static	
29540	Strapping, ankle	
50390	Aspiration of renal cyst by needle	
71010	Chest x-ray, single view, frontal	

PROCEDURES

71020	Chest x-ray, two views, frontal & lateral	
71030	Chest x-ray, complete, four views	
73070	Elbow x-ray, AP & lateral views	
73090	Forearm x-ray, AP & lateral views	
73100	Wrist x-ray, AP & lateral views	
73510	Hip x-ray, complete, two views	
73600	Ankle x-ray, AP & lateral views	

LABORATORY

80019	19 clinical chemistry tests	
80048	Basic metabolic panel	
80061	Lipid panel	
82270	Blood screening, occult; feces	
82947	Glucose screening--quantitative	
82951	Glucose tolerance test, three specimens	
83718	HDL cholesterol	
84478	Triglycerides test	
85007	Manual differential WBC	
85018	Hemoglobin	
85651	Erythrocyte sedimentation rate--non-auto	
86580	TB Mantoux test	
87072	Culture by commercial kit, nonurine...	
87076	Culture, anaerobic isolate	
87077	Bacterial culture, aerobic isolate	
87086	Urine culture and colony count	
87430	Strep test	X
87880	Direct streptococcus screen	

INJECTIONS

90471	Immunization administration	
90703	Tetanus injection	
96372	Injection	
92516	Facial nerve function studies	
93000	Electrocardiogram--ECG with interpretation	
93015	Treadmill stress test, with physician...	
96900	Ultraviolet light treatment	
99070	Supplies and materials provided	

FAMILY CARE CENTER
285 Stephenson Blvd.
Stephenson, OH 60089
614-555-0000

☐ DANA BANU, M.D.
☐ ROBERT BEACH, M.D.
☒ PATRICIA MCGRATH, M.D.
☐ JESSICA RUDNER, M.D.
☐ JOHN RUDNER, M.D.
☐ KATHERINE YAN, M.D.

NOTES

Next appt. 1 week from today, 2:00 pm, 15 minutes

REFERRING PHYSICIAN	NPI	AUTHORIZATION #

DIAGNOSIS
487.1 Influenza

PAYMENT AMOUNT
$20 copay, check #3419

ENCOUNTER FORM

11/14/2016	**2:30 pm**
DATE	TIME
Michael Syzmanski	**SYZMAMI0**
PATIENT NAME	CHART #

OFFICE VISITS - SYMPTOMATIC				PROCEDURES		
NEW				71020	Chest x-ray, two views, frontal & lateral	
99201	OF--New Patient Minimal			71030	Chest x-ray, complete, four views	
99202	OF--New Patient Low			73070	Elbow x-ray, AP & lateral views	
99203	OF--New Patient Detailed			73090	Forearm x-ray, AP & lateral views	
99204	OF--New Patient Moderate			73100	Wrist x-ray, AP & lateral views	
99205	OF--New Patient High			73510	Hip x-ray, complete, two views	
ESTABLISHED				73600	Ankle x-ray, AP & lateral views	
99211	OF--Established Patient Minimal			**LABORATORY**		
99212	OF--Established Patient Low			80019	19 clinical chemistry tests	
99213	OF--Established Patient Detailed			80048	Basic metabolic panel	
99214	OF--Established Patient Moderate			80061	Lipid panel	
99215	OF--Established Patient High	X		82270	Blood screening, occult; feces	X
PREVENTIVE VISITS				82947	Glucose screening--quantitative	
NEW				82951	Glucose tolerance test, three specimens	
99381	Under 1 Year			83718	HDL cholesterol	
99382	1 - 4 Years			84478	Triglycerides test	
99383	5 - 11 Years			85007	Manual differential WBC	
99384	12 - 17 Years			85018	Hemoglobin	
99385	18 - 39 Years			85651	Erythrocyte sedimentation rate--non-auto	
99386	40 - 64 Years			86580	TB Mantoux test	
99387	65 Years & Up			87072	Culture by commercial kit, nonurine...	
ESTABLISHED				87076	Culture, anaerobic isolate	
99391	Under 1 Year			87077	Bacterial culture, aerobic isolate	
99392	1 - 4 Years			87086	Urine culture and colony count	
99393	5 - 11 Years			87430	Strep test	
99394	12 - 17 Years			87880	Direct streptococcus screen	
99395	18 - 39 Years			**INJECTIONS**		
99396	40 - 64 Years			90471	Immunization administration	
99397	65 Years & Up			90703	Tetanus injection	
PROCEDURES				96372	Injection	
12011	Simple suture--face--local anes.			92516	Facial nerve function studies	
29125	App. of short arm splint; static			93000	Electrocardiogram--ECG with interpretation	
29540	Strapping, ankle			93015	Treadmill stress test, with physician...	
50390	Aspiration of renal cyst by needle			96900	Ultraviolet light treatment	
71010	Chest x-ray, single view, frontal			99070	Supplies and materials provided	

FAMILY CARE CENTER
285 Stephenson Blvd.
Stephenson, OH 60089
614-555-0000

☒ DANA BANU, M.D.
☐ ROBERT BEACH, M.D.
☐ PATRICIA MCGRATH, M.D.

☐ JESSICA RUDNER, M.D.
☐ JOHN RUDNER, M.D.
☐ KATHERINE YAN, M.D.

NOTES

REFERRING PHYSICIAN	NPI	AUTHORIZATION #

DIAGNOSIS
455.6 Hemorrhoids

PAYMENT AMOUNT
$20 copay, check #3119

FAMILY CARE CENTER
285 Stephenson Boulevard
Stephenson, OH 60089-4000
614-555-0000

PATIENT INFORMATION FORM

Patient				
Last Name Robertson	First Name Stewart	MI	Sex X M __ F	Date of Birth 12/21/1975
Address 109 West Central Ave.	City Stephenson		State OH	Zip 60089

Home Ph # (614) 022-3111 Cell Ph # (614) 022-3279		Marital Status Divorced		Student Status
SS# 920-39-4567	Email srobertson@abc.com		Allergies	
Employment Status Full-time	Employer Name Nichols Hardware	Work Ph # (614) 789-0200	Primary Insurance ID# 920394567 Group 63W	
Employer Address 12 Central Ave.	City Stephenson		State OH	Zip 60089
Referred By Dr. Janet Wood		Ph # of Referral (614) 459-3700		

Responsible Party (Complete this section if the person responsible for the bill is not the patient)

Last Name	First Name	MI	Sex __ M __ F	Date of Birth / /
Address	City	State Zip		SS#
Relation to Patient __ Spouse __ Parent __ Other	Employer Name		Work Phone # ( )	
Spouse, or Parent (if minor):			Home Phone # ( )	

Insurance (If you have multiple coverage, supply information from both carriers)

Primary Carrier Name OhioCare HMO	Secondary Carrier Name
Name of the Insured (Name on ID Card) Stewart Robertson	Name of the Insured (Name on ID Card)
Patient's relationship to the insured X Self __ Spouse __ Child	Patient's relationship to the insured __ Self __ Spouse __ Child
Insured ID # 920394567	Insured ID #
Group # or Company Name Group 63W	Group # or Company Name
Insurance Address 147 Central Ave., Haleville, OH 60890	Insurance Address
Phone # 614-555-0101	Copay $ 20	Phone #	Copay $
	Deductible $		Deductible $

Other Information   Routine Physical

Is patient's condition related to: Reason for visit:
__ Employment   __ Auto Accident (if yes, state in which accident occurred: ___)   __ Other Accident
Date of Accident: /   /   Date of First Symptom of Illness: /   /

Financial Agreement and Authorization for Treatment

I authorize treatment and agree to pay all fees and charges for the person named above. I agree to pay all charges shown by statements, promptly upon their presentation, unless credit arrangements are agreed upon in writing.

I authorize payment directly to FAMILY CARE CENTER of insurance benefits otherwise payable to me. I hereby authorize the release of any medical information necessary in order to process a claim for payment in my behalf.

Signed: Stewart Robertson   Date: 12/9/2016

ENCOUNTER FORM

12/17/2016
DATE

8:00 am
TIME

Stewart Robertson
PATIENT NAME

ROBERST0
CHART #

OFFICE VISITS - SYMPTOMATIC		
NEW		
99201	OF--New Patient Minimal	
99202	OF--New Patient Low	
99203	OF--New Patient Detailed	
99204	OF--New Patient Moderate	
99205	OF--New Patient High	
ESTABLISHED		
99211	OF--Established Patient Minimal	
99212	OF--Established Patient Low	
99213	OF--Established Patient Detailed	
99214	OF--Established Patient Moderate	
99215	OF--Established Patient High	
PREVENTIVE VISITS		
NEW		
99381	Under 1 Year	
99382	1 - 4 Years	
99383	5 - 11 Years	
99384	12 - 17 Years	
99385	18 - 39 Years	
99386	40 - 64 Years	X
99387	65 Years & Up	
ESTABLISHED		
99391	Under 1 Year	
99392	1 - 4 Years	
99393	5 - 11 Years	
99394	12 - 17 Years	
99395	18 - 39 Years	
99396	40 - 64 Years	
99397	65 Years & Up	
PROCEDURES		
12011	Simple suture--face--local anes.	
29125	App. of short arm splint; static	
29540	Strapping, ankle	
50390	Aspiration of renal cyst by needle	
71010	Chest x-ray, single view, frontal	

PROCEDURES		
71020	Chest x-ray, two views, frontal & lateral	
71030	Chest x-ray, complete, four views	
73070	Elbow x-ray, AP & lateral views	
73090	Forearm x-ray, AP & lateral views	
73100	Wrist x-ray, AP & lateral views	
73510	Hip x-ray, complete, two views	
73600	Ankle x-ray, AP & lateral views	
LABORATORY		
80019	19 clinical chemistry tests	
80048	Basic metabolic panel	
80061	Lipid panel	
82270	Blood screening, occult; feces	
82947	Glucose screening--quantitative	
82951	Glucose tolerance test, three specimens	
83718	HDL cholesterol	
84478	Triglycerides test	
85007	Manual differential WBC	
85018	Hemoglobin	
85651	Erythrocyte sedimentation rate--non-auto	
86580	TB Mantoux test	
87072	Culture by commercial kit, nonurine...	
87076	Culture, anaerobic isolate	
87077	Bacterial culture, aerobic isolate	
87086	Urine culture and colony count	
87430	Strep test	
87880	Direct streptococcus screen	
INJECTIONS		
90471	Immunization administration	
90703	Tetanus injection	
96372	Injection	
92516	Facial nerve function studies	
93000	Electrocardiogram--ECG with interpretation	X
93015	Treadmill stress test, with physician...	
96900	Ultraviolet light treatment	
99070	Supplies and materials provided	

FAMILY CARE CENTER
285 Stephenson Blvd.
Stephenson, OH 60089
614-555-0000

- ☐ DANA BANU, M.D.
- ☒ ROBERT BEACH, M.D.
- ☐ PATRICIA MCGRATH, M.D.
- ☐ JESSICA RUDNER, M.D.
- ☐ JOHN RUDNER, M.D.
- ☐ KATHERINE YAN, M.D.

NOTES

REFERRING PHYSICIAN
Janet Wood, M.D.

NPI

AUTHORIZATION #

DIAGNOSIS
v70.0

PAYMENT AMOUNT
$20 copay, check #416

ENCOUNTER FORM

12/17/2016	**4:00 pm**
DATE	TIME
Michael Syzmanski	**SYZMAMI0**
PATIENT NAME	CHART #

OFFICE VISITS - SYMPTOMATIC
NEW

99201	OF--New Patient Minimal	
99202	OF--New Patient Low	
99203	OF--New Patient Detailed	
99204	OF--New Patient Moderate	
99205	OF--New Patient High	

ESTABLISHED

99211	OF--Established Patient Minimal	
99212	OF--Established Patient Low	**X**
99213	OF--Established Patient Detailed	
99214	OF--Established Patient Moderate	
99215	OF--Established Patient High	

PREVENTIVE VISITS
NEW

99381	Under 1 Year	
99382	1 - 4 Years	
99383	5 - 11 Years	
99384	12 - 17 Years	
99385	18 - 39 Years	
99386	40 - 64 Years	
99387	65 Years & Up	

ESTABLISHED

99391	Under 1 Year	
99392	1 - 4 Years	
99393	5 - 11 Years	
99394	12 - 17 Years	
99395	18 - 39 Years	
99396	40 - 64 Years	
99397	65 Years & Up	

PROCEDURES

12011	Simple suture--face--local anes.	**X**
29125	App. of short arm splint; static	
29540	Strapping, ankle	
50390	Aspiration of renal cyst by needle	
71010	Chest x-ray, single view, frontal	

PROCEDURES

71020	Chest x-ray, two views, frontal & lateral	
71030	Chest x-ray, complete, four views	
73070	Elbow x-ray, AP & lateral views	
73090	Forearm x-ray, AP & lateral views	
73100	Wrist x-ray, AP & lateral views	
73510	Hip x-ray, complete, two views	
73600	Ankle x-ray, AP & lateral views	

LABORATORY

80019	19 clinical chemistry tests	
80048	Basic metabolic panel	
80061	Lipid panel	
82270	Blood screening, occult; feces	
82947	Glucose screening--quantitative	
82951	Glucose tolerance test, three specimens	
83718	HDL cholesterol	
84478	Triglycerides test	
85007	Manual differential WBC	
85018	Hemoglobin	
85651	Erythrocyte sedimentation rate--non-auto	
86580	TB Mantoux test	
87072	Culture by commercial kit, nonurine...	
87076	Culture, anaerobic isolate	
87077	Bacterial culture, aerobic isolate	
87086	Urine culture and colony count	
87430	Strep test	
87880	Direct streptococcus screen	

INJECTIONS

90471	Immunization administration	
90703	Tetanus injection	
96372	Injection	
92516	Facial nerve function studies	
93000	Electrocardiogram--ECG with interpretation	
93015	Treadmill stress test, with physician...	
96900	Ultraviolet light treatment	
99070	Supplies and materials provided	

FAMILY CARE CENTER
285 Stephenson Blvd.
Stephenson, OH 60089
614-555-0000

☐ DANA BANU, M.D.
☐ ROBERT BEACH, M.D.
☒ PATRICIA MCGRATH, M.D.

☐ JESSICA RUDNER, M.D.
☐ JOHN RUDNER, M.D.
☐ KATHERINE YAN, M.D.

NOTES

REFERRING PHYSICIAN	NPI	AUTHORIZATION #

DIAGNOSIS
870.8

PAYMENT AMOUNT
$20 copay, check #3139

ENCOUNTER FORM

1/4/2017
DATE

9:00 am
TIME

Luther Jackson
PATIENT NAME

JACKSLU0
CHART #

OFFICE VISITS - SYMPTOMATIC
NEW

99201	OF--New Patient Minimal	
99202	OF--New Patient Low	
99203	OF--New Patient Detailed	
99204	OF--New Patient Moderate	
99205	OF--New Patient High	

ESTABLISHED

99211	OF--Established Patient Minimal	
99212	OF--Established Patient Low	X
99213	OF--Established Patient Detailed	
99214	OF--Established Patient Moderate	
99215	OF--Established Patient High	

PREVENTIVE VISITS
NEW

99381	Under 1 Year	
99382	1 - 4 Years	
99383	5 - 11 Years	
99384	12 - 17 Years	
99385	18 - 39 Years	
99386	40 - 64 Years	
99387	65 Years & Up	

ESTABLISHED

99391	Under 1 Year	
99392	1 - 4 Years	
99393	5 - 11 Years	
99394	12 - 17 Years	
99395	18 - 39 Years	
99396	40 - 64 Years	
99397	65 Years & Up	

PROCEDURES

12011	Simple suture--face--local anes.	
29125	App. of short arm splint; static	
29540	Strapping, ankle	
50390	Aspiration of renal cyst by needle	
71010	Chest x-ray, single view, frontal	

PROCEDURES

71020	Chest x-ray, two views, frontal & lateral	
71030	Chest x-ray, complete, four views	
73070	Elbow x-ray, AP & lateral views	
73090	Forearm x-ray, AP & lateral views	
73100	Wrist x-ray, AP & lateral views	
73510	Hip x-ray, complete, two views	
73600	Ankle x-ray, AP & lateral views	

LABORATORY

80019	19 clinical chemistry tests	
80048	Basic metabolic panel	
80061	Lipid panel	
82270	Blood screening, occult; feces	
82947	Glucose screening--quantitative	
82951	Glucose tolerance test, three specimens	
83718	HDL cholesterol	
84478	Triglycerides test	
85007	Manual differential WBC	
85018	Hemoglobin	
85651	Erythrocyte sedimentation rate--non-auto	
86580	TB Mantoux test	
87072	Culture by commercial kit, nonurine...	
87076	Culture, anerobic isolate	
87077	Bacterial culture, aerobic isolate	
87086	Urine culture and colony count	
87430	Strep test	
87880	Direct streptococcus screen	

INJECTIONS

90471	Immunization administration	
90703	Tetanus injection	
96372	Injection	
92516	Facial nerve function studies	
93000	Electrocardiogram--ECG with interpretation	
93015	Treadmill stress test, with physician...	
96900	Ultraviolet light treatment	
99070	Supplies and materials provided	

FAMILY CARE CENTER
285 Stephenson Blvd.
Stephenson, OH 60089
614-555-0000

- [X] DANA BANU, M.D.
- [ ] ROBERT BEACH, M.D.
- [ ] PATRICIA MCGRATH, M.D.
- [ ] JESSICA RUDNER, M.D.
- [ ] JOHN RUDNER, M.D.
- [ ] KATHERINE YAN, M.D.

NOTES

REFERRING PHYSICIAN

NPI

AUTHORIZATION #

DIAGNOSIS
485 bronchopneumonia

PAYMENT AMOUNT
$20 copay, check #1291

ENCOUNTER FORM

1/4/2017
DATE

9:00 am
TIME

Jill Simmons
PATIENT NAME

SIMMOJI0
CHART #

OFFICE VISITS - SYMPTOMATIC		
NEW		
99201	OF--New Patient Minimal	
99202	OF--New Patient Low	
99203	OF--New Patient Detailed	
99204	OF--New Patient Moderate	
99205	OF--New Patient High	
ESTABLISHED		
99211	OF--Established Patient Minimal	X
99212	OF--Established Patient Low	
99213	OF--Established Patient Detailed	
99214	OF--Established Patient Moderate	
99215	OF--Established Patient High	
PREVENTIVE VISITS		
NEW		
99381	Under 1 Year	
99382	1 - 4 Years	
99383	5 - 11 Years	
99384	12 - 17 Years	
99385	18 - 39 Years	
99386	40 - 64 Years	
99387	65 Years & Up	
ESTABLISHED		
99391	Under 1 Year	
99392	1 - 4 Years	
99393	5 - 11 Years	
99394	12 - 17 Years	
99395	18 - 39 Years	
99396	40 - 64 Years	
99397	65 Years & Up	
PROCEDURES		
12011	Simple suture--face--local anes.	
29125	App. of short arm splint; static	
29540	Strapping, ankle	
50390	Aspiration of renal cyst by needle	
71010	Chest x-ray, single view, frontal	

PROCEDURES		
71020	Chest x-ray, two views, frontal & lateral	
71030	Chest x-ray, complete, four views	
73070	Elbow x-ray, AP & lateral views	
73090	Forearm x-ray, AP & lateral views	
73100	Wrist x-ray, AP & lateral views	
73510	Hip x-ray, complete, two views	
73600	Ankle x-ray, AP & lateral views	
LABORATORY		
80019	19 clinical chemistry tests	
80048	Basic metabolic panel	
80061	Lipid panel	
82270	Blood screening, occult; feces	
82947	Glucose screening--quantitative	
82951	Glucose tolerance test, three specimens	
83718	HDL cholesterol	
84478	Triglycerides test	
85007	Manual differential WBC	
85018	Hemoglobin	
85651	Erythrocyte sedimentation rate--non-auto	
86580	TB Mantoux test	
87072	Culture by commercial kit, nonurine...	
87076	Culture, anaerobic isolate	
87077	Bacterial culture, aerobic isolate	
87086	Urine culture and colony count	
87430	Strep test	X
87880	Direct streptococcus screen	
INJECTIONS		
90471	Immunization administration	
90703	Tetanus injection	
96372	Injection	
92516	Facial nerve function studies	
93000	Electrocardiogram--ECG with interpretation	
93015	Treadmill stress test, with physician...	
96900	Ultraviolet light treatment	
99070	Supplies and materials provided	

FAMILY CARE CENTER
285 Stephenson Blvd.
Stephenson, OH 60089
614-555-0000

- ☐ DANA BANU, M.D.
- ☒ ROBERT BEACH, M.D.
- ☐ PATRICIA MCGRATH, M.D.
- ☐ JESSICA RUDNER, M.D.
- ☐ JOHN RUDNER, M.D.
- ☐ KATHERINE YAN, M.D.

NOTES

REFERRING PHYSICIAN

NPI

AUTHORIZATION #

DIAGNOSIS
034.0 strep sore throat

PAYMENT AMOUNT

ENCOUNTER FORM

1/4/2017	**9:30 am**
DATE	TIME
Nancy Stern	**STERNNA0**
PATIENT NAME	CHART #

OFFICE VISITS - SYMPTOMATIC

NEW

99201	OF--New Patient Minimal	
99202	OF--New Patient Low	
99203	OF--New Patient Detailed	
99204	OF--New Patient Moderate	
99205	OF--New Patient High	

ESTABLISHED

99211	OF--Established Patient Minimal	
99212	OF--Established Patient Low	
99213	OF--Established Patient Detailed	
99214	OF--Established Patient Moderate	
99215	OF--Established Patient High	

PREVENTIVE VISITS

NEW

99381	Under 1 Year	
99382	1 - 4 Years	
99383	5 - 11 Years	
99384	12 - 17 Years	
99385	18 - 39 Years	
99386	40 - 64 Years	
99387	65 Years & Up	

ESTABLISHED

99391	Under 1 Year	
99392	1 - 4 Years	
99393	5 - 11 Years	
99394	12 - 17 Years	
99395	18 - 39 Years	
99396	40 - 64 Years	X
99397	65 Years & Up	

PROCEDURES

12011	Simple suture--face--local anes.	
29125	App. of short arm splint; static	
29540	Strapping, ankle	
50390	Aspiration of renal cyst by needle	
71010	Chest x-ray, single view, frontal	

PROCEDURES

71020	Chest x-ray, two views, frontal & lateral	
71030	Chest x-ray, complete, four views	
73070	Elbow x-ray, AP & lateral views	
73090	Forearm x-ray, AP & lateral views	
73100	Wrist x-ray, AP & lateral views	
73510	Hip x-ray, complete, two views	
73600	Ankle x-ray, AP & lateral views	

LABORATORY

80019	19 clinical chemistry tests	
80048	Basic metabolic panel	
80061	Lipid panel	
82270	Blood screening, occult; feces	
82947	Glucose screening--quantitative	
82951	Glucose tolerance test, three specimens	
83718	HDL cholesterol	X
84478	Triglycerides test	
85007	Manual differential WBC	X
85018	Hemoglobin	
85651	Erythrocyte sedimentation rate--non-auto	
86580	TB Mantoux test	
87072	Culture by commercial kit, nonurine...	
87076	Culture, anaerobic isolate	
87077	Bacterial culture, aerobic isolate	
87086	Urine culture and colony count	X
87430	Strep test	
87880	Direct streptococcus screen	

INJECTIONS

90471	Immunization administration	
90703	Tetanus injection	
96372	Injection	
92516	Facial nerve function studies	
93000	Electrocardiogram--ECG with interpretation	X
93015	Treadmill stress test, with physician...	
96900	Ultraviolet light treatment	
99070	Supplies and materials provided	

FAMILY CARE CENTER
285 Stephenson Blvd.
Stephenson, OH 60089
614-555-0000

☐ DANA BANU, M.D.	☐ JESSICA RUDNER, M.D.
☐ ROBERT BEACH, M.D.	☐ JOHN RUDNER, M.D.
☒ PATRICIA MCGRATH, M.D.	☐ KATHERINE YAN, M.D.

NOTES

REFERRING PHYSICIAN	NPI	AUTHORIZATION #

DIAGNOSIS
v70.0 routine physical examination

PAYMENT AMOUNT
$20 copay, check #1022

ENCOUNTER FORM

1/4/2017
DATE

9:30 am
TIME

Debra Syzmanski
PATIENT NAME

SYZMADE0
CHART #

OFFICE VISITS - SYMPTOMATIC
NEW

99201	OF--New Patient Minimal	
99202	OF--New Patient Low	
99203	OF--New Patient Detailed	
99204	OF--New Patient Moderate	
99205	OF--New Patient High	

ESTABLISHED

99211	OF--Established Patient Minimal	
99212	OF--Established Patient Low	
99213	OF--Established Patient Detailed	
99214	OF--Established Patient Moderate	
99215	OF--Established Patient High	

PREVENTIVE VISITS
NEW

99381	Under 1 Year	
99382	1 - 4 Years	
99383	5 - 11 Years	
99384	12 - 17 Years	
99385	18 - 39 Years	
99386	40 - 64 Years	
99387	65 Years & Up	

ESTABLISHED

99391	Under 1 Year	
99392	1 - 4 Years	
99393	5 - 11 Years	
99394	12 - 17 Years	
99395	18 - 39 Years	
99396	40 - 64 Years	X
99397	65 Years & Up	

PROCEDURES

12011	Simple suture--face--local anes.	
29125	App. of short arm splint; static	
29540	Strapping, ankle	
50390	Aspiration of renal cyst by needle	
71010	Chest x-ray, single view, frontal	

PROCEDURES

71020	Chest x-ray, two views, frontal & lateral	
71030	Chest x-ray, complete, four views	
73070	Elbow x-ray, AP & lateral views	
73090	Forearm x-ray, AP & lateral views	
73100	Wrist x-ray, AP & lateral views	
73510	Hip x-ray, complete, two views	
73600	Ankle x-ray, AP & lateral views	

LABORATORY

80019	19 clinical chemistry tests	
80048	Basic metabolic panel	
80061	Lipid panel	
82270	Blood screening, occult; feces	
82947	Glucose screening--quantitative	
82951	Glucose tolerance test, three specimens	
83718	HDL cholesterol	X
84478	Triglycerides test	
85007	Manual differential WBC	X
85018	Hemoglobin	
85651	Erythrocyte sedimentation rate--non-auto	
86580	TB Mantoux test	
87072	Culture by commercial kit, nonurine...	
87076	Culture, anerobic isolate	
87077	Bacterial culture, aerobic isolate	
87086	Urine culture and colony count	X
87430	Strep test	
87880	Direct streptococcus screen	

INJECTIONS

90471	Immunization administration	
90703	Tetanus injection	
96372	Injection	
92516	Facial nerve function studies	
93000	Electrocardiogram--ECG with interpretation	X
93015	Treadmill stress test, with physician...	
96900	Ultraviolet light treatment	
99070	Supplies and materials provided	

FAMILY CARE CENTER
285 Stephenson Blvd.
Stephenson, OH 60089
614-555-0000

[X] DANA BANU, M.D.
[ ] ROBERT BEACH, M.D.
[ ] PATRICIA MCGRATH, M.D.

[ ] JESSICA RUDNER, M.D.
[ ] JOHN RUDNER, M.D.
[ ] KATHERINE YAN, M.D.

NOTES

REFERRING PHYSICIAN | NPI | AUTHORIZATION #

DIAGNOSIS
v70.0 routine physical examination

PAYMENT AMOUNT
$20 copay, check #3219

ENCOUNTER FORM

1/4/2017
DATE

10:15 am
TIME

Sheila Giles
PATIENT NAME

GILESSH0
CHART #

OFFICE VISITS - SYMPTOMATIC		
NEW		
99201	OF--New Patient Minimal	
99202	OF--New Patient Low	
99203	OF--New Patient Detailed	
99204	OF--New Patient Moderate	
99205	OF--New Patient High	
ESTABLISHED		
99211	OF--Established Patient Minimal	X
99212	OF--Established Patient Low	
99213	OF--Established Patient Detailed	
99214	OF--Established Patient Moderate	
99215	OF--Established Patient High	
PREVENTIVE VISITS		
NEW		
99381	Under 1 Year	
99382	1 - 4 Years	
99383	5 - 11 Years	
99384	12 - 17 Years	
99385	18 - 39 Years	
99386	40 - 64 Years	
99387	65 Years & Up	
ESTABLISHED		
99391	Under 1 Year	
99392	1 - 4 Years	
99393	5 - 11 Years	
99394	12 - 17 Years	
99395	18 - 39 Years	
99396	40 - 64 Years	
99397	65 Years & Up	
PROCEDURES		
12011	Simple suture--face--local anes.	
29125	App. of short arm splint; static	
29540	Strapping, ankle	
50390	Aspiration of renal cyst by needle	
71010	Chest x-ray, single view, frontal	

PROCEDURES		
71020	Chest x-ray, two views, frontal & lateral	
71030	Chest x-ray, complete, four views	
73070	Elbow x-ray, AP & lateral views	
73090	Forearm x-ray, AP & lateral views	
73100	Wrist x-ray, AP & lateral views	
73510	Hip x-ray, complete, two views	
73600	Ankle x-ray, AP & lateral views	
LABORATORY		
80019	19 clinical chemistry tests	
80048	Basic metabolic panel	
80061	Lipid panel	
82270	Blood screening, occult; feces	
82947	Glucose screening--quantitative	
82951	Glucose tolerance test, three specimens	
83718	HDL cholesterol	
84478	Triglycerides test	
85007	Manual differential WBC	
85018	Hemoglobin	
85651	Erythrocyte sedimentation rate--non-auto	
86580	TB Mantoux test	
87072	Culture by commercial kit, nonurine...	
87076	Culture, anaerobic isolate	
87077	Bacterial culture, aerobic isolate	
87086	Urine culture and colony count	
87430	Strep test	
87880	Direct streptococcus screen	
INJECTIONS		
90471	Immunization administration	X
90703	Tetanus injection	X
96372	Injection	
92516	Facial nerve function studies	
93000	Electrocardiogram--ECG with interpretation	
93015	Treadmill stress test, with physician...	
96900	Ultraviolet light treatment	
99070	Supplies and materials provided	

FAMILY CARE CENTER
285 Stephenson Blvd.
Stephenson, OH 60089
614-555-0000

- ☐ DANA BANU, M.D.
- ☒ ROBERT BEACH, M.D.
- ☐ PATRICIA MCGRATH, M.D.
- ☐ JESSICA RUDNER, M.D.
- ☐ JOHN RUDNER, M.D.
- ☐ KATHERINE YAN, M.D.

NOTES

REFERRING PHYSICIAN

NPI

AUTHORIZATION #

DIAGNOSIS
v03.7 tetanus immunization

PAYMENT AMOUNT

ENCOUNTER FORM

1/4/2017	10:30 am
DATE	TIME
Pauline Battistuta	**BATTIPA0**
PATIENT NAME	CHART #

OFFICE VISITS - SYMPTOMATIC
NEW

99201	OF--New Patient Minimal	
99202	OF--New Patient Low	
99203	OF--New Patient Detailed	
99204	OF--New Patient Moderate	
99205	OF--New Patient High	

ESTABLISHED

99211	OF--Established Patient Minimal	X
99212	OF--Established Patient Low	
99213	OF--Established Patient Detailed	
99214	OF--Established Patient Moderate	
99215	OF--Established Patient High	

PREVENTIVE VISITS
NEW

99381	Under 1 Year	
99382	1 - 4 Years	
99383	5 - 11 Years	
99384	12 - 17 Years	
99385	18 - 39 Years	
99386	40 - 64 Years	
99387	65 Years & Up	

ESTABLISHED

99391	Under 1 Year	
99392	1 - 4 Years	
99393	5 - 11 Years	
99394	12 - 17 Years	
99395	18 - 39 Years	
99396	40 - 64 Years	
99397	65 Years & Up	

PROCEDURES

12011	Simple suture--face--local anes.	
29125	App. of short arm splint; static	
29540	Strapping, ankle	
50390	Aspiration of renal cyst by needle	
71010	Chest x-ray, single view, frontal	

PROCEDURES

71020	Chest x-ray, two views, frontal & lateral	
71030	Chest x-ray, complete, four views	
73070	Elbow x-ray, AP & lateral views	
73090	Forearm x-ray, AP & lateral views	
73100	Wrist x-ray, AP & lateral views	
73510	Hip x-ray, complete, two views	
73600	Ankle x-ray, AP & lateral views	

LABORATORY

80019	19 clinical chemistry tests	
80048	Basic metabolic panel	
80061	Lipid panel	
82270	Blood screening, occult; feces	
82947	Glucose screening--quantitative	
82951	Glucose tolerance test, three specimens	
83718	HDL cholesterol	
84478	Triglycerides test	
85007	Manual differential WBC	
85018	Hemoglobin	
85651	Erythrocyte sedimentation rate--non-auto	
86580	TB Mantoux test	
87072	Culture by commercial kit, nonurine...	
87076	Culture, anerobic isolate	
87077	Bacterial culture, aerobic isolate	
87086	Urine culture and colony count	
87430	Strep test	
87880	Direct streptococcus screen	

INJECTIONS

90471	Immunization administration	
90703	Tetanus injection	
96372	Injection	
92516	Facial nerve function studies	
93000	Electrocardiogram--ECG with interpretation	
93015	Treadmill stress test, with physician...	
96900	Ultraviolet light treatment	
99070	Supplies and materials provided	

FAMILY CARE CENTER
285 Stephenson Blvd.
Stephenson, OH 60089
614-555-0000

- ☐ DANA BANU, M.D.
- ☐ ROBERT BEACH, M.D.
- ☒ PATRICIA MCGRATH, M.D.
- ☐ JESSICA RUDNER, M.D.
- ☐ JOHN RUDNER, M.D.
- ☐ KATHERINE YAN, M.D.

NOTES

upper respiratory infection

REFERRING PHYSICIAN	NPI	AUTHORIZATION #

DIAGNOSIS
465.9

PAYMENT AMOUNT

MEDICARE
246 WEST MAIN ST.
CLEVELAND, OH 60120

PROVIDER REMITTANCE
THIS IS NOT A BILL
A PAYMENT SUMMARY AND AN EXPLANATION OF
CODES ARE AT THE END OF THIS STATEMENT

FAMILY CARE CENTER
285 STEPHENSON BLVD.
STEPHENSON, OH 60089-4000

PAGE: 1 OF 1
DATE: 12/30/2016
ID NUMBER: 3470629

PROVIDER: PATRICIA MCGRATH, M.D.

PATIENT: BATTISTUTA ANTHONY   CLAIM: 234567890

FROM DATE	THRU DATE	PROC CODE	UNITS	AMOUNT BILLED	AMOUNT ALLOWED	DEDUCT	COPAY/ COINS	PROV PAID	REASON CODE
10/27/16	10/27/16	99212	1	54.00	37.36	.00	.00	29.89	
10/27/16	10/27/16	82947	1	25.00	5.48	.00	.00	4.38	
	CLAIM TOTALS			79.00	42.84	.00	.00	34.27	

PATIENT: BATTISTUTA ANTHONY   CLAIM: 234567891

FROM DATE	THRU DATE	PROC CODE	UNITS	AMOUNT BILLED	AMOUNT ALLOWED	DEDUCT	COPAY/ COINS	PROV PAID	REASON CODE
11/11/16	11/11/16	99212	1	54.00	37.36	.00	.00	29.89	
11/11/16	11/11/16	82951	1	63.00	16.12	.00	.00	12.90	
11/11/16	11/11/16	87086	1	51.00	11.28	.00	.00	9.02	
	CLAIM TOTALS			168.00	64.76	.00	.00	51.81	

PROVIDER: KATHERINE YAN, M.D.

PATIENT: JONES ELIZABETH   CLAIM: 234567892

FROM DATE	THRU DATE	PROC CODE	UNITS	AMOUNT BILLED	AMOUNT ALLOWED	DEDUCT	COPAY/ COINS	PROV PAID	REASON CODE
10/3/16	10/3/16	99213	1	72.00	51.03	.00	.00	40.82	
	CLAIM TOTALS			72.00	51.03	.00	.00	40.82	

PAYMENT SUMMARY		TOTAL ALL CLAIMS		EFT INFORMATION	
TOTAL AMOUNT PAID	126.90	AMOUNT CHARGED	319.00	NUMBER	3470629
PRIOR CREDIT BALANCE	.00	AMOUNT ALLOWED	158.63	DATE	12/30/16
CURRENT CREDIT DEFERRED	.00	DEDUCTIBLE	.00	AMOUNT	126.90
PRIOR CREDIT APPLIED	.00	COPAY	.00		
NEW CREDIT BALANCE	.00	COINSURANCE	.00		
NET DISBURSED	126.90	AMOUNT APPROVED	158.63		

STATUS CODES:
A - APPROVED   AJ - ADJUSTMENT   IP - IN PROCESS   R - REJECTED   V - VOID

CHAMPVA
240 CENTER ST.
COLUMBUS, OH 60220

PROVIDER REMITTANCE
THIS IS NOT A BILL
A PAYMENT SUMMARY AND AN EXPLANATION OF
CODES ARE AT THE END OF THIS STATEMENT

FAMILY CARE CENTER
285 STEPHENSON BLVD.
STEPHENSON, OH 60089-4000

PAGE:	1 OF 1
DATE:	12/30/2016
ID NUMBER:	76374021

PROVIDER: JOHN RUDNER, M.D.

PATIENT: FITZWILLIAMS JOHN   CLAIM: 123456789

FROM DATE	THRU DATE	PROC CODE	UNITS	AMOUNT BILLED	AMOUNT ALLOWED	DEDUCT	COPAY/ COINS	PROV PAID	REASON CODE
10/3/16	10/3/16	99212	1	54.00	37.36	.00	15.00	22.36	
10/3/16	10/3/16	82270	1	19.00	4.54	.00	.00	4.54	
		CLAIM TOTALS		73.00	41.90	.00	15.00	26.90	

****************** CHECK #76374021 IN THE AMOUNT OF $26.90 IS ATTACHED ******************

PAYMENT SUMMARY

TOTAL AMOUNT PAID	26.90
PRIOR CREDIT BALANCE	.00
CURRENT CREDIT DEFERRED	.00
PRIOR CREDIT APPLIED	.00
NEW CREDIT BALANCE	.00
NET DISBURSED	26.90

TOTAL ALL CLAIMS

AMOUNT CHARGED	73.00
AMOUNT ALLOWED	41.90
DEDUCTIBLE	.00
COPAY	15.00
OTHER REDUCTION	.00

STATUS CODES:
AJ - ADJUSTMENT   IP - IN PROCESS   R - REJECTED   V - VOID

MEDICAID
246 WEST MAIN ST.
CLEVELAND, OH 60120

PROVIDER REMITTANCE
THIS IS NOT A BILL
A PAYMENT SUMMARY AND AN EXPLANATION OF
CODES ARE AT THE END OF THIS STATEMENT

FAMILY CARE CENTER
285 STEPHENSON BLVD.
STEPHENSON, OH 60089-4000

PAGE:	1 OF 1
DATE:	12/30/2016
ID NUMBER:	137291449

PROVIDER. ROBERT DEACH, M.D.

PATIENT: PALMER CHRISTOPHER   CLAIM: 56789012

FROM DATE	THRU DATE	PROC CODE	UNITS	AMOUNT BILLED	AMOUNT ALLOWED	DEDUCT	COPAY/ COINS	PROV PAID	REASON CODE
11/11/16	11/11/16	99201	1	66.00	35.58	.00	10.00	25.58	
11/11/16	11/11/16	87430	1	29.00	16.01	.00	.00	16.01	
	CLAIM TOTALS			95.00	51.59	.00	10.00	41.59	

PAYMENT SUMMARY

TOTAL AMOUNT PAID	41.59
PRIOR CREDIT BALANCE	.00
CURRENT CREDIT DEFERRED	.00
PRIOR CREDIT APPLIED	.00
NEW CREDIT BALANCE	.00
NET DISBURSED	41.59

TOTAL ALL CLAIMS

AMOUNT CHARGED	95.00
AMOUNT ALLOWED	51.59
DEDUCTIBLE	.00
COPAY	10.00
OTHER REDUCTION	.00

EFT INFORMATION

NUMBER	137291449
DATE	12/30/16
AMOUNT	41.59

STATUS CODES:
A - APPROVED   AJ - ADJUSTMENT   IP - IN PROCESS   R - REJECTED   V - VOID

EAST OHIO PPO
10 CENTRAL AVENUE
HALEVILLE, OH 60890

PROVIDER REMITTANCE
THIS IS NOT A BILL
A PAYMENT SUMMARY AND AN EXPLANATION OF
CODES ARE AT THE END OF THIS STATEMENT

FAMILY CARE CENTER
285 STEPHENSON BLVD.
STEPHENSON, OH 60089-4000

PAGE:	1 OF 1
DATE:	12/30/2016
ID NUMBER:	376490713

PROVIDER: DANA BANU, M.D.

PATIENT: SYZMANSKI HANNAH   CLAIM: 78901234

FROM DATE	THRU DATE	PROC CODE	UNITS	AMOUNT BILLED	AMOUNT ALLOWED	DEDUCT	COPAY/ COINS	PROV PAID	REASON CODE
11/11/16	11/11/16	99383	1	224.00	201.60	.00	20.00	181.60	
	CLAIM TOTALS			224.00	201.60	.00	20.00	181.60	

PATIENT: SYZMANSKI MICHAEL   CLAIM: 89012345

FROM DATE	THRU DATE	PROC CODE	UNITS	AMOUNT BILLED	AMOUNT ALLOWED	DEDUCT	COPAY/ COINS	PROV PAID	REASON CODE
11/14/16	11/14/16	99215	1	163.00	146.70	.00	20.00	126.70	
11/14/16	11/14/16	82270	1	19.00	17.10	.00	.00	17.10	
	CLAIM TOTALS			182.00	163.80	.00	20.00	143.80	

PROVIDER: PATRICIA MCGRATH, M.D.

PATIENT: SYZMANSKI MICHAEL   CLAIM: 901234563

FROM DATE	THRU DATE	PROC CODE	UNITS	AMOUNT BILLED	AMOUNT ALLOWED	DEDUCT	COPAY/ COINS	PROV PAID	REASON CODE
12/17/16	12/17/16	99212	1	54.00	48.60	.00	20.00	28.60	
12/17/16	12/17/16	12011	1	202.00	181.80	.00	.00	181.80	
	CLAIM TOTALS			256.00	230.40	.00	20.00	210.40	

PAYMENT SUMMARY		TOTAL ALL CLAIMS		EFT INFORMATION	
TOTAL AMOUNT PAID	535.80	AMOUNT CHARGED	662.00	NUMBER	376490713
PRIOR CREDIT BALANCE	.00	AMOUNT ALLOWED	595.80	DATE	12/30/16
CURRENT CREDIT DEFERRED	.00	DEDUCTIBLE	.00	AMOUNT	535.80
PRIOR CREDIT APPLIED	.00	COPAY	60.00		
NEW CREDIT BALANCE	.00	COINSURANCE	0.00		
NET DISBURSED	535.80				

REASON CODES:
AJ - ADJUSTMENT   IP - IN PROCESS   R - REJECTED   V - VOID

OHIOCARE HMO
147 CENTRAL AVENUE
HALEVILLE, OH 60890

FAMILY CARE CENTER
285 STEPHENSON BLVD.
STEPHENSON, OH 60089-4000

PAGE:	1 OF 1
DATE:	12/30/2016
ID NUMBER:	767729

OHIOCARE HMO CAPITATION STATEMENT
MONTH OF NOVEMBER 2016

PROVIDERS
BANU DANA
BEACH ROBERT
MCGRATH PATRICIA
RUDNER JESSICA
RUDNER JOHN
YAN KATHERINE

MEMBER NUMBER	MEMBER NAME	CONTRACT NUMBER	CONTRACT STATUS
0003602149	FAMILY CARE CENTER	YG34906	APPROVED

AMOUNT OF PAYMENT $2,500.00
EFT STATUS: SENT 12/30/16 2:46PM
TRANSACTION #767729

CiMO glossary

a

access rights   security option that determines the areas of the program a user can access, and whether the user has rights to enter or edit data

accounting cycle   the flow of financial transactions in a business

accounts receivable (AR)   monies that are flowing into a business

adjudication   series of steps that determine whether a claim should be paid

adjustments   changes to patients' accounts that alter the amounts charged or paid

administrative safeguards   administrative policies and procedures designed to protect electronic health information outlined by the HIPAA Security Rule

aging report   a report that lists the amount of money owed to the practice, organized by the amount of time the money has been owed

audit/edit report   a report from a clearinghouse that lists errors to be corrected before a claim can be submitted to the payer

audit trail   a report that traces who has accessed electronic information, when information was accessed, and whether any information was changed

Auto Log Off   feature of Medisoft that automatically logs a user out of the program after a period of inactivity

autoposting   an automated process for entering information from a remittance advice (RA) into a practice management program

b

backup data   a copy of data files made at a specific point in time that can be used to restore data

billing cycle   regular schedule of sending statements to patients

breach   the acquisition, access, use, or disclosure of unsecured PHI in a manner not permitted under the HIPAA Privacy Rule

c

capitated plan   an insurance plan in which prepayments made to a physician cover the physician's services to a plan member for a specified period of time

capitation   payment to a provider that covers each plan member's health care services for a certain period of time

capitation payments   payments made to physicians on a regular basis for providing services to patients in a managed care plan

case   a grouping of transactions that share a common element

charges   amounts a provider bills for the services performed

chart   a folder that contains all records pertaining to a patient

chart number   a unique number that identifies a patient

clean claims   claims with all the correct information necessary for payer processing

clearinghouse   a company that receives claims from a provider, prepares them for processing, and transmits them to the payers in HIPAA-compliant format

coding   the process of translating a description of a diagnosis or procedure into a standardized code

coinsurance   percentage of charges that an insured person must pay for health care services after payment of the deductible amount

CMS-1500 (08/05)   the mandated paper insurance claim form

collection agency   an outside firm hired to collect on delinquent accounts

collection list   a tool for tracking activities that need to be completed as part of the collection process

collection tracer report   a tool for keeping track of collection letters that were sent

computer-assisted coding   assigning preliminary diagnosis and procedure codes using computer software

consumer-driven health plan (CDHP)   a type of managed care in which a high-deductible, low-premium insurance plan is combined with a pretax savings account to cover out-of-pocket medical expenses

copayment   A fixed fee paid by the patient at the time of an office visit

cycle billing   a type of billing in which statement printing and mailing is staggered throughout the month

d

database   a collection of related bits of information

day sheet   a report that provides information on practice activities for a twenty-four-hour period

deductible   amount due before benefits start

diagnosis physician's opinion of the nature of the patient's illness or injury

diagnosis code a standardized value that represents a patient's illness, signs, and symptoms

documentation a record of health care encounters between the physician and the patient, created by the provider

e

electronic data interchange (EDI) the exchange of routine business transactions from one computer to another using publicly available communications protocols

electronic funds transfer (EFT) the electronic routing of funds between banks

electronic health record (EHR) a computerized lifelong health care record for an individual that incorporates data from providers who treat the individual

electronic medical records (EMRs) the computerized records of one physician's encounters with a patient over time

electronic prescribing the use of computers and handheld devices to transmit prescriptions in digital format

electronic remittance advice (ERA) an electronic document that lists patients, dates of service, charges, and the amount paid or denied by the insurance carrier

encounter form a list of the procedures and charges for a patient's visit

established patient a patient who has been seen by a provider in the practice in the same specialty within three years

evidence-based medicine medical care based on the latest and most accurate clinical research

explanation of benefits (EOB) document from a payer that shows how the amount of a benefit was determined

f

fee-for-service health plan that repays the policyholder for covered medical expenses

fee schedule a document that specifies the amount the provider bills for provided services

filter a condition that data must meet to be selected

g

guarantor an individual who may not be a patient of the practice, but who is financially responsible for a patient account

h

health information technology (HIT) technology that is used to record, store, and manage patient health care information

Health Information Technology for Economic and Clinical Health Act (HITECH) part of the American Recovery and Reinvestment Act of 2009 that provides financial incentives to physicians and hospitals to adopt EHRs and strengthens HIPAA privacy and security regulations

health maintenance organization (HMO) a managed health care system in which providers agree to offer health care to the organization's members for fixed payments

health plan a plan, program, or organization that provides health benefits

HIPAA (Health Insurance Portability and Accountability Act of 1996) federal act that set forth guidelines for standardizing the electronic data interchange of administrative and financial transactions, exposing fraud and abuse in government programs, and protecting the security and privacy of health information

HIPAA Electronic Transaction and Code Sets standards regulations requiring electronic transactions such as claim transmission to use standardized formats

HIPAA Privacy Rule regulations for protecting individually identifiable information about a patient's health and payment for health care that is created or received by a health care provider

HIPAA Security Rule regulations outlining the minimum administrative, technical, and physical safeguards required to prevent unauthorized access to protected health care information

i

insurance aging report a report that lists how long a payer has taken to respond to insurance claims

k

knowledge base a collection of up-to-date technical information

m

managed care a type of insurance in which the carrier is responsible for both the financing and the delivery of health care

medical coder a person who analyzes and codes patient diagnoses, procedures, and symptoms

medical necessity treatment provided by a physician to a patient for the purpose of preventing, diagnosing, or treating an illness, injury, or its symptoms in a manner that is appropriate and is provided in accordance with generally accepted standards of medical practice

medical record a chronological record of a patient's medical history and care that includes information that the patient provides, as well as the physician's assessment, diagnosis, and treatment plan

Medisoft Program Date date the program uses to record when a transaction occurred

MMDDCCYY format the way dates must be keyed in Medisoft, in which "MM" stands for the month, "DD" stands for the day, "CC" represents the century, and "YY" stands for the year

modifier a two-digit character that is appended to a CPT code to report special circumstances involved with a procedure or service

MultiLink codes groups of procedure code entries that relate to a single activity

n

National Provider Identifier (NPI) a standard identifier for health care providers consisting of ten numbers

navigator buttons buttons that simplify the task of moving from one entry to another

new patient a patient who has not received services from the same provider or a provider of the same specialty within the same practice for a period of three years

NSF check a check that is not honored by a bank because the account it was written on does not have sufficient funds to cover it

o

Office Hours break a block of time when a physician is unavailable for appointments with patients

Office Hours calendar an interactive calendar that is used to select or change dates in Office Hours

Office Hours patient information the area of the Office Hours window that displays information about the patient who is selected in the provider's daily schedule

once-a-month billing a type of billing in which statements are mailed to all patients at the same time each month

p

packing data the deletion of vacant slots from the database

patient aging report a report that lists a patient's balance by age, date and amount of the last payment, and telephone number

patient day sheet a summary of patient activity on a given day

patient information form a form that includes a patient's personal, employment, and insurance data needed to complete an insurance claim

patient ledger a report that lists the financial activity in each patient's account

patient statement a list of the amount of money a patient owes, the procedures performed, and the dates the procedures were performed

payer private or government organization that insures or pays for health care on behalf of beneficiaries

payment day sheet a report that lists all payments received on a particular day, organized by provider

payment plan an agreement between a patient and a practice in which the patient agrees to make regular monthly payments over a specified period of time

payment schedule a document that specifies the amount the payer agrees to reimburse the provider for a service

payments monies received from patients and insurance carriers

personal health records (PHRs) private, secure electronic files that are created, maintained, and owned by the patient

physical safeguards mechanisms required to protect electronic systems, equipment, and data from threats, environmental hazards, and unauthorized intrusion

policyholder a person or entity who buys an insurance plan; the insured

practice analysis report a report that analyzes the revenue of a practice for a specified period of time

practice management program (PMP) a software program that automates many of the administrative and financial tasks in a medical practice

preferred provider organization (PPO) managed care network of health care providers who agree to perform services for plan members at discounted fees

premium the periodic amount of money the insured pays to a health plan for insurance coverage

primary insurance carrier the first carrier to whom claims are submitted

procedure medical treatment provided by a physician or other health care provider

procedure code a code that identifies a medical service

procedure day sheet a report that lists all the procedures performed on a particular day, in numerical order

prompt payment laws state laws that mandate a time period within which clean claims must be paid; if they are not, financial penalties are levied against the payer

protected health information (PHI) information about a patient's health or payment for health care that can be used to identify the person

provider selection box   a selection box that determines which provider's schedule is displayed in the provider's daily schedule

provider's daily schedule   a listing of time slots for a particular day for a specific provider that corresponds to the date selected in the calendar

purging data   the process of deleting files of patients who are no longer seen by a provider in a practice

r

rebuilding indexes   a process that checks and verifies data and corrects any internal problems with the data

recalculating balances   the process of updating balances to reflect the most recent changes made to the data

record of treatment and progress   a physician's notes about a patient's condition and diagnosis

referring provider   a physician who recommends that a patient see a specific other physician

remainder statements   statements that list only those charges that are not paid in full after all insurance carrier payments have been received

remittance advice (RA)   an explanation of benefits transmitted by a payer to a provider

restoring data   the process of retrieving data from backup storage devices

s

selection boxes   fields within the Search dialog box that are used to select the data that will be included in a report

sponsor   in TRICARE, the active-duty service member

standard statements   statements that show all charges regardless of whether the insurance has paid on the transactions

statement   a list of all services performed for a patient, along with the charges for each service

t

technical safeguards   automated processes used to protect data and control access to data

tickler   a reminder to follow up on an account

u

uncollectible account   an account that does not respond to collection efforts and is written off the practice's expected accounts receivable

w

walkout statement   a document listing charges and payments that is given to a patient after an office visit

workflow   a set of activities designed to produce a specific outcome

write-off   a balance that has been removed from a patient's account

x

X12-837 Health Care Claim (837P)   HIPAA standard format for electronic transmission of a professional claim from a provider to a health plan

Coding. *See also* CPT codes; ICD-9-CM
      codes
    color, in transaction entry, 183
    computer-assisted, 42
    defined, 11
    impact of health information
        technology (HIT) on, 42–44
    reviewing compliance with, 13–15
Coinsurance, 6
Collection agencies, 348–350
Collection list, 353–361
    tickler in, 353, 357–361
    using, 353–357
Collection List button, 71
Collection process, 18–20, 343–368
    collection agencies in, 348–350
    collection letters, 361–366
    day sheets, 19
    importance of, 344
    laws governing patient
        collections, 347–348
    laws governing timely payment of
        insurance claims, 344
    medical practice financial policy, 8,
        20, 344–347
    monthly report, 19
    nonsufficient funds (NSF)
        checks, 204–205
    outstanding balances, 20
    patient collections, 344–367
    payment plans in, 115,
        347–348, 350
    practice management
        programs, 353–367
    writing off uncollectible
        accounts, 350–352
Collection reports
    Collection tracer report, 366–367
    overdue balance report for patients
        with appointments, 401–402
    patient, 361–366
Color coding, in transaction
    entry, 183
Comment tab
    for case notes, 160
    in editing claims, 230
    statement, 284
Computer-assisted coding, 42
Computerized medical records
    (CMRs). *See* Electronic health
    records (EHRs)
Computerized patient records (CPRs).
    See Electronic health records
    (EHRs)
Computers. *See* Health information
    technology (HIT)
Condition tab, 155–158
Confidentiality. *See* Privacy
Consumer Credit Protection Act,
    347–348
Consumer-driven health plan
    (CDHP), 7
Copayment, 7, 8–10, 149, 191–197

Copayment report, 317
Copy Address button, 111
Copy feature, Copy Case button, 139
CPT codes. *See also* Procedure codes
    described, 65
    for entering charges, 178–179
    MultiLink codes, 181–182
    sample, 12
    as standards, 46
Create Claims dialog box, 221–223
Create Statement dialog box, 279–282
Crossover claims, 151
Current Procedural Terminology (CPT),
    12–13, 65. *See also* CPT codes
Custom report(s), 327–332
Custom Report List button, 71
Cycle billing, 287

d

Databases
    defined, 64
    Medisoft®, 64–65
Dates, in Medisoft®, 76–81, 177–178,
    304–306
Day sheets, 19, 307–313
    defined, 307
    patient day sheet, 19, 308–311
    payment day sheet, 312–313
    procedure day sheet, 311–312
Death/Status box, 156
Deductible, 6
Delete feature, 76
    for appointments in Office
        Hours, 392–393
    for cases, 139
    purging data, 92–93
    for transaction information, 181
Department of Health and Human
    Services (HHS), 51
Deposit dialog box, fields in, 255–257
Deposit List dialog box, 253–260
    entering capitation payments, 270–277
    entering deposits, 258–260
    fields in, 253–255
Details button, 183
Diagnosis, 11
Diagnosis Code List button, 71
Diagnosis codes, 11–12. *See also*
        ICD-9-CM codes
    Diagnosis tab for cases, 153–155
    for entering charges, 179–180
    in Medisoft® database, 64–65
Dialog boxes. *See specific types of
        dialog boxes*
Dictation, 41
Documentation, 10–13
    diagnosis, 11–12
    impact of health information
        technology (HIT) on, 41–44
    procedure, 12–13

e

Early and Periodic Screening,
    Diagnosis, and Treatment
    (EPSDT), 151, 162
EDI Report, 237–239
EDI tab, 160–163
Edit Case button, 138, 163–164
Edit feature
    for appointments in Office
        Hours, 392–393
    for case information, 138, 163–164
    Edit menu, 66
    for information on established
        patients, 126–127, 138, 163–164
    for insurance claims, 227–231
    for patient statements, 282–283
    for transaction information,
        184–185
Edit Patient Notes in Final Draft
    button, 72
Edit Statement dialog box, 282–283
EHRs. *See* Electronic health records
    (EHRs)
Electronic claims, 29–30, 232–236
    attachments, sending, 237–239
    audit/edit report, 30
    changing status of claims, 231–232
    clearinghouses for, 29–30
    in Medisoft®
        creating cases for imported
            transactions, 165
        importing transactions, 165
    standards for, 44–46, 232–233
    steps in submitting, 232–236
    transmitting, 237–239
Electronic data interchange (EDI), 45,
    154, 160–163, 232–236
Electronic encounter form (EEF), 42
Electronic funds transfer (EFT), 45
Electronic health records (EHRs)
    advantages, 39–41
        efficiency, 40–41
        quality, 39–40
        safety, 39
    core functions, 33–38
        administrative processes, 38
        decision support, 37
        electronic communication and
            connectivity, 37
        health information and data,
            33–34
        order management, 35
        patient support, 38
        reporting and population
            management, 38
        results management, 34–35
    creating cases for imported
        transactions, 165
    defined, 13, 32, 34
    functions of EHR programs, 32–38
    importing transactions, 165, 205

practice management program
(PMP) and, 13
sample, 35
transferring appointment
information, 403
transferring patient
information, 127–128
viewing data transfer reports, 333
Electronic medical records (EMRs), 32,
34, 38
Electronic patient records (EPRs). *See*
Electronic health records (EHRs)
Electronic prescribing, 35, 36
Electronic remittance advice (ERA), 32,
250–252
Emergencies
Condition tab, 156
emergency contact information, 114
Employer drop-down list, 114
Employer information, 114, 118–121, 143
EMRs (electronic medical records),
32, 34
Encounter form, 13, 14, 174
electronic, 42
Enter Deposits button, 72
EPSDT (Early and Periodic
Screening, Diagnosis, and
Treatment), 151, 162
Errors
common claim, 252
computers in reduction of, 39
electronic medical record (EMR)
and, 39
Established patients
creating new case for, 138
defined, 5, 109
editing information on, 126–127,
138, 163–164
searching for patient
information, 121–126
Evidence-based medicine, 39–40
Exiting Medisoft®, 72, 85–87
Exiting Office Hours, 381
Explanation of benefits (EOB), 16–18

f

F8 function key, 119
Fair Debt Collection Practices Act of
1977, 347
Fee-for-service plans, 6
Fee schedule
defined, 248
in third-party reimbursement,
248–250, 252
Field box, 122–124, 125
Field Value box, 125
File maintenance utilities, 89–94
backing up data, 85–87
packing data, 90–92
purging data, 92–93

rebuilding indexes, 90
recalculating patient balances, 93–94
restoring backup files, 87–89
File menu, 65, 66
Filters
Create Claims dialog box, 221–223
defined, 221
selecting, in printing
statements, 287–288
Final Enforcement Rule, 46
Find Report box, 325
Follow-up appointments, 386–388
Forms. *See also* Report(s)
Acknowledgment of Receipt of
Notice of Privacy Practices, 48
CMS-1500 (08/05), 46, 216, 217–219
encounter form, 13, 14, 42, 174
Notice of Privacy Practices, 47
patient information form, 8–10, 14

g

General tab, 282–283
Guarantor (insured), 112

h

Hackers, 49–50
Health information technology (HIT),
27–51. *See also* Electronic claims
advantages of computer use, 28
advantages of electronic health
records, 39–41
defined, 28
functions of practice management
programs, 28–32
claims and billing, 29–30
reimbursement, 30–32
scheduling, 28–29
functions of electronic health record
programs, 32–38
HIPAA and, 44–51
HITECH Act of 2009 and, 40–41, 51,
94–97
impact on documentation and
coding, 41–44
medical office applications of, 28–38.
See also Medisoft®; Office Hours
privacy requirements for, 46–48, 49,
50–51, 345
security requirements for, 49–50,
94–97
Health Information Technology for
Economic and Clinical Health
Act (HITECH), 40–41, 51, 94–97
Health insurance. *See* Medical
insurance
Health Insurance Portability and
Accountability Act of 1996
(HIPAA), 44–51, 232–233

Health maintenance organizations
(HMOs), 7
Health Net, 51
Health plans, 5–7. *See also* Medical
insurance
Health savings accounts, 7
Help feature, 69, 72, 81–85
built-in, 81, 82–85
hints, 81
online, 82, 83–85
reports, 324, 325
HIPAA (Health Insurance Portability
and Accountability Act of
1996), 44–51, 232–233
HIPAA Electronic Transaction and
Code Sets Standards, 44–46,
232–233
HIPAA Privacy Rule, 46–48, 49,
50, 345
HIPAA Security Rule, 49–50, 94–97
HITECH Act of 2009, 40–41, 51, 94–97
Home health claims, 163

i

ICD-9-CM codes. *See also* Diagnosis
codes
for charges, 179–180
described, 64–65
development of, 11–12
as standards, 46
Identification cards, insurance, 8, 10
IDE Number, 162
Indemnity plans, reimbursement
from, 248
Indexes, rebuilding, 90
Indicator code, 158
Institute of Medicine, 33, 39
Insurance. *See* Medical insurance
Insurance aging report, 326
Insurance analysis report, 317
Insurance carrier database, 64
Insurance Carrier List button, 71
Insurance Carrier List dialog box, 76
Insurance Coverage Percents by
Service Classification box, 149
Insurance identification card, 8, 10
Insured (guarantor), 112
*International Classification of Diseases
9th Revision, Clinical
Modification* (ICD-9-CM),
11–12, 46, 64–65, 179–180.
See also ICD-9-CM codes

k

Karnofsky Performance Status
Scale, 156
Knowledge base, 82–85

credits

Walkthrough: (Woman in lab coat on verso page behind green background): © Design Pics Inc./Alamy RF
(Woman in professional attire): © Thinkstock/CORBIS RF; 1: © Getty RF; 2: © Comstock/PunchStock RF;
3, 4: © Glow Images/Super Stock RF; 5: © Masterfile RF; 6: © Corbis RF; 7: © Istock RF; 8: © Corbis RF;
9: © Istock RF; 10: © Getty RF; 11: © Corbis RF; 12: © Getty RF; 13: © Glow Images/Super Stock RF;
14: © Getty RF; 15: Gino Cieslik; Mouse: © Yuri Arcurs/Getty Images